HJHP (Red)

The Process of
Patient Education

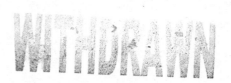
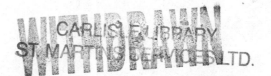
0801666708

The Process of Patient Education

BARBARA KLUG REDMAN, RN, Ph.D

Executive Director,
American Nurses Association,
American Nurses Foundation,
Washington, DC

SEVENTH EDITION
Illustrated

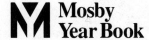

Mosby
Year Book

St. Louis Baltimore Boston Chicago London Philadelphia Sydney Toronto

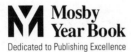
Mosby
Year Book
Dedicated to Publishing Excellence

Editor: Terry Van Schaik
Developmental Editor: Jeanne Rowland
Project Manager: Patricia Tannian
Production Editor: Barbara Jeanne Wilson
Designer: Gail Morey Hudson

SEVENTH EDITION

Printed in the United States of America

Mosby–Year Book, Inc.
11830 Westline Industrial Drive, St. Louis, Missouri 63146

Library of Congress Cataloging in Publication Data

Redman, Barbara Klug.
  The process of patient education / Barbara Klug Redman.—7th ed.
    p.   cm.
  Includes bibliographical references and index.
  ISBN 0-8016-6670-8
  1. Patient education.   2. Nurse and patient.   I. Title.
  [DNLM: 1. Nurse-Patient Relations.   2. Nursing Care.   3. Patient
Education.   WY 87 R318p]
RT90.R43   1992
615.5'07—dc20
DNLM/DLC
for Library of Congress ·   92-12909
                                                       CIP

93 94 95 96 97 GW/DC 9 8 7 6 5 4 3 2 1

To

Darlien and Harlan Klug

In grateful appreciation

for years of sustenance of various kinds

Preface

This book is written for all health care providers who want to know more about how to teach patients and families. Since the book began as a text in nursing, and since nursing has such a rich philosophic and conceptual heritage in patient education, much of the background is still drawn from that field. Students should be ready to use the book when they recognize the need for learning in their patients, when they have enough knowledge to be able to teach the subject matter, and when they are competent in their interactions with patients.

The book was inspired by students who were interested in and excited about teaching patients. It has been nourished over the years by extensive contact with providers who develop and manage programs of patient education.

After a beginning statement about the relevance of patient education in health care, the chapters are organized around elements of the teaching-learning process and delivery systems for patient education. Examples given are not meant to be exhaustive; they are only illustrative of the process. It will be advantageous if the student already has a basic understanding of the psychology of learning, because this complex subject must be abbreviated in a book of this size. Recent events in health care require a fresh look at ethics; therefore this edition includes a new section on ethics in Chapter 11.

Barbara Klug Redman

Contents

Appendixes

The Process of
Patient Education

CHAPTER 1

The place of patient education in health care

Many will agree that patients need assistance with understanding their health situations, making health care decisions, and changing health behaviors. Patient and family education has become an integral part of safe, cost-effective, quality patient care. Providers will encounter many questions and deal with issues such as the following: Does the patient want to learn? How important is it that the patient learn? What should he or she know and be able to do? What is the best way to teach patients? How does the provider know whether the patient has learned? What are the roles of the various health team members in patient education? What resources must health care agencies provide to ensure that education is delivered?

It is important to understand teaching as a tool of health care, what it is expected to accomplish, and the many ways in which providers can function as teachers. Such a perspective helps to delineate the role of patient education. Chapter 1 develops this perspective, and the following chapters focus on the process of teaching-learning.

HISTORIC, PHILOSOPHIC, AND LEGAL BACKGROUND
Nursing background

In the middle and late nineteenth century, English leaders in nursing saw the importance of teaching families about sanitation, cleanliness, and care of the sick. In that era the sick were usually cared for by their families. Nurses extended their services as they began to educate families in health care. Early visiting nurses in the United States, who were similarly motivated, joined others to fight disease and poverty among immigrants. Basic to these health education efforts was the realization that health could not be legislated or mandated successfully. These same tenets remain important today.

Statements by the National League of Nursing Education reflect concern with preparing twentieth-century nurses for their teaching tasks. The following comment[26] shows such a concern as early as 1918:

Another limitation of the ordinary training is that it deals only or mainly with disease, neglecting almost entirely the preventive and educational factors which are such an essential element in the many new branches of public health work, such as school and visiting nursing, infant welfare, industrial welfare, and hospital social service.*

The 1937 curriculum guide comments, "The nurse is essentially a teacher and an agent of health in whatever field she may be working."[27] In 1950 some of the areas common to all nursing curricula were identified as "teaching, contributing subject matter, psychology (especially principles of learning) . . . knowledge of principles of learning and teaching . . . [and] teaching skills."[28] Note that each of the foregoing statements exhibits interest in the scientific bases of the teaching-learning process and relates its importance to the nursing curricula. These recommendations represent the thinking of the nursing leaders; however, actual trans-

---

*National League of Nursing Education: *Standard curriculum for schools of nursing,* Baltimore, 1918, The Waverly Press, p 6.

lation of these thoughts into schools of nursing and then into nursing practice seems to have occurred much more slowly.

Since this early work, nursing has continued to develop conceptual models to explain the phenomena with which the discipline is concerned. These models focus in varying degrees on the following four concepts basic to nursing models: person, environment, health, and nursing, as well as the interrelationships among these concepts. Generally nursing models may be classified as developmental frameworks that focus on the forward movement of the personality and skills for meeting needs; as system frameworks that focus on the nurse learning to coordinate and function within his or her system and to negotiate with external systems; and as interactionist frameworks, that focus on the symbolic meanings and values in all interactions.

Books that analyze various proposals suggested by authors who are nurses are helpful.[12] Table 1-1 represents excerpts from several models that focus on the patient's need for education.

In addition to the theorists identified previously, Benner and Wrubel's book on the primacy of caring provides a useful perspective for teaching.[8] These authors note that people seek care when they experience a disruption, a loss, or a concern; they want to have the symptom removed or explained in ways that will minimize the disruption or alleviate the worry. Clearly, a difference exists between disease (the manifestation of aberration at the tissue, cellular, or organ levels) and illness (the human experience of loss or dysfunction), yet each affects the other. Curing the disease does not automatically cure the illness. Each patient is unique. Caring involves listening to their stories of illnesses and symptoms, being with them in an engaged manner, providing comfort and support, enabling them to grieve, and maintaining the belief in their goals. The nurse becomes an interpreter of the situation for the patient, guiding, coaching, and helping shape the illness experience for the patient. Understanding the meaning of the illness for the patient is a form of healing, even when no treatment is available and no cure is possible.

General background

A number of factors have converged to bring health teaching into prominence. The greater effort in this century to maintain health rather than just

TABLE 1-1. Elements of selected nursing models that are instructive for patient education[12]

Model author	Elements of model instructive for patient education
Peplau	Nursing helps patients gain intellectual and interpersonal competencies beyond those that they have at the point of illness. Nursing is an educative instrument that facilitates the patient's ability to transform symptom-bound energy into problem-solving energy.
Henderson	Function of the nurse is to assist the individual, sick or well, in performance of activities that he or she would perform unaided if he or she had the necessary strength, will, or knowledge to do so.
Orem	When the patient's self-care agency is inadequate to meet the therapeutic self-care demand, a self-care deficit occurs. Nursing assists patients to develop self-care abilities.
Neuman	Nurses teach individuals and communities how to respond to stressors.
Allen (McGill Model)	Nursing engages the client/family in the search for healthy being by structuring appropriate learning experiences that use pertinent health information by giving the client/family opportunities to share, discuss, and test appropriate plans of action.
Watson	Nursing includes a commitment to caring as a moral ideal. Two of the ten carative factors used by nurses are the use of problem-solving techniques for decision making and the promotion of interpersonal teaching-learning.

treat disease has enlarged the sphere of knowledge a person needs and has changed attitudes about health. Shortened hospital stays with early ambulation require preparation for the convalescence of the patient at home. Since the incidence of long-term illnesses and disabilities has increased, the patient and the family need to understand the illness and its treatment. The consumer movement and the general movement of society toward social leveling also play a part.

Recent additions to social thought on patient education reflect more strident themes, such as control and patients' rights. Some believe that medicine has become a major institution of social control by making the labels "healthy" and "ill" relevant to an ever-increasing part of human existence. Anything shown to have a negative effect on the workings of the body, and to a lesser extent the mind, may now be labeled an "illness" and jurisdictionally a "medical problem." Further, the patient's moral character is defined by how the patient handles the disease.[39] It follows that patient education could be one means of effecting control.

In the same vein, Myra Levine has charged that a large percentage of that which is called "teaching" is actually a communication of the rules of behavior as dictated by the rituals the nurse has been taught to value. The intransigent patient is one who either rejects the rules or fails to understand them in the same way that the nurse understands them.[24]

People who are classified as ignorant by their educators tend to think of themselves in this way and discredit their practical experiential knowledge. Education has focused on disseminating medical information to patients; it is assumed that patients do not contribute to their own knowledge.[11]

Breslow suggests that during the era 1925-1975, the technology of medicine escalated so rapidly that the idea of personal responsibility for health and the corollary patient education was almost eliminated.[9] More recently emphasis on cost containment in health care has led to earlier discharges from the hospital and more use of complex technologies in the patient's home. These patterns of care require patient education.

Significant changes have been occurring in medical ethics basic to patient education and in statements of support for patient education by physician groups. In July 1980 the American Medical Association's House of Delegates approved a new version of Principles of Medical Ethics, which indicates that a physician shall make relevant information available to patients and the public.[3] In commentary on this revision, Veatch underlines this document's basic shift of position from the Hippocratic ethics. Traditionally the physician has considered honesty with patients secondary to the more fundamental commitment of protecting the patient from harm. The new statement implicitly recognizes the rights of patients and recognizes the role of the lay person in determining ethics appropriate in the professional role. Clearly, the traditional paternalism of the profession is in conflict with society.[37]

More recently, the New York Academy of Medicine endorsed a statement that the physician community and the leadership of academic medical centers have an ethical obligation to include patient education as a service function and that programs in patient education should be expanded.[29] In addition, the American College of Physicians has reaffirmed its position (promulgated in 1979) that patients be provided essential information about prescribed drugs, that is, reasons the drugs have been ordered, ways in which they should be taken, common side effects and how to deal with them, and warnings about serious problems that demand the prompt cessation of drug use and the seeking of medical attention.[1]

This analysis is consistent with Pellegrino's view that the right of self-determination in a democratic society is so fundamental that to limit it, even in ordinary medical transactions, is an injustice. The usual objections, which are fear of inducing anxiety in the patient, the patient's inability to participate in decisions, the technical nature of medical knowledge, and the possibility of litigation, do not justify concealment except in special circumstances. Disclosure permits the physician to serve as technical expert and adviser; the most important revision is to consider the patient's personal values. The definition of health is highly personal. The professional can make a valid claim for technical authority but no longer for moral authority. In a pluralistic society, patients have the right to their own moral agency if they wish to exercise it.[31] Because medicine is not an accomplished science, physicians who assume complete autonomy for medical decision making are putting themselves in a strained ethical position.[10] Most of a physician's daily decisions do not involve situations that have been tested in double-blind randomized clinical trials. Indeed, in an estimated 90% of medical conditions, either no specific remedy exists or the effectiveness of treatment is unknown.[32] Thus, given the arbitrary nature of many clinical decisions, unilaterally ordering a patient to comply with a decision without considering the person's values and preferences seems unjustifiable to Brody.[10]

The discipline of medical phenomenology begins with an understanding of illness as it is lived by the patient and not just as an objective entity located somewhere anatomically, or one that perturbs a defined physiologic process. The person who is ill experiences a sense of disorder or a loss of control and begins to view health as problematic. When people experience illness, they seek an explanation that reintegrates the experience and makes it seem less disorderly, a cure, and a prediction. However, medical diagnosis is a categorization, not an explanation; treatment often does not result in cure; and prognosis is always statistical and rarely tells a particular person what will happen to him or her.[5]

Collegial and contractual models of medical care have been added to older ones. The consumerist perspective in which the physician and patient bargain over the terms of the relationship, with neither automatically in charge, conflicts with the traditional sociologic concept of the patient's sick role as the basis for the relationship. In the traditional concept the physician is in charge and the patient is obligated to cooperate with the regimen. One study of members of the public and physicians showed substantial minorities expressing beliefs and reporting actions congruent with the consumerist perspective. Information control with a wide competence gap between patient and provider formed the traditional pattern of relationship; the consumerist concept turns on a narrowed competence gap.[14]

Holistic health care embodies a number of the precepts of the consumerist ethic: (1) comprehensive programs that address physical, psychologic, and spiritual needs of those who come for help, (2) programs that meet unique needs of each individual, (3) therapeutic approaches that mobilize the individual's capacity for self-healing and independence rather than remedies that promote further dependence, (4) emphasis on education and self-care rather than on treatment or dependence, and (5) the view that the setting where health care takes place is also a place for education, volunteer work, and socializing. The holistic health care movement is part of a broad movement to create humane, democratic alternatives to large, impersonal, unresponsive services and institutions. It had its beginnings in the commitment to participatory democracy that animated the civil rights, youth, and women's movements of the 1960s.[13]

The legal base for medicine has long included the patient education area of practice. As early as 1898, instructing a diabetic patient in the care of an injured limb was considered a duty, and failure to supply these instructions was abandonment. Today, other duties include giving explicit instruction in the use of prescribed medication, providing follow-up care, and informing the patient that he or she has a condition requiring continual treatment.[18]

In regard to disclosure, in *Canterbury v Spence* and subsequent cases, the trend has been to disregard community or national standards of disclosure and to substitute the needs of a reasonably prudent patient. Such a rule is likely to lead to either greater disclosure or greater liability. It is permissible to withhold information if the disclosure will cause physiologic or psychologic harm to the extent that the effectiveness of the procedure will be impaired; however, it is not permissible to withhold information merely to negate the possibility that the patient will refuse treatment or make a "wrong" decision.[19]

The Patient's Bill of Rights, developed and approved by the American Hospital Association,[2] appears on pp. 6 and 7. It has been suggested that once a hospital adopts the Bill of Rights as policy, the provisions can be the basis for legal action in the same manner as are the hospital's bylaws and rules of nursing practice.[30] Now, courts may use the bill as a higher standard of hospital conduct. The position of nursing regarding the compliance of physicians with the Patient's Bill of Rights may well include involvement in upholding the hospital's policy.[16]

The case of *Darling v Charleston Community Hospital* established liability of a hospital that failed to perform treatment consistent with its own standard of care. If a patient education program is available to all patients admitted to a hospital, if the community knows it is offered, and if it is part of the standards of care drafted by the medical staff of the hospital, then liability is likely if the standard of care is breached and if that breach is the proximate cause of injury to the patient. It is the responsibility of the hospital that establishes such a program to monitor the professional care in patient education. Under the doctrine of respondeat superior, a hospital can be held liable for negligent actions of its employees.[25] Hospital policy, procedure manuals, job descriptions, and testimony from experts could be used.

Revision of many nurse practice acts has made explicit the inclusion of patient education, in addition to increasing the independence of the nurse.

In the 1970s several pieces of federal legislation affirmed a degree of commitment to health education, often affecting patient education. The Health Maintenance Organization Act of 1973 stipulates that HMOs must provide health education to their subscribers. The 1974 National Health Planning and Resources Development Act establishes public education in preventive health care and effective use of health care services as one of the nation's 10 health planning goals; the 1976 National Consumer and Health Information Act

provides funds to assist health care agencies in the integration of patient education into their health care services.[34] Through the Joint Commission for the Accreditation of Healthcare Organizations, standards for the incorporation of patient education into the care of patients serve as criteria for the accreditation of agencies.[17]

GOALS OF HEALTH TEACHING

What health teaching can accomplish is a key issue. Alternative approaches to change in health behavior, such as legislation and environmental controls, ultimately depend on educating the public. In addition, issues such as family planning and seeking early diagnosis are important for improved health and welfare; however, they are privately controlled and are, therefore, not completely cognizant of other approaches designed to effect behavioral change.[33] It is possible to prevent, promote, maintain, or modify a number of health-related behaviors by teaching the patients.

Every person who receives health care has some need to learn. Major objectives of teaching are often classified by phases of health care. Providers teach about health care services, growth and development, nutrition and hygiene, safety, first aid, preparation for childbearing, and other such topics to help people maintain health and prevent disease. During the phase of diagnosis and treatment, patients and their families learn about the disease, the need for care and treatment, and the hospital or clinic environment. During the follow-through phase, they need to understand care at home, including medications and diet, activity, continuing rehabilitation, and prevention of recurrence or complications.

Put in the broader framework of health education, primary health education, according to Watts, means instructing people how to avoid contracting preventable diseases, how to change life-styles, and how to control their environments. The people are educated in school, on the job, and by mass media. Secondary health education instructs people how to detect illness at early stages and prevent its progress. It is carried out in clinics, in community set-

---

A PATIENT'S BILL OF RIGHTS

The American Hospital Association presents a Patient's Bill of Rights with the expectation that observance of these rights will contribute to more effective patient care and greater satisfaction for the patient, his physician, and the hospital organization. Further, the Association presents these rights in the expectation that they will be supported by the hospital on behalf of its patients, as an integral part of the healing process. It is recognized that a personal relationship between the physician and the patient is essential for the provision of proper medical care. The traditional physician-patient relationship takes on a new dimension when care is rendered within an organizational structure. Legal precedent has established that the institution itself also has a responsibility to the patient. It is in recognition of these factors that these rights are affirmed.

1. The patient has the right to considerate and respectful care.
2. The patient has the right to obtain from his physician complete current information concerning his diagnosis, treatment, and prognosis in terms the patient can be reasonably expected to understand. When it is not medically advisable to give such information to the patient, the information should be made available to an appropriate person in his behalf. He has the right to know, by name, the physician responsible for coordinating his care.
3. The patient has the right to receive from his physician information necessary to give informed consent prior to the start of any procedure and/or treatment. Except in emergencies, such information for informed consent should include but not necessarily be limited to the specific procedure and/or treatment, the medically significant risks involved, and the probable duration of incapacitation. Where medically significant alternatives for care or treatment exist, or when the patient requests information concerning medical alternatives, the patient has the right to such information. The patient also has the right to know the name of the person responsible for the procedures and/or treatment.
4. The patient has the right to refuse treatment to the extent permitted by law and to be informed of the medical consequences of his action.
5. The patient has the right to every consideration of his privacy concerning his own medical care program. Case discussion, consultation, examination, and treatment are confidential and should be conducted discreetly. Those not directly involved in his care must have the permission of the patient to be present.

From American Hospital Association: *A patient's bill of rights,* Chicago, 1980, The Association.

---

tings, and by the mass media. Tertiary health education instructs patients about their illnesses, treatments, and available health services. It is carried out in hospitals, hospices, rehabilitation centers,[38] and, increasingly, at home. Some might see tertiary health education as patient education; others might see it as encompassing any of these goals and provided to people entering care, already under care, or receiving any of the various personal services related to health care.[29]

Strong forces in the health care field (including the consumer movement, which is demonstrating a growing and widespread dissatisfaction with the results of enormous expenditures on therapeutic medicine) have thrust health education forward to a higher priority. These forces have introduced goals for changing patient behavior. For example, individuals must be responsible for their own health; it is a moral obligation. This means exercising regularly, improving nutrition, going to the

A PATIENT'S BILL OF RIGHTS—cont'd

6. The patient has the right to expect that all communications and records pertaining to his care should be treated as confidential.

7. The patient has the right to expect that within its capacity a hospital must make reasonable response to the request of a patient for services. The hospital must provide evaluation, service, and/or referral as indicated by the urgency of the case. When medically permissible, a patient may be transferred to another facility only after he has received complete information and explanation concerning the needs for and alternatives to such a transfer. The institution to which the patient is to be transferred must first have accepted the patient for transfer.

8. The patient has the right to obtain information as to any relationship of his hospital to other health care and educational institutions insofar as his care is concerned. The patient has the right to obtain information as to the existence of any professional relationships among individuals, by name, who are treating him.

9. The patient has the right to be advised if the hospital proposes to engage in or perform human experimentation affecting his care or treatment. The patient has the right to refuse to participate in such research projects.

10. The patient has the right to expect reasonable continuity of care. He has the right to know in advance what appointment times and physicians are available and where. The patient has the right to expect that the hospital will provide a mechanism whereby he is informed by his physician or a delegate of the physician of the patient's continuing health care requirements following discharge.

11. The patient has the right to examine and receive an explanation of his bill regardless of source of payment.

12. The patient has the right to know what hospital rules and regulations apply to his conduct as a patient.

No catalog of rights can guarantee for the patient the kind of treatment he has a right to expect. A hospital has many functions to perform, including the prevention and treatment of disease, the education of both health professionals and patients, and the conduct of clinical research. All these activities must be conducted with an overriding concern for the patient, and, above all, the recognition of his dignity as a human being. Success in achieving this recognition assures success in the defense of the rights of the patient.

dentist, practicing family planning, establishing a harmonious family life, and submitting to screening examinations. After fulfilling these obligations, individuals have the "right" to expect help with information, accessible services of good quality, and minimal financial barriers.[20] Acceptance of this responsibility by consumers is an essential strategy for reducing the demand for health care, resulting in financial savings for all.

Self-care in health, which has become a political movement, refers to activities undertaken without professional assistance although informed by technical knowledge and skills derived from the pool of both professional and lay experience. Initiatives such as the formation of mutual aid groups and the measurement of success in care by patient-derived criteria are congruent with the lay definition of self-care. In recent years health technology has been designed for lay use, allowing people to monitor themselves for bladder infections, pregnancy, bowel cancer, and high blood pressure. The bulk of lay self-care involves coping with common symptoms and managing self-limiting and chronic illnesses. Its legal status is vague.[23]

The self-care movement is characterized by a strong "antiestablishment" thrust. It began outside the traditional, or formal, medical delivery system. Its goals include helping the public protect itself against the abuses of medical services provided by institutions, allowing individuals to determine their own risk mix, and restoring a more appropriate control over professional and technologic domination. An estimated 85% of health care is now self-provided. Purposeful self-care is necessary as a part of the health care system to avoid overloading services.[22] Educational support is obviously a necessary part of the self-care movement. The model promotes an organizational approach and a philosophy that nurtures self-reliance, responsibility, and initiative.

DEFINITIONS OF TEACHING

The definition of *teaching* as "activities that allow the teacher to help students learn" is broad yet useful because it emphasizes active learning by the student as the primary goal. An equally broad view is that teaching, like any other interpersonal influence, is aimed at changing the way in which other persons can or will behave. Teaching involves a controlled introduction of new objects, events, or information into the learner's environment.

Teaching is a special form of communication that encompasses and expresses knowledge about a particular subject, a communication specially structured and sequenced to produce learning. Some authors believe teaching is limited to activities designed to change behavior in the learner; they think that other interaction is outside the realm of teaching. Although it is true that a change in behavior is often an intended result, it is not always easy to observe the change immediately. Therefore many believe that the intention of teaching is to initiate learning; however, it does not always succeed. This interpretation is consistent with our lack of knowledge about exactly how and to what extent teaching contributes to or causes learning.

Bartlett has defined *patient education* as a planned learning experience using a combination of methods such as teaching, counseling, and behavior modification techniques that influence patients' knowledge and health behavior.[7] Others believe, philosophically, that teaching meets patients' desires for new information and new skills and that whatever patients do with this knowledge is their own affair.

Perhaps it is most useful for health practitioners to view all interaction with patients as contributing to the broad process and objectives of teaching-learning. Each time providers are with patients, they are assessing patient needs. Often these needs can be met by providing patients with information, clarifying their thinking, reflecting their feelings, or teaching them a skill. Also providers can communicate nonverbally and by example about such topics as health and good hygiene practices.

Not only are clear definitions of teaching needed, but it is also necessary for providers to hold a positive perspective about health care, including education in their practices. Few studies describe the degree to which providers include education in their daily interactions with patients. The health care climate in the United States has changed considerably since the introduction of the prospective payment system in 1983. Surveys done before that date are likely to reflect different conditions in care.

Of the several surveys available,* all report that nurses place a high value on patient education and believe that it is an important component of their jobs. However, in one survey,[21] nurses rated the overall achievement of patient education activities below the good rating. In another study,[6] nurses reported that patients did not have enough knowledge to care for themselves when they left the hospital and that too much information regarding patients' conditions was withheld from them. A study done in a single institution showed that only 25% of the nurses believed that patients were adequately taught before being discharged, with 90% believing that there was not enough time to educate patients. In yet another study[37] 50% of the patients were able to recall a particular occasion when they had received teaching, and nurses were identified as the

---

*References 6, 15, 21, 35, 36.

source of this information twice as often as were physicians. Although there is compelling evidence that physicians influence their patients' behavior patterns, most evidence also reveals that physicians usually do not take advantage of opportunities to do so in daily practice.[4]

SUMMARY

Although old philosophic positions emphasizing patient education exist, there is now a firm position that education is an essential component of health care.

REFERENCES

1. American College of Physicians: Drug information for patients, *Ann Intern Med* 104:121, 1986.
2. American Hospital Association: *A patient's bill of rights*, Chicago, 1972, The Association.
3. American Medical Association: *Principles of medical ethics*, Chicago, 1980, The Association.
4. American Medical Association, Council on Scientific Affairs: Education for health: a role for physicians and the efficacy of health education efforts, *JAMA* 263:1816-1819, 1990.
5. Baron RJ: An introduction to medical phenomenology: I can't hear you while I'm listening, *Ann Intern Med* 103:606-611, 1985.
6. Barrett C, and others: Nurses' perceptions of their health educator role, *J Nurs Staff Devel* 6:283-286, 1990.
7. Bartlett EE: At last, a definition, *Patient Educ Couns* 7:323-324, 1985.
8. Benner P, Wrubel J: *The primary of caring*, Menlo Park, Calif, 1989, Addison-Wesley.
9. Breslow L: Patient education in historical perspective, *Bull NY Acad Med* 61:115-121, 1985.
10. Brody DS: The patient's role in clinical decision-making, *Ann Intern Med* 93:718-722, 1980.
11. Fahrenfort M: Patient emancipation by health education: an impossible goal?, *Patient Educ Couns* 10:25-37, 1987.
12. Fitzpatrick JJ, Whall AL: *Conceptual models of nursing*, ed 2, Norwalk, Conn, 1989, Appleton & Lange.
13. Gordon JS: Holistic health centers, *J Holistic Med* 3(1):72-85, 1981.
14. Haug MR, Lavin B: Practitioner or patient—who's in charge?, *J Health Soc Behav* 22:212-229, 1981.
15. Honan S and others: The nurse as patient educator: perceived responsibilities and factors enhancing role development, *J Cont Educ* 19:33-37, 1988.
16. Hospitals must adapt patients' bill of rights or courts will tell them what it means, lawyer warns, *Mod Hosp* 120:33, 1973.
17. Joint Commission for the Accreditation of Health Care Organizations: *Accreditation manual for hospitals*, Chicago, 1991, The Commission.
18. Jowers LV: Medicolegal aspects of diabetes, *J Leg Med* 3:25-28, 1975.
19. Knapp TA, Huff, RL: Emerging trends in the physician's duty to disclose: an update of *Canterbury v Spence, J Leg Med* 3:41-45, 1975.
20. Knowles JH: Responsibility for health, *Science* 198:1413, 1977.
21. Kruger S: The patient educator role in nursing, *Appl Nurs Res* 4:19-24, 1991.
22. Levin LS: Self-care: an emerging component of the health care system, *Hosp Health Serv Admin* 23:17-25, 1978.
23. Levin LS, Idler EL: Self-care in health, *Annu Rev Public Health* 4:181-201, 1983.
24. Levine ME: The intransigent patient, *Am J Nurs* 70:2106-2111, 1970.
25. McCaughrin WC: Legal precedents in American law for patient education, *Patient Couns Health Educ* 2:135-141, 1979.
26. National League of Nursing Education: *Standard curriculum for schools of nursing*, Baltimore, 1918, The Waverly Press.
27. National League of Nursing Education: *A curriculum guide for schools of nursing*, New York, 1937, The League.
28. National League of Nursing Education: *Nursing organization curriculum conference*, Glen Gardner, NJ, 1950, Libertarian Press.
29. New York Academy of Medicine: The role of academic medicine in patient education: report of findings and recommendations, *Bull NY Acad Med* 61:219-223, 1985.
30. Patients' bill of rights could expose hospitals to liability, expert warns at AWH meeting, *Mod Hosp* 120:26, 1973.
31. Pellegrino ED: *Humanism and the physician*, Knoxville, 1979, University of Tennessee Press.
32. Pickering G: Therapeutics: art or science? *JAMA* 242:649-653, 1979.
33. Roberts B: Research in educational aspects of health programmes, *Int J Health Educ* 13(suppl I): Jan-March 1970.
34. Stanton MP: Patient education in the hospital health-care setting, *Patient Educ Couns* 5:14-22, 1983.
35. Stanton MP: Nurses' attitudes toward patient education, *Nurs Success Today* 3(3):16-21, 1986.
36. Tilley JD, Gregor FM, Thiessen V: The nurse's role in patient education: incongruent perceptions among nurses and patients, *J Adv Nurs* 12:291-301, 1987.
37. Veatch RM: Professional ethics: new principles for physicians?, *Hastings Center Rep* 10(3):16-19, 1980.
38. Watts AC, Breindel CL: Health education: structural vs. behavioral perspectives, *Health Pol Educ* 2:47-57, 1981.
39. Zola IK: Medicine as an institution of social control, *Sociol Rev* 20:487-503, 1972.

CHAPTER 2

A process model for patient education

Patient education is the deliberative process of creating behavioral and cognitive change in patients. Patient education is accomplished by assessing the patient's need and readiness for learning, by initiating activities that are designed to create cognitive and behavioral change in the learner, and by evaluating the results. A rich complexity of models of motivation, teaching, and learning is used within this overall process model.

The process model that supplies the organizational framework for this book was derived from the Tyler model in the field of education. It asks the following questions: (1) What are the purposes of patient education? (2) How can learning experiences be selected to achieve these purposes? (3) How can the learning experiences be organized for effective instruction? and (4) How can learning experiences be evaluated?[4] Each of these steps has a number of submodels.

The purpose of this chapter is to describe the relationships among the various parts of the teaching-learning process. These parts will be separated for a more thorough examination in succeeding chapters. In addition, a general health education planning model, PRECEDE,[3] is described. Although it is meant to be an independent model, elements of it can provide a valuable addition to the process model described in this book.

IDENTIFYING NEED FOR TEACHING

The process of teaching-learning often begins when an individual needs to know something or needs to know how to do something. This person may be a community member, an inpatient, an outpatient, or a family member of someone who needs care. He or she may request information about promoting health and preventing disease, about a health facility, or about the disease or treatment. Also the physician or other members of the health team may recognize that a particular patient needs information even though the patient may not be aware of the need.

How does the provider recognize the patient's need to learn? A patient may ask a direct question such as "Why does my baby clench his fist that way?," "What will happen to me when they do the x-ray?," or "How do I use these crutches?" A member of the family may ask, "Why does my father cry when I come to visit him?" The women's club may wish to be informed about home nursing and may ask a community health nurse to address the group. A group of obstetricians may agree on a postpartum teaching program to be given to all their patients after delivery. Or a community may suffer from high infant mortality and indicate a need to learn about the problem and its prevention.

It is easy to identify an opportunity for teaching when the request is direct. It is more difficult to infer patients' needs by observing their physical condition and behavior or by anticipating their needs from the treatment plan. For example, if a nurse notices that the skin on the feet of a diabetic patient is dry and cracking, it is necessary to ask if the patient is carrying out foot care, and, if not, why not. Patients who do not ask questions do not necessarily understand the consequences of the illness. Caregivers must become proficient in helping patients to identify their needs. Often, at the end of the assessment process, a diagnostic statement is made that will focus the interaction. An example might be lack of skill in baby care related to lack of child care experience.

WHAT CAN BE LEARNED

Since learning requires motivation, a realistic goal cannot be achieved without first capturing the learner's interest. Individuals who are not convinced that they need to learn a particular skill will not be receptive. Providers must try to convince these patients that they need to learn. Sometimes lack of motivation is a result of difficulty in adapting to an illness; sometimes it is the result of differences in value systems or in concepts of health and illness between the professional health worker and the client. The provider may be convinced that an individual needs to learn about the importance of immunizations; however, the person's values may be fatalistic—"I will get the disease if I am meant to"—so that the person views immunization as useless. Value systems vary according to cultural groups and socioeconomic class.

The learner's abilities and the demands of the situation also determine learning goals. Patients need a certain degree of independence today because chronic illness is prevalent and health care providers can provide only a minimum of supervision. It is important for a parent to be able to care for a new baby, recognizing common signs of illness. Other patients and their families are asked to assume considerably more responsibility than previously because dialysis, intravenous chemotherapy and antibiotic therapy, total parenteral and enteral nutrition, and care of ventilator-dependent individuals are provided at home. Individuals vary in their readiness for health education because of their general educational backgrounds, intellectual abilities, or attitudes toward acceptance of responsibility. Therefore some patients and families would not be capable of understanding the purpose of hemodialysis or the method of performing the procedure. They might not be emotionally stable enough to live with this responsibility. Therefore

goals or objectives of health learning can vary a great deal. In addition, the special concerns brought by illness or suspicion of illness can alter the individual's emotional stability and therefore his or her interest in learning.

That which a person is to learn is stated in the form of an objective, such as "how to give yourself an injection." To further delineate new behaviors, subobjectives are stated: "how to use sterile technique in giving an injection"; "how to measure dosage of medication accurately within 0.1 ml"; "how to identify sites for injection"; "how to redirect the needle if blood is aspirated." All these behaviors and others are necessary in order to realize the main objective: how to give an injection to oneself. If patient educators force themselves to identify in precise terms the behavior to be acquired, they will have a clearer notion of the content, the sequence of content, and the teaching methods that will most likely be successful. In health care the scheduling of work time and the variety of professionals who contribute to care make it necessary for many members of the staff to interact with the patient and to teach. Therefore communication of teaching goals must be absolutely clear.

STIMULATION OF LEARNING

Goals of learning have been classified into three domains: cognitive (understandings), affective (attitudes), and psychomotor (motor skills).[1] Providers commonly teach material pertaining to all three domains. Patients learn to understand (cognitive domain) how diabetes affects their bodies, how insulin controls diabetes, and many other intellectual concepts that are necessary for them to live healthfully with diabetes. Most important to this goal is an attitude of acceptance (affective domain) of their disease and a willingness to become responsible in caring for themselves. They must also learn motor skills (psychomotor domain), such as giving an injection.

Each of the domains responds best to particular methods of teaching. Facts and concepts are basic to intellectual learning and are taught by written materials and audiovisual aids, presenting the concepts, lectures, and discussion. Proper attitudes toward an illness do not always follow an educated perspective about the illness. For example, accepting responsibility for following a medical regimen in diabetes does not necessarily result from learning how diabetes affects the body. Providers can help patients and family develop healthy attitudes toward the illness by empathizing, setting an example, counseling, and helping them take action. Motor skills are best learned through a demonstration of the skills, with subsequent practice until the skills are perfected.

Group learning can save a great deal of teacher time and can provide an opportunity for people to profit from each other's experiences. Commonly, groups are taught topic areas such as prenatal, postnatal, diabetes, oncology, and pulmonary care in whatever site care is given.

The teacher plans to use both real and vicarious (substitute) experiences to encourage learning. The combination usually depends on the goals, the patient's experiences, and the ability to profit from vicarious experiences. People who do not read well have difficulty following directions from written sources and frequently cannot interpret diagrams. They may be able to imitate skills demonstrated in a movie and learn better in a hands-on experience.

EVALUATION OF LEARNING

Teaching involves assessing the needs of the patient, the family, or the community member, planning the lesson, and teaching. It also includes ascertaining whether the desired behavioral change has occurred, which is accomplished by observing the patient's behavior, and by oral and written questioning. The teacher and the learner should constantly assess their progress. In this way their efforts can be redirected if necessary. Evaluation is also done at the end of a lesson or at the end of a series of lessons to determine what the patient has retained.

When teaching is done during a phase of health care, it is important to keep a written record that documents the teaching plan and learning evalua-

tion. This is particularly important when teaching is a major form of therapy, such as it is in the initial orientation and regulation of a patient's diabetes. Accumulation of health information, skills, and attitudes occurs throughout an individual's life. Records describing this development in a clinic, hospital, or public health situation can be most helpful in furthering development.

HOW THE PROCESS IS SYNTHESIZED IN PRACTICE

The process of teaching can be summarized as follows:

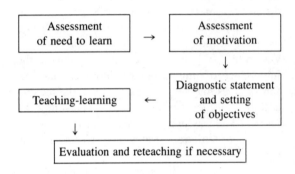

A few words must be said about the use of processes in practice and about the way the teaching process fits with the nursing process. It is impossible not to use a process in professional practice. The amount of data that must be synthesized to do purposeful intervention requires a categorizing system because people cannot keep any more than seven items in their short-term memories. Little is known about how process is actually used by practitioners, but what seems clearest is that it does not flow in an orderly, sequential fashion, as shown in the preceding diagram. Data about physician decision making may be instructive.

One study shows that most of the clinical workup is used by physicians to test specific hypotheses they form early in their contact with the patient. The number of hypotheses at any one time seems to be four, plus or minus one, and those are ranked according to probability, seriousness, treatability, and novelty, as well as by other criteria. Adhering to a strict routine of problem solving can help to compensate for the characteristic in human thinking of becoming wedded to a hypothesis even though it is incorrect.[2] The implications for use of the teaching process may be that (1) one starts at the beginning of the process but subsequently skips from step to step, and (2) the elements do serve as check points to ensure that the relevant variables that affect the teaching-learning activity have been considered. Although teaching does not have a complete set of commonly used diagnostic categories, the objectives can serve such a purpose. In addition, as nursing diagnostic categories are refined and expanded, they are useful but incomplete in categorizing patient learning needs. Indeed, in medicine, diagnosis may never be known, and it is not unheard of to have started and completed the treatment plan without a named diagnosis.

The teaching process can be seen as parallel to the nursing process in that each has an assessment, diagnosis, intervention, and evaluation phase (Table 2-1). Since learning about health is pertinent to nursing practice, some general screening questions should be part of the general nursing assessment; for example, what do patients know and how do they see their present problems? If at any time during care the ongoing assessment indicates a patient learning problem that teaching can alleviate,

a more refined assessment of need and readiness is made, and that problem is dealt with through the teaching process.

Of course, the most cogent question concerns the quality of use of either the nursing process or the teaching process and whether (at least in the psychosocial realm) fine points used in the process make any difference in patient outcome. I believe that there are gross errors in the practice of patient education that make a difference. Errors in practice are probably made in this order: (1) omission of assessment of the patient's need to learn, so that no activity in patient education is initiated; (2) omission of any given step: for example, omitting the assessment of readiness, the setting of goals, or the systematic evaluation, but not omitting the actual intervention. Of course, it is impossible not to have at least implicit goals when one teaches, but the goals may not be related to a particular patient's readiness and the instruction may not be constructed to meet those goals.

With adequate practice, providers can become proficient in thinking through the required steps of the teaching process. They can become sensitive to expressions of readiness that may be part of an ordinary conversation with the patient and learn to organize care to elicit measurements of readiness. The teaching that many patients require can be done

TABLE 2-1. Relationship of teaching process to nursing process

Assessment	Diagnosis	Goals	Intervention	Evaluation
NURSING PROCESS				
General screening questions to detect patient's need to learn; if positive, use teaching process	One of the problem statements may be a need to learn or a nursing diagnosis	Learning goals are a subset of the goals	Teaching intervention may be delivered with other intervention	Evaluating whether the nursing care outcome was met
TEACHING PROCESS				
Refined assessment of need to learn and readiness	Learning diagnosis	Setting of learning goals	Teaching	Evaluating learning

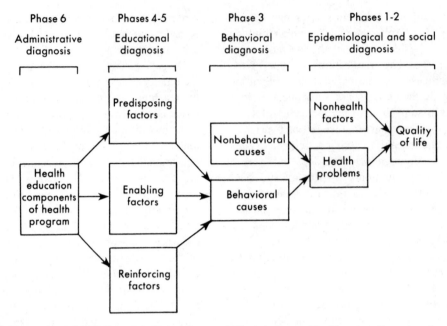

FIGURE 2-1. PRECEDE model. (From Greene LW and others: *Health education planning: a diagnostic approach,* Mountain View, Calif, 1980, Mayfield.)

in the same amount of time that the nursing process takes if it is done at the proper level of proficiency.

PRECEDE MODEL

The PRECEDE[3] (which stands for "predisposing, reinforcing, and enabling causes in educational diagnosis and evaluation") is a health education planning model depicted in Figure 2-1. It is based on the proposition that because health and health behavior are determined by several factors, health education efforts must be multidimensional. The model suggests a sequential process starting with consideration of desired outcomes and working back to original causes, in the following phases:

Phase 1: Consider the quality of life for the group or individual involved.

Phase 2: Identify specific health problems that appear to be contributing to the social problems noted in Phase 1 and select the problem most deserving of scarce educational resources.

Phase 3: Identify the specific health-related behaviors that appear to be linked to the health problem that deserves more attention.

Phase 4: Categorize the factors that seem to have direct impact on the behavior selected in Phase 2 into:

Predisposing factors: a person's attitudes, beliefs, values, and perceptions, which facilitate or hinder personal motivation for change,

Enabling factors: barriers created mainly by societal forces or systems, and

Reinforcing factors: related to the feedback the learner receives from others, the result of which may be to encourage or to discourage behavior change

Phase 5: Decide exactly which of these factors are to be the focus of the intervention.

Phase 6: Select interventions and assess administrative problems and resources.
Phase 7: Evaluate.

SUMMARY

Patient education requires providers to make judgments about what patients need to know and do, what they are capable of learning, how they can best be taught, and what they have learned. Since knowledge of human behavior is at best tentative (particularly with regard to motivation and learning processes), teachers must be aware of the extent of evidence about the teaching-learning process. This research is the topic in succeeding chapters.

STUDY QUESTIONS

1. Read Royle and Green's article, "Right atrial catheters: a patient and family education program" (*Can Nurse* 81[3]:51-54, March 1985). Identify these parts of the teaching-learning process:
   a. Assessing readiness for learning
   b. Determining learning goals (objectives)
   c. Preparing a plan for teaching, and also preparing teaching materials
   d. Carrying out the teaching
   e. Evaluating in terms of desired learning

2. T. Berry Brazelton has written: "Demonstrating the behavior of a newborn baby to an inexperienced mother can be both exciting and revealing. The mother's comments as the baby performs are likely to be meaningful in terms of her past experience and present expectations. As her baby goes from sleep to crying in an all-too-short period, the examiner might describe the speed of the state change without labeling it with a value judgment. The mother may then feel it safe to say: 'I just get frantic when he cries and I don't know how to stop him.' The pediatrician or nurse practitioner can then join her, recognizing her anguish and offering to participate with her by saying, 'Well, I don't know how either yet but we can work on it together.' A tacit but powerful alliance between the two is struck, with the baby's behavior a common ground for open communication."*

   Label the parts of the teaching-learning process, as in question 1 above.

REFERENCES

1. Bloom BS, editor: *Taxonomy of educational objectives: The classification of educational goals. Handbook I: Cognitive domain*, New York, 1977, Longman.
2. Elstein AS and others: Methods and theory in the study of medical inquiry, *J Med Educ* 47:85-92, 1972.
3. Green LW: *Health education planning: a diagnostic approach,* Palo Alto, Calif, 1980, Mayfield.
4. Tyler R: *Basic principles of curriculum and instruction,* Chicago, 1950, University of Chicago Press.

*Brazelton TB: Demonstrating infants' behavior, *Children Today* 10(4):5, 1981.

CHAPTER 3

Assessment of motivation to learn and the need for patient education

Motivation is a term that describes forces acting on or within an organism that initiate, direct, and maintain behavior. Motivation also explains differences in the intensity and direction of behavior. In the teaching-learning situation, motivation addresses the willingness of the learner to embrace learning. The term *readiness* describes evidence of motivation at a particular time. This chapter discusses theories of motivation in general, with specific application to health. It also describes assessment of motivation as part of the teaching-learning process and presents teaching practices that stimulate and develop motivation.

MOTIVATION THEORY

Six general theories of motivation can be used to direct learning in a variety of situations.[50]

Reinforcers. In behavioral learning theory the concept of motivation is tied closely to reinforcement of repeated behaviors. For example, behaviors that have been reinforced in the past are more likely to be repeated than behaviors that have not been reinforced or that have been punished. Reinforcement histories and schedules of reinforcement help explain why some individuals learn better than others.

Needs. Satisfaction of needs for food, shelter, love, and maintenance of positive self-esteem explains the concept of motivation for other theorists. People differ in the degree of importance they attach to each of these needs; the well-known Maslow's hierarchy[31] predicts which needs individuals will try to satisfy at any given moment.

Cognitive dissonance. Cognitive dissonance theory holds that people experience tension or discomfort when a deeply held value or belief is challenged by a psychologically inconsistent belief or behavior. To resolve the discomfort, patients may change a behavior or a belief, or they may develop justifications or excuses that resolve the inconsistency.

Attribution. In order to make sense of the world, individuals will often try to identify causes to explain why something has happened to them. People are particularly motivated to conduct attributional searches in ambiguous, extraordinary, unpredictable, or uncontrollable situations. Attributions may occur after a diagnosis, an exacerbation of chronic illness, an accidental injury, or the relief or cure of a symptom or illness. We know that attributions can have powerful effects on psychologic adjustment, behavior, and morbidity. In a study of patients with myocardial infarctions, attributions of patients and their spouses (Why did this happen to me?) significantly predicted whether the family considered themselves rehabilitated. People make attributions about disease severity and treatment efficacy. They use these ideas to regulate self-management of their diseases.[29] So, it is always important to know patients' beliefs about the cause of their present situation because their actions are guided by these attributions. Fielding notes that frequently physicians and patients do not hold the same causal attributions about myocardial infarction. Physicians tend to focus on the patients' medications, encouraging them to stop smoking, and helping them reduce cholesterol levels. Physicians provide less help for patients with problems such as stress, worry, and overwork—problems that the patients attribute to the illness.[11]

A concept central to attribution theory is locus of control. Those with an internal locus of control in a situation attribute success or failure to their own efforts or abilities. Those with an external locus of control believe that success or failure depends on luck, task difficulty, or other people's actions. Clinical studies are being done with locus of control, because different intervention methods may be required to deal with these very different notions about causality of events. One study involving individuals undergoing dental surgery showed that patients with high internal locus of control adjusted poorly in surgery when given general, marginally relevant information about the impending operation. However, the patients adjusted well if they viewed a tape that gave them specific information about the procedures and the sensations they could expect. The reverse was true of patients with a high external locus of control.[1] Among older, white individuals at a public hypertension screening clinic, those with a greater locus of control were more inclined to seek informational pamphlets on heart disease.[54]

A study of individuals with diabetes showed surprising outcomes. "Internals" had more diabetic information but seemed to incur more problems with the disease as it progressed than did "externals." The major features of diabetes and its treatment are still too poorly understood to permit adequate therapeutic recommendations for many patients. Therefore people with internal locus of control may find themselves surveying a situation in which the environment cannot be completely controlled. This might cause them to relinquish some of the control they would normally exercise. For people with external locus of control, the mode of coping is compliance with authority (physician), which may be the more adaptive set of responses.[30]

Personality. Motivation in personality theory describes a general tendency to strive toward certain types of goals such as affiliation or achievement.

Motivation is a relatively stable characteristic. An extreme motivation to avoid failure is learned helplessness, which causes people to believe that they are doomed to failure no matter what. This behavior can arise from an inconsistent and unpredictable use of rewards and punishments by teachers. The problem can be avoided or alleviated by giving learners opportunities to realize success in small steps and by giving them immediate, positive feedback with consistent expectations and follow-through. Coping styles may also be part of personality. Some people are vigilant and seek information from all available sources. If these people find discrepancies in the information they receive, they will feel anxious. Others use a coping style of avoidance. They want little information because it constitutes a source of stress.

Expectancy. Expectancy theories of motivation hold that a person's motivation to realize a goal depends on the perceived chance of success as well as how much value that person places on success. Learners' tasks should be neither too easy nor too difficult. Learners try to live up to expectations in the environment. The theory of reasoned action is related to theories of expectancy. The theory posits that volitional behavior is predicted by the person's intention to perform the behavior. Intention is, in turn, a function of beliefs about the consequences of the behavior and norms about the behavior that are held by significant others.[37]

Ideas and emotions are motivators and are nearly always influenced by the environment. Recent summaries of research have shown a powerful relationship between perceived self-efficacy and adequate performance. How people judge their capabilities to produce and regulate events in their lives affects their motivation, their thought patterns, their behavior, and their emotions. Those who believe that they will not be able to cope well dwell on their personal deficiencies and imagine that potential difficulties will be more formidable than they really are. There are notable increases in self-efficacy when people's experiences contradict their fears and when they gain new skills in managing threatening activities. Repeated failures lower self-efficacy, especially if failure occurs early in the course of events and does not reflect lack of effort or adverse external circumstances.[2]

Judgments about self-efficacy are based on the following sources of information: performance attainments (the most influential), vicarious experiences of observing performance of others, verbal persuasion and other social influences, and physiologic states. These courses of information are effective in cardiac rehabilitation programs. The goal is to reestablish the patient's sense of physical efficacy. The program uses the treadmill to demonstrate adequate performance to patient and spouse; it uses examples of former patients who lead active lives; it persuades patients of their capabilities, by explaining the meaning of physiologic efficacy information sources so that patients will not misread them. Self-efficacy probes during the course of treatment can provide helpful guides for implementing a program of personal change. Adopting attainable subgoals that lead to more impressive future goals can provide the patient with clear markers of progress to verify a growing sense of self-efficacy.[2]

Finally, humanistic interpretations of motivation emphasize personal freedom, choice, self-determination, and a striving for personal growth. Although generally not expressed as a theory in the scientific sense, humanists make important assumptions that cause us to reflect on learners' resolutions to become motivated and to make their own decisions about whether to pursue a course of action.

HEALTH BELIEFS AND BEHAVIOR FACTORS AFFECTING CHANGE

The previous discussion of theories of motivation makes it clear that health beliefs energize people to learn as well as provide them with direction for health actions. Health beliefs are frequently cultural, and it is not unusual for patients and providers to hold different beliefs. One model of beliefs is known to predict motivation to take health action.

Health belief model

The Health Belief Model, developed in the early 1950s, affirms that people are not likely to take a health action unless (1) they believe that they are susceptible to the disease in question; (2) they believe that the disease would have serious effects on their lives if they should contract it; (3) they believe that certain actions can reduce their likelihood of contracting the disease or reduce the severity of it; and (4) they believe that taking the action is not as great a threat as the threat that is implicit in the disease.[46] The model is an example of the value-expectancy approach to predicting behavior.

A major addition to the model has been the concept of motivation. Apparently, it is necessary for some factor to serve as a cue to trigger action. The required intensity of the cue presumably varies with differences in the level of perceived susceptibility and severity.[45] Examples of triggers that are believed to affect timing include interpersonal crisis, symptoms that will not allow the patient to participate in a valued social activity, or the nature and severity of the symptoms. Samples of the modified model for preventive health behavior and for explaining sick-role behavior may be seen in Figures 3-1 and 3-2.[7] Recently, it has been suggested that self-efficacy should be incorporated as an additional element in the model to increase its predictability with complex behavior patterns.[47]

Studies show that it is possible to modify the perceived threat of disease (that is, the combination of perceived susceptibility and severity) as well as the perceived efficacy of professional intervention and that such modifications lead to predictable changes in health behavior.[7,45]

The Health Belief Model was originally formulated to explain why persons would or would not undertake health actions; it was later applied to predictions of compliance with prescribed therapies. A body of research findings now exists linking the model to compliance with regimens for hypertension, end stage renal disease, middle ear infection, asthma, obesity, and behaviors such as taking medication, adhering to dietary restrictions, following exercise prescriptions, and keeping clinic appointments.[5] Janz and Becker recently reviewed studies of the model since 1974, dealing with prevention, sick-role behaviors, and clinic use. Across the various study designs and behaviors, perceived barriers proved to be the most powerful of the dimensions. Perceived susceptibility was a stronger contributor to understanding preventive behavior than it was to understanding sick-role behavior. The reverse was true for perceived benefits. Although it was weakly associated with preventive behaviors, perceived severity was strongly related to sick-role behaviors.[22]

Some limitations of the model (important for those who would use it in health education) must be explained. A balance is required between vulnerability, severity, and the psychologic benefit and cost ratio. Perceived severity can cause the patient to reach dysfunctional levels. There is some evidence of a threshold level, but neither theory nor

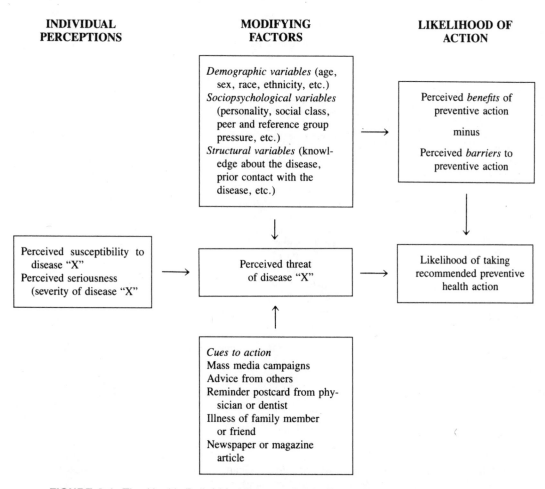

INDIVIDUAL PERCEPTIONS

MODIFYING FACTORS

LIKELIHOOD OF ACTION

Demographic variables (age, sex, race, ethnicity, etc.)
Sociopsychological variables (personality, social class, peer and reference group pressure, etc.)
Structural variables (knowledge about the disease, prior contact with the disease, etc.)

Perceived *benefits* of preventive action

minus

Perceived *barriers* to preventive action

Perceived susceptibility to disease "X"
Perceived seriousness (severity of disease "X"

Perceived threat of disease "X"

Likelihood of taking recommended preventive health action

Cues to action
Mass media campaigns
Advice from others
Reminder postcard from physician or dentist
Illness of family member or friend
Newspaper or magazine article

FIGURE 3-1. The Health Belief Model as predictor of preventive health behavior. (From Becker MH and others: *Am J Public Health* 64:205-216, 1974.)

READINESS TO
UNDERTAKE
RECOMMENDED
SICK-ROLE BEHAVIOR

MODIFYING
AND ENABLING
FACTORS

SICK-ROLE
BEHAVIORS

Motivations
Concern about (salience of)
   health matters in general
Willingness to seek and
   accept medical direction
Intention to comply
Positive health activities

*Value of illness threat
   reduction*
Subjective estimates of:
   Susceptibility or resuscep-
      tibility (including belief
      in diagnosis)
   Vulnerability to illness in
      general
   Extent of possibly bodily
      harm*
   Extent of possible inter-
      ference with social
      roles*
Presence of (or past ex-
   perience with) symptoms

Demographic (very young or
   old)
Structural (cost, duration,
   complexity, side effects,
   accessibility of regimen;
   need for new patterns of
   behavior
Attitudes (satisfaction with
   visit, physician, other staff,
   clinic procedures and
   facilities)
Interaction (length, depth,
   continuity, mutuality of
   expectation, quality, and
   type of doctor-patient
   relationship; physician
   agreement with patient;
   feedback to patient)
Enabling (poor experience
   with action, illness or
   regimen; source of advice
   and referral)

Likelihood of
Compliance with prescribed
   regiment (e.g., drugs, diet,
   exercise, personal and
   work habits, follow-up
   tests, referrals and follow-
   up appointments, entering or continuing a
   treatment program)

*Probability that compliant
   behavior will reduce the
   threat*
Subjective estimates of:
   The proposed regimen's
      safety
   The proposed regimen's
      efficacy (including
      "faith in doctors and
      medical care" and
      "chance of recovery")

*At motivating, but not inhibiting, levels

FIGURE 3-2. Summary Health Belief Model for predicting and explaining sick-role behaviors. (From Becker MH: *Health Educ Monogr* 2:409-419, 1974.)

TABLE 3-1. Sample questions from scales to measure beliefs of diabetic patients

	Response scale				
Question	Strongly agree (SA)	Agree (A)	Undecided (U)	Disagree (D)	Strongly disagree (SD)
Perceived Susceptibility (sequelae of noncompliance)					
My diabetes is well controlled.	(SA)	(A)	(U)	(D)	(SD)
My diabetes would be worse if I did nothing about it.	(SA)	(A)	(U)	(D)	(SD)
I believe that my diet (medications) will help prevent diseases (complications) related to diabetes.	(SA)	(A)	(U)	(D)	(SD)
Diabetes can be a serious disease if you don't control it.	(SA)	(A)	(U)	(D)	(SD)
Perceived Severity					
My diabetes is no problem to me as long as I feel all right.	(SA)	(A)	(U)	(D)	(SD)
My diabetes will have a bad effect on my future health.	(SA)	(A)	(U)	(D)	(SD)
My diabetes will cause me to be sick a lot.	(SA)	(A)	(U)	(D)	(SD)
I believe I will always need my diabetes diet (medications).	(SA)	(A)	(U)	(D)	(SD)
Perceived Benefits					
I believe I can control my diabetes.	(SA)	(A)	(U)	(D)	(SD)
I believe that my diet (medications) will control my diabetes.	(SA)	(A)	(U)	(D)	(SD)
If I change my eating habits it will probably help me.	(SA)	(A)	(U)	(D)	(SD)
My medicine makes me feel better.	(SA)	(A)	(U)	(D)	(SD)
Perceived Barriers					
I would have to change too many habits to follow my diet (medication).	(SA)	(A)	(U)	(D)	(SD)
It has been difficult following the diet prescribed for me.	(SA)	(A)	(U)	(D)	(SD)
I cannot understand what the doctor told me about my diet.	(SA)	(A)	(U)	(D)	(SD)
Taking my medication interferes with my normal daily activities.	(SA)	(A)	(U)	(D)	(SD)

From Becker M, Janz N, *The Diabetes Educator*, vol 2, Chicago, 1985, American Association of Diabetes Educators, p 46; Given CW, Given BA, Gallin RS, Condon JW: *Res Nurs Health* 6:127-141, 1983.

BSE QUESTIONNARE ITEMS

Perceived seriousness

Q1. When you go to your physician for examination, about how often does *the doctor* examine your breasts?

_____ never _____ most of the time
_____ sometimes _____ always

Q2. One of the reasons I don't do self-exams is I'm not concerned about breast cancer.

_____ yes _____ no

Q3. How serious would it be to get breast cancer?

serious ___: ___: ___: ___: ___: ___:
_____ not serious

Perceived susceptibility

Q4. If I had to think about the possibility that I might someday get breast cancer, I would rate my chances as compared with other women as: (circle one)

a. average b. above average c. below average
(more likely I (less likely I
would get it) would get it)

Q5. Whenever I hear of a friend or relative (or public figure) getting breast cancer, it makes me realize that I could get it too.

agree ___: ___: ___: ___: ___: ___: disagree

Q6. Do you have a *family* history of *breast* cancer?

_____ yes _____ no _____ I don't know

Q7. I know a close friend/relative who has had breast cancer:

_____ yes _____ no

Q8. Have you had any *personal* history of breast *lumps?*

_____ yes _____ no

Perceived benefit of action

Q9. If a woman gets breast cancer and it is detected and treated early, what are the chances that it can be cured? (circle one)

15% chance 33% 50% 67% 85% 99%

Q10. Even though breast tumors can be discovered, they seldom can be totally removed. (circle one)

disagree 1 2 3 4 agree

Q11. After a doctor finds out that a woman actually has breast cancer, what do you think is done to treat the disease? (NOTE: This item was scored "has" or "does not have" knowledge of treatment.)

Q12. If you found a breast lump, do you know where to turn for help?

_____ yes _____ no

Barriers to action

Q13. Even though it's a good idea, I find having to examine my breasts an embarrassing thing to do. (circle one)

disagree 1 2 3 4 agree

Q14. Examining my breasts often makes/would make me worry unnecessarily about breast cancer. (circle one)

disagree 1 2 3 4 agree

Q15. The BSE is too complex to remember. (circle one)

disagree 1 2 3 4 agree

Q16. If I lost a breast, I would feel less feminine. (circle one)

disagree 1 2 3 4 agree

Q17. Is it possible to surgically *replace* a breast removed because of cancer?

_____ yes _____ no _____ I don't know

General health motivation

Which of the following things do you do to take care of your health?

regularly seldom

Q18. Have Pap smear

___: ___: ___: ___: ___:

Q19. Have blood pressure checked

___: ___: ___: ___: ___:

Q20. How many times during the past year did you go to a doctor for a general check-up—that is, *not* because of a specific illness or condition? Don't include eye doctors or dentists. How many times? _____

From Rutledge DN, Davis GT: *Oncol Nurs Forum* 15:175-179, 1988.

BSE QUESTIONNARE ITEMS—cont'd

Modifying variables

Q21. Socioeconomic status (Green's index based on income, education, occupation).

Q22. Do you have any method of reminding yourself to do breast self-exams?

_____ no _____ yes (please list your method)

Q23. How confident are you in your own ability to do a breast self-examination? (place a check)

confident ___: ___: ___: ___: ___: ___:

_____ not confident

Q24. Were you taught BSE:

_____ individually (you and an instructor only)

_____ in a group setting (with other women)

_____ impersonally (you alone, no instructor present)

_____ not at all

Q25. In learning BSE, did you practice on yourself or on a breast model?

_____ yes   _____ no

Q26. Does your doctor ask you if you are doing monthly BSE?

_____ yes   _____ no

Q27. Are you encouraged to do BSE?

_____ yes   _____ no

If yes, by: _____ friends _____ spouse

_____ other relative

Q28. Age _____

---

research has disclosed what the optimal levels of readiness are. Little is known about the stability of the beliefs.[6] Perceived severity is the most doubtful of the elements, although it seems to be more useful in illness than in preventive behavior.

The causal roles of the beliefs have not been studied. The beliefs are more prevalent in whites than in other racial groups, in people of high socioeconomic status than in those of low socioeconomic status, in women than in men, and in the relatively young than in the old. However, we do not know why.[46] The relationship among the elements—that is, whether they are additive, multiplicative, or interactive—is not clear. Some evidence shows them to be relatively independent.[29] Significant elements missing from the model are a study of the social environment (including lay referral and social support), the physician-patient interaction, the patient's perception of symptoms, the lay construction of illness, and the sick role.[25]

The perceptions and beliefs that make up the Health Belief Model are alterable and can be used as part of a framework of assessment for educational diagnosis. Sample questions from scales to measure the beliefs of patients with diabetes are shown in Table 3-1 and for breast self-examination,[48] in the box on pp. 22 and 23.[17] The model does not imply or prescribe strategies for changing health behavior. A paucity of rigorous research evaluates the efficacy of different interventions that modify Health Belief Model dimensions to achieve desired health behaviors.[22] Sometimes, providing corrective factual information will prove sufficient. In other cases, motive-arousing appeals from sources credible to the patient will be necessary, as may be environmental and structural changes in the health care delivery system.[5] Others have found insufficient evidence that elements of the model are reliable clinical predictors of compliance.

More recently, Jones found that an intervention based on the Health Belief Model increased by 50% the likelihood that hypertensive patients using the emergency department would keep a follow-up appointment. The intervention consisted of a standardized assessment of the patient's perceptions of hypertension followed by a 10- to 25-minute educational session designed to increase the patient's awareness of his or her susceptibility to complications in hypertension, the seriousness of complications, and the benefits derived from a follow-up appointment.[23]

The Health Belief Model may not apply equally to all diseases; however, investigators are using it to analyze teaching materials available for a field. Prewitt found that AIDS educational materials available in 1988 were heavily focused on susceptibility; however, they were not explicit regarding the sexual behaviors that made individuals susceptible. The materials also focused on the severity of the disease but did not emphasize the benefits of preventive health behavior. The AIDS educational materials also did not mention the many known obstacles that hinder taking action.[42]

Systems of health belief and behavior

There are many accounts of the health beliefs of cultures throughout the world. The information an individual or group will learn regarding health depends in part on the orientation of the culture to such issues as whether human nature is good or evil, how independent of nature humans can be, whether the basic orientation is present, past, or future, whether an individual's cultural role is primarily active or passive, and how the individual is bound to other individuals.[27]

For example, in most technologically underdeveloped areas, the limited future time orientation makes educating for disease prevention difficult. Therefore preventive programs are combined with those that meet immediate needs.

In a recent study of working-class mothers in Boston, at least half were found to hold fatalistic views about illness causation and were prepared to accept blame only under restricted circumstances involving direct risk taking. This finding contrasts with a prominent theme of modern preventive medicine: the need for people to assume greater responsibility for their own health.[41]

Horn identifies cultural beliefs that should be incorporated into pregnancy prevention models.[20] Her in-depth interviews with Native American Indian, black, and white teenage women indicate cultural differences in beliefs about prevention of pregnancy, the significance of becoming a mother at an early age, and their knowledge of the kinds of support available to women within their social network. All of the subjects were knowledgeable about contraceptives. The Native American Indians did not believe that contraception should be used until after the first baby was born. They believed that intrauterine devices marked the baby. Black subjects believed that contraceptive pills and intrauterine devices were not acceptable because they altered the menstrual cycle. The white subjects followed their religious views. The Native American Indians placed a high value on early pregnancy. For blacks, becoming a mother at a young age had a fairly high level of acceptance in the group studied. Both groups felt that they would be supported in their pregnancies. For the whites studied, early pregnancy was not valued, and they felt that they would not be supported during a pregnancy.

Behavioral ethnicity often entails general styles of interaction, attitudes toward authority figures, sex-role allocations, and ways of expressing emotion or asking for help. These ethnic styles often translate in the health realm into ways of presenting symptoms, expectations of provider behavior, understanding of terms, and responses to diagnostic and treatment regimens. The authority accorded professional standards of health and medical care in the culture has contributed to making patients' own experience of their illness seem incorrect, irrelevant, or inferior. The health professional needs to know these beliefs in general and to elicit the patient's own model of the problem by asking the following questions:

1. What do you think has caused your problem?
2. Why do you think it started when it did?
3. What do you think your sickness does to you? How does it work?
4. How bad (severe) do you think your illness is? Do you think it will last a long time, or will it be better soon in your opinion?
5. What kind of treatment would you like to have?

6. What are the most important results you hope to get from treatment?

7. What are the chief problems your illness has caused you?

8. What do you fear most about your sickness?[19]

Preventive health behavior has assumed increased importance in the past few years as society has tried to control health care costs. A Harris poll found that the people most likely to engage in health-promoting behavior had incomes of more than $25,000 per year, were college educated, were currently in excellent health, and felt that they had a great deal of control over their future health. Table 3-2 from that survey shows reported compliance with the health-seeking behaviors chosen on the basis of consensus among experts of a documented relationship between compliance and prevention of disease.[60]

Belief differences in provider-patient relationship

Later chapters will return to the topic of the provider-patient relationship as the prime objective-setting and instructional medium. A strong belief exists in certain groups that dominance on the part of providers in the patient-provider relationship has frustrated the natural readiness of patients to learn because the goals were not theirs.

A study of provider-parent communication in an assessment center for preschool handicapped children in England found that the two groups had divergent goals and subscribed to divergent models about the child's ailment.[52] Particularly regarding the relationship of etiology to cure, parents wanted to know "why" in the sense of what was wrong with the way the child's mind and body worked and "why" in the sense of why this damage should have happened to their child—how it came about. Parents were anxious to have the cause discovered because they believed that then a cure could be found; however, staff was not able to clarify this misperception. Contrary to expectations, when the parents received the medical assessment report, they did not agree with the staff's models of normality, abnormality, or the causes. Half of the parents remembered little of the report, and staff

TABLE 3-2. Reported compliance with health-seeking behaviors

Health-seeking behaviors	Percent of adult compliance	
	1983	1984
Avoid smoking/bed	88	89
Moderate alcohol	88	87
Socialize regularly	83	85
Not smoking	70	72
Avoid drive/drink	72	72
Blood pressure screen	82	85
Avoid home accidents	72	84
Smoke detector	67	74
Control stress	68	74
Dental examination	71	72
Obey speed limit	61	58
Adequate vitamins/minerals	63	57
Consume fiber	59	58
Restrict fat	55	59
7-8 hours sleep	64	63
Restrict sodium	53	54
Restrict sugar	51	52
Restrict cholesterol	42	43
Exercise strenuously	34	33
Maintain weight	23	23
Wear seatbelts	19	27

From Young R: *Health Med* 3(2/3):6-17, 1985.

would not provide a written note to be studied at the parents' leisure.

Oakley's studies of childbirth, viewed from a feminist perspective, found a considerable gap between expectation and reality in the pain involved with birth and the amount of technical medical intervention offered. She felt that this was a deliberate misrepresentation based on cultural expectations of women, that it contributed to the risk of postpartum depression, and that prenatal classes had been colonized by the medical point of view.[40]

Table 3-3, reproduced from a text on women's health care by Fogel and Woods,[13] depicts the attitudinal differences between traditional and new systems of health care in structure and process. Imagine how different the definitions of motivation

TABLE 3-3. Comparison of structure and process of the relationship between nurse and client in traditional versus new systems

Dimension	Traditional system	New system
Power structure in relationship between nurse and client	Nurse seen as authority figure, more powerful than client.	Nurse and client have egalitarian, collaborative relationship. Power balanced between nurse and client.
Information exchange	Nurse maintains stratification in relationship by withholding some information from client; makes judgments about how much information client can "handle" or "needs to know." Minimal information obtained from client.	Information exchanged freely between nurse and client. Nurse recognizes client is expert in self-care; nurse is expert in processes used to facilitate client's health.
Decision making	Nurse may make some decisions that she judges client is unable to make. Usually this is subtle (e.g., only limited alternatives may be presented).	Client clearly the decider for self-care. Nurse is consultant. Client chooses from available alternatives.
Integration of client in system	Client clearly not a part of the "provider" system. Client passive recipient of prescriptions for health.	Client is component of system in which professionals and other clients strive for health. Client has an active role and makes prescriptions for own health based on information about self-care.
View of women	Woman seen as a "role." Problems of population of women are defined on the basis of their reproductive roles in society.	Woman seen as individual, in social network also viewed as part of population of women with emergent health care requirements.

From Fogel CI, Woods NF: *Health care of women: a nursing perspective,* St Louis, 1981, Mosby–Year Book.

would be in these two systems. Motivation is dependent on the roles of provider and patient in the decision-making process about health and also on the way that goals are set.

Perhaps the best philosophy is that every patient is ready to learn something. It is up to the provider to discover what the patient wants to learn and then build on the area of motivation that exists. Beliefs and behaviors become crucial at certain stages in the health-illness cycle. An example of a crucial stage is when the individual seeks care, either preventive or diagnostic.

Seeking care

The behavior that persons display when they seek care has been studied because it is viewed by

health professionals as important for a satisfactory outcome. Many diseases can be treated best with early diagnosis. People with chronic illness may function inefficiently for long periods of time because they fail to seek treatment. Such a pattern creates economic and social loss for the family.

Differences by sex in preventive health behavior have been recorded. In our culture, men engage in more risk-taking behavior and take preventive health care measures less frequently than do women. Women avoid risks and take more preventive action, particularly those actions associated with medical intervention. These behavioral differences are consistent with certain aspects of the socialization and adult role patterns deemed appropriate for each sex in our society. Ironically, it is women's positive orientation toward medical care that may be responsible for the one class of risk-taking behavior in which women clearly predominate: women are more frequent users than men of psychotropic medications, the most common substances obtained by entry into the medical system.[38]

Available evidence indicates that seeking health care is influenced by many factors and by the interplay among them. A single factor, such as ignorance, is often not solely responsible for delay or promptness in seeking medical care. Denial may play a part. Economic ability to pay for care is bound up with health beliefs and with values about the priority of health among many motivations. The individual's, the family's, and the culture's answers to the following questions help to determine whether care will be sought: What is the meaning attached to a symptom located at a particular body site? How are hospitals, health personnel, surgery, and the body itself viewed? Does the family support the health action psychologically and financially? How do people view their responsibility for their own health? How important is the individual? What kinds of care facilities are acceptable for use? All these factors influence the way in which people select, perceive, and interpret information and services available to them.

Certainly the development of anxiety helps to determine action in seeking health care. Mild anxiety is useful because it causes the individual to act. However, greater degrees of anxiety interfere with adaptive action. Fear of negative reactions from high-status medical personnel may prevent some individuals from going to the physician with an "insignificant" symptom. Between 1946 (when the method for breast self-examination was introduced) and 1963, women delayed less often in seeking care for breast cancer. It is believed that part of this change may have occurred because women had a valid "confirmation tool" that was viewed in a positive light by the caregiver; therefore they were free to act. In a sense, the patient believes that the caregiver has granted approval; therefore the patient now has permission to ask for

an examination. Negative attitudes toward symptoms exhibited by health personnel can influence and override the individual's personal bias or knowledge. Health education should provide sufficient information about health and care systems that will encourage individuals to seek help when dysfunction is suspected.

Often, people have no clear understanding of their disorder and will wait for symptoms that they consider worthy of medical attention and treatment. These symptoms may include cough, fever, pain, bleeding, and nervousness. The person may just note a frequent symptom in a particular location.[61] Many chronically ill patients are old, and some of them tolerate functional impairments unnecessarily because they erroneously associate their symptoms with aging rather than with illness and therefore fail to adhere to their medical regimen.

Evidence now available questions the assumption that individuals at most times during their lives are really asymptomatic. Medically, there is little to distinguish many minor disorders that are brought to the provider's attention from those that are ignored, tolerated, or self-medicated.[61] This sort of "illness" is often ignored. The presence of clinical symptoms is the statistical norm. On the average, a person may have a new "illness" episode every 6 days. The question usually asked is: What makes people delay in getting medical aid? It might be more fruitful to ask: What on earth makes people consult?[43]

One study found that the crux of the decision to seek health care was based in the patient's unwillingness to accommodate the symptoms any further. Usually this decision was not made at the time the patient was most physically ill. Incentives to seek aid originated with interpersonal crises, a perceived interference with vocational or physical activity, social or personal relationships, or sanctioning. When the physician paid little attention to the specific trigger, the patient usually stopped seeking treatment.[61] The patient often responds to symptoms by taking prescribed or over-the-counter medicine. A British study found that although 91% of the adults reported having had symptoms during the 2 weeks before the interview, only 16% had consulted a physician during that time. Of the adults, 55% said they had used some medicine during the 24 hours before the interview.[10]

A social psychologic model of the process of seeking help has been described by Mechanic. The following seven groups of variables appear to be particularly important[33]:

1. Number and persistence of symptoms
2. The individual's ability to recognize symptoms
3. Perceived seriousness of symptoms
4. The extent of social and physical disability resulting from the symptoms
5. The cultural background of the defining person, group, or agency in terms of emphasis on qualities such as tolerance or stoicism
6. Available information and medical knowledge
7. Availability of sources of help and their social and physical accessibility

Note that a number of the variables are the same as those in the Health Belief Model, or it has been suggested that they be included in it.

One study broke down the phases of patients seeking help and discovered that different factors mediate delay in each of three phases. Patients who experienced extremely painful symptoms and those who had not read about their symptoms quickly appraised a symptom as a sign of illness. Patients with long-standing symptoms and those who feared possible severe consequences procrastinated in seeking health care after deciding that they were ill. The time period between deciding to seek care and getting it was shorter for persons who were not concerned about the cost of treatment, who were experiencing pain, and who were certain that the illness could be cured. Patients with the shortest total delays were those who did not have a personal problem competing for attention and who were experiencing a painful symptom.[49]

Providers have assumed that the physical symptoms of those patients seeking care accurately reflect the extent of tissue abnormality. However, recent evidence indicates that the symptoms of or-

ganic disease vary widely among patients with the same tissue abnormality. For example, myocardial ischemia may not generate a report of chest pain for the following reasons: (1) the patient is hyposensitive to visceral sensation; (2) the patient is coping with the threat of heart disease by denying pain; or (3) the patient misunderstands the cause and significance of a vague or ambiguous cardiac sensation. Also, many symptomatic patients have no demonstrable electrocardiographic findings, and numerous patients with arrhythmias do not report symptoms. Between 10% and 30% of patients with angina-like pain that is severe enough to warrant coronary angiography are without significant coronary stenosis. Similarly, the existence of a peptic ulcer is only weakly related to symptoms, arthritic pain cannot be predicted from spine x-ray study, dyspnea reported by asthmatic patients corresponds poorly to objective measures of airway obstruction, and symptoms of diabetes correlate better with depression levels than with glycosylated hemoglobin levels. Do these patterns occur because patients acknowledge and selectively attend only those symptoms that alert them to an aberration in health and body? Or is something additional occurring?[3]

MOTIVATING FACTORS IN THE PATIENT

Beliefs regarding health as well as a background of physical and mental skills and attitudes play a part as the patient experiences a health crisis. The situation places special stresses on the patient as well as the family, and it affects the patient's motivation to learn. Models of the psychosocial adaptation to illness suggest some variations in motivation during this process. The hospital (a setting in which patients may find themselves during some of this process) supports them during the adaptation period. However, the hospital creates stresses of its own.

Psychosocial adaptation to illness

The threat of illness and the later confirmation of it precipitate a series of redefinitions of the self. It is a process that allows a person to adapt to illness. The patient's adaptation to the illness will

TABLE 3-4. Stages of psychosocial adaptation to illness

Disbelief	Development of awareness	Reorganization	Resolution and identity change
CRATE*			
This begins when person learns by diagnosis or change in function (symptoms) that he or she has a particular condition. He or she may express denial by "I don't have it," a claim to have something else, avoidance by forgetting or refusing to do things required of him or her, attempts to control treatment, or diverting attention to other issues. Nurse should allow patient to deny but does not join him or her in the denial.	Patient becomes less able to maintain denial, more aware of what has happened to him or her and the implications of it. Dependence on others causes conflict yielding anger, at first diffuse and later more specifically focused on being sick. Anger may be expressed openly, projected, or directed inward in depression. Nurse should avoid joining patient in his or her anger. Nurse assumes responsibility for care so that patient is free to deny.	Patient accepts increased dependence. There is reorganization of feelings between family members. Nurse is safety valve when family cannot accept patient.	Patient resolves his or her loss; he or she begins to acknowledge changes in how he or she sees himself or herself. He or she begins to identify with others who have same problem. Nurse encourages patient to express his or her views of himself or herself. Goal of this process is for patient to be better able to live with his or her illness, rather than repressing it. If he or she has chronic illness, he or she is likely to undergo this process again and again.

Transition from health to illness	Accepted illness	Convalescence	
LEDERER†			
Apprehension and anxiety are present. Many patients ignore symptoms and use denial to allay anxieties, reinforced by plunge into health. Denial may be expressed by minimizing importance of symptoms by identifying them with common, benign, or trivial indispositions. Some patients meet anxiety aggressively and are irascible and ill humored. Others allay anxiety by passivity and are compliant. Patient is driven by his or her symptoms to seek diagnosis and therapy but is anxious and so displays vacillating behavior, reflecting indecision. Urgent requests for diagnostic examinations are rapidly alternated with failure to appear for examination.	Patient has accepted diagnosis and initial therapeutic procedures. He or she views himself as ill and abandons pretenses of health. He or she is preoccupied with symptoms and illness, is greatly concerned with functioning of his or her body, and is dependent. He or she assumes that physician and nurse share these preoccupations and is highly subjective in judging things. In people who have elaborate defenses against regression and expression of "accepted illness." These people continue to deny and do not follow medical advice; rather, they challenge it. This phase ends gradually after pathologic process has been reversed or arrested.	There is return of physical strength and reintegration of personality. This stage may be prolonged if previous life pattern was not satisfying or if person believes he or she cannot return to a life that will be satisfying. Some patients wrench themselves quickly from dependency and overdo. This stage has been likened to adolescence. Nurse must not encourage dependency with protection.[28]	

*Crate MA: *Am J Nurs* 65:72-76, Oct. 1965.
†Lederer HE: *J Soc Issues* 84(4):415, 1952.

Continued.

TABLE 3-4. Stages of psychosocial adaptation to illness—cont'd

Symptom experience	Assumption of sick role	Medical care contact	Dependent patient role	Recovery or rehabilitation
SUCHMAN‡				
Decision that something is wrong is made in these ways: 1. Physical experience (pain, discomfort, change of appearance) 2. Cognitive aspect (interpretation of physical experience) 3. Emotional response of fear or anxiety There is often denial of illness or "flight of health."	Person decides that he or she is sick and needs professional care. He or she seeks symptom alleviation, information and advice, and temporary acceptance of his or her condition by family and friends. How they react has much to do with his or her ability to enter sick role. Patient wants confirmation of his or her feelings and permission to suspend normal obligations.	Patient seeks professional medical diagnosis and course of treatment. He or she seeks authoritative sanction to become "legitimately" ill or return to normal activities. If he or she refuses to accept diagnosis or treatment, this stage is prolonged as he or she searches for another diagnosis. Patients who perceive their symptoms as less serious use self-treatment rather than going to the physician.	There is decision to transfer control to physician and to accept and follow prescribed treatment—to be a "patient"; 74% of people studied felt this task to be difficult for them.	Person relinquishes patient role. For many with chronic illnesses or physical impairments, this is a long and demanding stage with recurring episodes of illness. Person reestablishes relationships changed by illness.

Stage I: Denial	Stage II: Resistance	Stage III: Affirmation	Stage IV: Integration
MATSON AND BROOKS§			
"It's not true; it can't be happening to me." Concealing symptoms. Seeking an authority who will deny the diagnosis. Refusing help. Holding to past life and values.	"It won't get me down!" Searching for a cure or treatment. Active in programs seeking other patients. Reluctant to accept help. Initial recognition of change in life-orientation.	"I guess I have to face it." Grieving for loss of former self. Publicly explaining about multiple sclerosis. Learning to accept help. Subjectively rearranging priorities in life.	"I know it's there, but I don't think much about it." Living with it. Spending time and energy on other matters. Accepting help when necessary. Integration of life style with new values.

‡ Suchman EA: *Health Hum Behav* 6:114-128, 1965.
§ Matson RR, Brooks NA: *Soc Sci Med* 11:245-250, 1977.

TABLE 3-5. The Fredette model for improving cancer patient education: a summary

Period	Adaptation stage	Content	Strategies
1	Existential plight: impact distress, disbelief, shock	Talk about the cancer as it relates to: harms, threats, resources. Discuss disease: personal aspects, family, social concerns.	Be present whenever diagnosis and therapy are discussed by physician. Move out of denial/avoidance. Use one-on-one approach, pamphlets, discussion—short frequent sessions; provide what is asked for.
2	Existential plight proper, developing awareness	Correct misinformation. Expand knowledge base. Reexplain concepts formerly blocked. Explain treatment plan. Teach self-care. Teach about coping strategies, especially information seeking.	Continue one-on-one. Be accepting of anger and crying. Watch for a "teachable moment." Have short frequent sessions. Toward end of period, use simple audio-visuals always followed by discussion.
3	Mitigation, reorganization, restitution	Strengthen coping. Introduce new ideas and options about disease, treatment side effects, and treatments for side effects. Reteach facts presented in earlier period. Teach anxiety reduction methods. Model expression of feelings. Use "I can cope" program.	Use pamphlets, videotapes, films, self-learning packages, longer sessions, group education. Continue to reserve time for questions/discussion. Include family.
4	Accommodation, resolution and identity change	Discuss new identity, further therapy, treatment of side effects, second opinions, work, sexuality, interpersonal issues, fear of recurrences, coping with a chronic illness, living as a cancer survivor. Teach stress reduction. Use "Living with Cancer" program.	Use group teaching, support groups, all other methods. Encourage all free expression.
5	Decline and deterioration, stages of dying	Answer questions asked. Interpret what is happening in the illness. Explain/discuss options. Validate patient's right of choice. Stress hope for comfort rather than cure.	Use one-on-one. Take clues from patient as to when and what to teach.
6	Preterminality and terminality, stages of dying	The dying process The grieving process Spiritual-existential concerns Physical symptom management Psychologic symptom management Interpersonal/communication problems Need for open, honest communication	Use one-on-one. Include family. Use short verbal explanations. Use periods of acceptance and physical comfort. Take clues from patient. Have patience with "middle knowledge phenomenon."[14]

From Fredette SL: *Cancer Nurs* 13:207-215, 1990.

vary according to his or her self-concept, the severity of the illness, the possible change in living patterns, and how the altered function has been perceived by the patient and his or her family. Effective professional care supports and guides the patient and family as they move through the stages of adaptation.[9,44] Teaching, properly timed, is a care skill that can facilitate adaptation.

A number of authors have described the process of psychosocial adaptation to illness. They agree on its general characteristics but focus on slightly different behavioral aspects and divide the process into different numbers of stages. Table 3-4 presents descriptions of models general to all illnesses.

Variations in patients' receptivity to teaching are suggested by these models. During the first stage, denial may interfere with patients' learning about their diagnosis and restrictions. The provider must expect to reinterpret this information for patients. In the stage of denial, patients suppress and distort information that has been presented in unambiguous terms, take a grandiose approach to their situation, and withdraw from role demands. For example, a patient might not speak about his or her heart attack, rationalizing that the pain must have been gas pains. The patient might deny the occurrence altogether ("This couldn't happen to me"). If during this stage of disbelief the caregiver tries to force the patient to look at the illness, the patient may resist.

In later stages of adaptation, people become better able to consider the illness, to hear facts about it, and to participate in their own care.[9] During these later stages, one can expect the patient to be more receptive to teaching regarding diagnosis, treatment, and the course of the illness.

In convalescence patients have three tasks: they must reassess their lives, bolster their self-images, and accept their dependence on others. Short hospital stays enable patients to go when adaptation must still be accomplished. Patients may have rapid mood swings, pain, restlessness, sleeplessness, and other problems for which family members are ill prepared and in which the roles of patients and family members are not clearly defined.[39]

Different disease processes might be expected to produce slightly different patterns of adaptation.

Lay consultation frequently mediates decisions to seek health care. They can support and assist patients to think more clearly about their predicaments; provide new information about symptoms, etiology, ways of coping, and treatments; and offer support for action.[15] Table 3-4 contains an example of the process found in patients with multiple sclerosis.[32] These patients may regress from an advanced stage of adaptation to an earlier one when exacerbation occurs, or they may remain forever in one stage if the disease does not progress. Because each new "attack" reminds patients of their vulnerability, it takes a long time to reestablish integration, and it has to be done with each exacerbation. This may account for the finding that as the disease (disability and symptoms) worsens, the self-concept gets better—in many cases, markedly better.[32] Table 3-5 presents a model of adaptation specific to cancer, drawing clear direction for appropriate patient education. The box on p. 33 indicates other disease-specific models of adaptation that have been developed for the family and patient undergoing heart transplant[35] and for burn recovery.[57]

GENERAL PRINCIPLES OF MOTIVATION

Basic principles of motivation exist that are applicable to learning in any situation.

The environment can be used to focus the patient's attention on what needs to be learned. Teachers who create warm and accepting yet business-like atmospheres will promote persistent effort and favorable attitudes toward learning in children.[26] This strategy should also be successful with adults. Interesting visual aids, such as booklets for new mothers, posters of postpartum exercises, or equipment for practicing the drawing of fluid into a syringe, motivate learners by capturing their attention and curiosity.

Incentives motivate learning. Incentives include privileges, such as leaving the ward, having special treats of food, and receiving praise from a health professional or a family member. The teacher de-

MODELS FOR PATIENTS UNDERGOING HEART TRANSPLANT OR BURN RECOVERY

HEART TRANSPLANT*

Stage 1: Immersion. During the waiting period for a donor, the partner pledges himself or herself to the welfare of the patient and focuses all cognitive activity on that goal; filters information; monitors the patient's physiologic state; and takes on roles and behaviors previously performed by the patient.

Stage 2: Passage. After transplant surgery, patient and partner move from a belief in the patient's return to normal, to recognition of the patient's permanent vulnerability.

Stage 3: Negotiation. Partners are in conflict between commitment to the patient with an uncertain future and the drive to attend their own survival. Frequently patients are not interested in seeking security. They want to enjoy a second chance at life, viewing themselves as healthy.

BURN†

Stage 1: Survival anxiety. The focus is on whether physical survival is possible. The patient has difficulty concentrating or following instructions and frequently withdraws. Educational efforts should focus on informing patients about the extent of their injuries and outlining the most likely course for recuperation.

Stage 2: Problem of pain. Cognitive and affective functioning is centered on pain and its relief.

Stage 3: Search for meaning. The patient constantly reexamines events leading up to and including the trauma, until a plausible cause and effect sequence is intellectually and emotionally tolerable. The provider listens nonjudgmentally and discusses alternate explanations with the patient.

Stage 4: Investment in recuperation. Patients understand and participate in treatment measures for recovery and autonomous functioning. Patients will judge themselves and their progress and may be depressed.

Stage 5: Acceptance of losses. Patients may go through this stage repeatedly as they struggle to develop a realistic concept of permanent losses as well as the assurance that postburn life can still offer them pleasure and value.

Stage 6: Investment in rehabilitation. This stage focuses cognitively and affectively on steps that will allow patients to resume as many of their preburn functions as they can.

Stage 7: Reintegration of identity. A continuing, new identity emerges; frequently, identity reintegration occurs with only supportive care by the staff.

*Mishel MH, Murdaugh CL: *Nurs Res* 36:332-338, 1987.
†Watkins PN and others: *J Burn Care Rehabil* 9:376-384, 1988.

termines an incentive that is likely to motivate an individual at a particular time. For some individuals and families, being able to care for their own health needs is incentive enough; they are eager to learn. For many patients, who are still startled that they have an illness, the provider needs to guide learning and reward appropriate behavior until the patients have a clearer view of their situation and become more self-motivating.

In the areas of prevention of disease and promotion of health without the threat of illness, self-motivation without rewards may not succeed. Patients must find satisfaction in learning based on the understanding that the goals are useful to them or, less commonly, based on the pure enjoyment of exploring new things. *This internal motivation is longer lasting and more self-directive than is external motivation, which must be repeatedly reinforced by praise or concrete rewards.* Some individuals—particularly children of certain ages and some adults—have little capacity for internal motivation and must be guided and reinforced constantly. The use of incentives is based on the principle that learning occurs more effectively when the individual experiences feelings of satisfaction. Caution should be exercised in using external rewards when they are not absolutely necessary; their use may be followed by a decline in internal (intrinsic) motivation.[16]

Learning is most effective when an individual is ready to learn, that is, when one wants to know something. The purpose of this chapter is to describe factors that affect readiness to learn about health so that the caregiver can use the state when it exists or analyze the reasons for its absence. Sometimes the patient's readiness to learn comes with time, and the caregiver's role is to encourage its development. If the desired change in behavior is urgent, the nurse may need to supervise directly to ensure that the desired behavior occurs. For example, patients with myocardial infarctions who have been instructed to temporarily limit physical activity might refuse to listen because they are not intellectually convinced that they have myocardial infarction, or they may not have accepted it emotionally. Patients may not be reliable in following instructions and therefore must be supervised and have the instructions repeated again and again.

Motivation is enhanced by the way in which the instructional material is organized. In general, the best organized material makes the information meaningful to the individual. One method of organization includes relating new tasks to those already known. For example, if patients know that caring for surgical wounds involves many of the same principles used in dressing superficial wounds with Band-Aids, they can easily connect the concepts. Other ways to relay meaning are to determine whether the persons being taught understand the final outcome desired and instruct them to compare and contrast ideas.[26]

None of these techniques will produce sustained motivation unless the goals are realistic for the learner. The basic learning principle involved is that *success is more predictably motivating than is failure.* Ordinarily, people will choose activities of intermediate uncertainty rather than those that are difficult (little likelihood of success) or easy (high probability of success). For goals of high value there is less tendency to choose more difficult conditions. Having learners assist in defining goals increases the probability that they will understand them and want to reach them.

However, patients and families sometimes have unrealistic notions about what they can accomplish. Possibly they do not understand the precision with which a skill must be carried out; they do not have the depth of knowledge necessary to provide adequate care (such as in the administration of insulin), or they do not have the skill, strength, or determination necessary to care adequately for an invalid relative. Nurses have this perspective and are responsible for assessing learners' abilities to meet the goals. The nurse may suggest that the family use the services of a home health aide to provide the skill and physical energy necessary in caring for the invalid. Patients with diabetes, for example, can be assisted in learning routines of general hygiene and insulin administration if persons with medical backgrounds are available to assess the effectiveness of their self-care. These limited goals may be intermediate to more advanced goals, or they may be all that the individual can accomplish. To identify realistic goals, providers must be skilled in assessing a patient's readiness or a patient's progress toward goals.

Sometimes the accepted goals of a health education program are beyond the readiness of a whole group of individuals who need to learn. This seemed to be the case in one study of medically indigent diabetics. This study suggested that the traditional teaching and therapeutic programs for the management of diabetes have been planned for the middle- or upper-class patient. For example, diets call for a generous amount of expensive protein foods and a three-meal pattern. The administration of insulin requires a concept of asepsis and the purchase of equipment and medicine. Keeping written records and understanding signs and symptoms imply abstract thinking. These may be unrealistic goals for some individuals.

Because learning requires change in beliefs and

behavior, it normally produces a mild level of anxiety, which is useful in motivating the individual; however, severe anxiety is incapacitating.[26] A high degree of stress is inherent in some of the situations health care providers encounter. During an emergency, teaching-learning is at a minimum because other goals are more important and because anxiety is high. Individuals with less severe health crises may also react with intense anxiety because they feel threatened by what has occurred. If anxiety is severe, the individuals' perception of what is going on around them is limited. They are oriented more toward gaining relief than toward attending to learning, and they show physical signs and symp-

TABLE 3-6. Motivation factors and strategies, by time periods

Time	Motivation factors	Motivational strategies
BEGINNING: When learning enters and starts learning process	**Attitudes**—toward the learning environment, teacher, subject matter, and self	Make the conditions that surround the subject positive. Positively confront the possible erroneous beliefs, expectations, and assumptions that may underlie a negative learner attitude.
	Needs—the basic needs within the learner at the time of learning	Reduce or remove components of the learning environment that lead to failure or fear. Plan activities to allow learners to meet esteem needs.
DURING: When learner is involved in the body or main content of the learning process	**Stimulation**—the stimulation processes affecting learner during the learning experience	Change style and content of the learning activity. Make learner reaction and involvement essential parts of the learning process, that is, problem solving, role playing, stimulation.
	Affect—the emotional experience of the learner while learning	Use learner concerns to organize content and to develop themes and teaching procedures. Use a group cooperative goal to maximize learner involvement and sharing.
ENDING: When learner is completing the learning process	**Competence**—the competence value for the learner that is a result of the learning behavior	Provide consistent feedback regarding mastery of learning. Acknowledge and affirm the learners' responsibility in completing the learning task.
	Reinforcement—the reinforcement value attached to the learning experience, for the learner	When learning has natural consequences, allow them to be congruently evident. Provide artificial reinforcement when it contributes to successful learning, and provide closure with a positive ending.

Modified from Wlodkowski RJ: *Educ Psychol* 16(2):101-110, 1981.

toms of anxiety. For this reason, mothers who are highly distressed because of their children's illness may be unable to learn skills with which to care for them. Providers must be able to identify anxiety and understand its effect on learning. They also have a responsibility to avoid causing severe anxiety in learners by setting ambiguous or unrealistically high goals for them.

It is important to help each learner set goals and to provide informative feedback regarding progress toward those goals. Setting a goal demonstrates an intention to achieve and activates learning from one day to the next. It also directs the learner's activities toward the goal and offers an opportunity to experience success.[26] Additional discussion of goals may be found in Chapter 4 and of reinforcement and feedback in Chapter 5.

Both affiliation and approval are strong motivators. People seek out others with whom to compare their abilities, opinions, and emotions. Affiliation can also result in direct anxiety reduction by the social acceptance and the mere presence of others. However, these motivators can also lead to conformity, competition, and other behaviors that may be seen as negative.[16]

Many behaviors result from a combination of motives. Table 3-6 organizes major motivational elements, each with a research and theory base, into a model useful for instruction. It recognizes that no grand theory exists; however, motivation is so necessary for learning that strategies should be planned to organize a continuous and interactive motivational dynamic for maximum effectiveness.[58]

These general principles of motivation are interrelated. A single teaching action can use many of them simultaneously. For example, having a display of teaching pamphlets available in the patient lounge of a maternity floor may focus the patients' attention on things to be learned, taking advantage of their natural curiosity about subjects such as breastfeeding or postpartum exercises. The content of these pamphlets is aimed at helping patients set and attain realistic goals and often is organized to relate new material to that which most women know. A display of teaching pamphlets can en-

courage questions as well as convey the staff's interest in the patients' learning.

Finally, let it be said that an enormous gap exists between knowing that health behavior is motivated and identifying the specific motivational components of any particular act. Providers must focus on learning patterns of motivation for an individual or group, with the realization that errors will be common.

ASSESSMENT OF MOTIVATION

Methods used to measure the need and motivation to learn also may be used as part of a general health assessment process or for a problem or a disease assessment. The assessment may discover the existence of an undesirable state thought to be amenable to treatment by patient education, or the measurements may pertain to the teaching process that has already begun, as is depicted below:

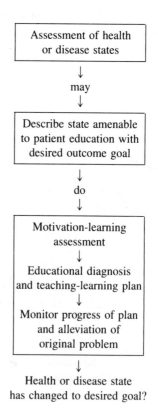

Assessment of health
or disease states

↓

may

↓

Describe state amenable
to patient education with
desired outcome goal

↓

do

↓

Motivation-learning
assessment

↓

Educational diagnosis
and teaching-learning plan

↓

Monitor progress of plan
and alleviation of
original problem

↓

Health or disease state
has changed to desired goal?

For example, while conducting an admission assessment, a provider might ask these questions: What do you know about your disease and treatment? How do you cope with symptoms? How do you manage stressful situations? How do you prefer to learn new information? What concerns you the most right now?[56] A second example is an assessment of parenting skill, done for the purpose of identifying parents at risk for child abuse or child neglect. One area of that assessment may be knowledge of normal growth and development.[24] It is of course necessary to have studies that show the validity of predictions in present observations. For example, one study showed that the absence of a positive maternal perception of the neonate (as measured by the Neonatal Perception Inventories) is associated with a high rate of subsequent psychosocial disorder.[8] This tool should of course minimize false negatives and false positives. Functions of measurements are as follows: (1) screen to identify those who have a problem or might develop one and those who should receive further assessment, (2) assess in detail, leading to diagnosis and intervention strategies, and (3) monitor—review the progress of those receiving treatment. Measurements may be done by staff or by patients and families. To be useful in a clinical setting, they should be as short as possible and easy to administer.

Studies will often be aimed at assessing the patient's self-care capability in a particular environment. In general, practitioners should hesitate to screen the patient unless useful actions are possible when the findings are positive. Measurements often can provide groundwork for program decisions—for example, decisions made for the diabetes care program as well as the patient education portion of that program.

Assessments should also be done to tailor an educational program and target it to the particular needs of a specific group of people who will receive it. For example, a "community needs" assessment structured by the health belief model was used to assess women who needed mammograms. The women in this particular community believed they were susceptible to breast cancer and were cognizant of the benefits of mammography. Fear of pain and radiation as well as embarrassment proved to be significant barriers for some of the women. Also, women over 65 rarely had physicians who recommended mammography; therefore the intervention included educating physicians and using senior citizen groups to encourage older women to be more aggressive in asking for referrals. Since the assessment also found a need to reach Spanish-speaking Hispanics, a bilingual mammography facility guide was developed.[36] The intervention was of course validated by an increase in the number of women obtaining mammography.

Before initiating an educational program, a public health department surveyed county residents by phone to determine their knowledge, attitudes, and practices regarding diabetes and glaucoma. While general knowlege of these illnesses was relatively widespread, knowledge of symptoms and risk factors (which are important for early detection) was deficient. Age, sex, level of education, and family history were significant predictors of knowledge that could be used in targeting educational programs. This baseline survey of a population can identify needed areas of emphasis and subgroups with special needs as well as provide a basis for evaluation of the program.[34] In a postpartum unit in which hospital stays were short, a systematic assessment of the patient's reaction to the birth experience, adaptation to the infant, and family's reaction to the infant were essential to identify those in need of additional teaching and assistance.[18] Finally, marketing research uses focus groups of consumers to identify trends in the way consumers think, feel, react, or make decisions about a particular topic. The focus groups are used to test a new service concept, to stimulate ideas about how service can be improved, and to provide consumer terminology for promotional material.[55]

Two examples follow of specialized measuring tools that may be used to assess the patient's need for education and his or her ability to learn. The Self-Efficacy Scale (Figure 3-3) measures cardiac patients' perceived ability to perform various physical tasks. The value of the method results from

10	20	30	40	50	60	70	80	90	100
Quite uncertain				Moderately certain					Certain

Walk (distance)	Can Do	Confidence
Walk one block	_____	_____
Walk two blocks	_____	_____
Walk one mile	_____	_____
Walk two miles	_____	_____
Walk three miles	_____	_____

FIGURE 3-3. Self-efficacy scale. (From Houston-Miller N: *J Cardiac Rehabil* 4:104-106, 1984.)

DIABETES IN PREGNANCY KNOWLEDGE SCREEN

Below are questions about diabetes during pregnancy. Answering these questions will help us determine your current knowledge about diabetes during pregnancy and enable us to provide the best care possible during your pregnancy. Many questions have more than one answer, therefore circle "I don't know" rather than guessing. By answering to the best of your knowledge, we will be able to counsel you most effectively about diabetes during your pregnancy.

1. Which of the following feelings may result from a reaction? (Circle all that might happen, not just those that have happened to you)
   A. Difficulty thinking
   B. Blurred vision
   C. Nervousness or shaky
   D. Numbness
   E. Sweating
   F. I don't know

2. What should you do if you have a reaction? (Circle all that apply)
   A. Walk it off
   B. Sit down and rest
   C. Eat crackers or cheese
   D. Drink milk
   E. I don't know

3. Glycosylated hemoglobin levels are drawn about once per month during pregnancy. Why are these levels taken?
   A. They measure previous blood sugar control
   B. They measure the amount of iron in your blood
   C. They measure how helpful your diet is in controlling your blood sugar
   D. I don't know

From Spirito A: *Diabetes Care* 13:712-718, 1990.

DIABETES IN PREGNANCY KNOWLEDGE SCREEN—cont'd

4. When planning vigorous exercise (e.g., swimming, playing tennis), what changes should you make in your daily diabetes routine? (Circle all that apply)
   A. Decrease insulin
   B. Carefully time when to do your exercising
   C. Increase amount of carbohydrates (e.g., bread, fruits) you eat
   D. Increase the amount of protein (e.g., meat, cheese) you eat
   E. I don't know

5. On days when you are sick, what steps should you take to control your diabetes?
   A. Increase the amount of water or other fluids
   B. Stop your insulin
   C. Call your doctor
   D. I don't know

6. The normal range for blood sugar during pregnancy is:
   A. 40-150 mg/dl
   B. 60-120 mg/dl
   C. 100-200 mg/dl
   D. I don't know

7. A specific meal plan has been devised for you by the dietitian. Which of the following statements about your meal plan are correct. (Circle all that apply)
   A. You should eat everything on your meal plan
   B. You can reduce the amount of food you eat if you're not hungry
   C. You should control the amount of food you eat all the time
   D. You can eat your meals any time during the day as long as you eat everything on your plan
   E. I don't know

8. Bedtime snacks are an important part of your meal plan because they help you avoid having reactions overnight. (Circle one)
   True or False

9. Margarine is mainly:
   A. Protein
   B. Carbohydrate
   C. Fat
   D. Mineral and vitamin
   E. I don't know

10. Rice is mainly:
    A. Protein
    B. Carbohydrate
    C. Fat
    D. Mineral and vitamin
    E. I don't know

11. If you don't feel like having the egg on your diet for breakfast, you can: (Circle two)
    A. Have extra toast
    B. Substitute one small chop
    C. Have an ounce of cheese instead
    D. Skip the egg, and don't eat anything else
    E. I don't know

12. If you have problems controlling your blood sugar during pregnancy, what are some of the possible effects on your baby after birth? (Circle all that apply)
    A. Could be born with low blood sugar (hypoglycemia)
    B. Could be a large baby making delivery more difficult
    C. Could have breathing problems after birth
    D. I don't know

13. What does glucagon do?
    A. It helps the liver release more sugar into the blood
    B. It makes the liver stop releasing sugar into the blood
    C. It helps the pancreas release more insulin
    D. It stops the pancreas from releasing insulin
    E. I don't know

14. After using glucagon, it's most important to:
    A. Drink plenty of fluids
    B. Get plenty of rest
    C. Eat a meal so your blood sugar doesn't drop
    D. None of the above
    E. I don't know

the close relationship that exists between self-efficacy and the probability that a given activity will be attempted. These scores can also be used to evaluate interventions, such as exercise testing when it is followed by explanation of test results by staff. This scale measures perceived self-efficacy for walking. Results likely would not hold true for dissimilar tasks.[21] Also, a brief test to assess the baseline knowledge of pregnant women with overt diabetes is shown (boxes on pp. 38 and 39); it could also be used to evaluate the outcomes of instruction.[51] This test should be used with other assessment devices. Knowledge is necessary but not sufficient for most positive health outcomes.

It is important to assess the mental abilities of some patients to make effective decisions. While mental status examinations have been used clinically for some time, recent studies have questioned the veracity of these screens. The principle of selective decision-making capacity declares that people may not be able to function competently in making financial decisions; however, they may be able to make decisions about medical treatment competently. Fitten and others have constructed an approach to assess a patient's ability to make particular decisions. Their vignette approach may be seen in the box on p. 40.[12] Table 3-7 suggests a list of behavioral descriptors of cognitive deficits.

Finally, tools for assessment of motivation and readiness to learn exist within the context of the patient-provider relationship. Rapport within this relationship is necessary to obtain evidence about motivation, and data from tools must be synthesized with data from interactions with the patient. In addition, teachers frequently stimulate motivation by questioning, by caring, and by helping the patient reach a learning goal as well as encouraging the sense of commitment a patient develops toward a caregiver.

Teachers must consciously activate motivation before learning and help the patient maintain it during learning. The construction of goals is important, especially ones that are specific, moderately difficult, and attained quickly. Such goals enhance motivation and encourage persistence be-

---

VIGNETTE FOR ASSESSING DECISION-MAKING CAPACITY

Mr./Ms. _____ , let's suppose for a minute that I am your doctor and you are my patient. Let's also imagine for a minute that you've been having a hard time sleeping. Let's suppose that you have told the nurses about this problem and that you would like some help with it. The nurses have told me about it and now I have come to talk to you about this.

Let us suppose I tell you that I want to give you a sleeping pill to take at bedtime. This medicine will likely help you sleep better for a while, but after two or three weeks, the effect of helping you sleep may begin to wear off. Let us suppose I also tell you that there could be some unpleasant side effects with taking the pills. For example, during the day these pills may slow down your thinking and learning, and if you take them for a while you could become dependent on them. That means, if you stop taking them you may become nervous and lose more sleep. You could, of course, choose not to take the sleeping pills. This would leave your present sleep problem about the same as it is now.

Do you have any questions about this story? I will repeat it for you. Now try to answer as many of the following questions about this story as you can.

1. Am I *really* your doctor?
2. Are you *really* my patient?
3. In this story, what problem are you having?
4. How do I plan to help you with your problem?
5. Why do I want to give you a sleeping pill?
6. Do you think this medicine may help?
7. Are there any problems in taking this medicine?
8. What are these problems?
9. What would happen if you chose not to take the medicine at all?
10. As the patient, would you take this medicine or not?
11. Can you tell me why?
Scoring criteria not provided.

From Fitten LJ, Lusky R, Hamann C: *J Am Geriatr Soc* 38:1097-1104, 1990.

TABLE 3-7. Possible behavioral indicators of cognitive deficits

Disorientation (Inability to identify time, place, or person)	Generalized confusion (Imprecisely defined state resulting from impairment of attention span, concentration, perception, orientation, and memory)	Memory deficit (Inability to recall recent or remote past events and inability to learn new information)
Unable to ask appropriate questions to familiarize self with environment ("Where's my call light?"; "What time is my test tomorrow?")	Evasive and vague answers	Unable to list medications
	Slowed verbal response	Unable to give correct recent medical history
	Emotional lability	
Unable to use cues in environment to maintain orientation	Restlessness and irritability	Unable to give appropriate past history related to family or employment
	Unable to follow instructions and procedures	
Unable to give information related to living arrangements, age, family, etc.	Unable to appropriately discuss reasons for admission	Unable to refer appropriately to comments given earlier in conversation
Unable to estimate passage of time during course of day	Disregard for own safety (careless smoking or handling of objects)	Repetitive statements, requests, and questions
Wanders and is unable to relocate room	Self-inflicted painful actions (pulls intravenous tubes out)	Demanding behavior
		Loses possessions
	Demonstrates poor social judgment	Evidence of confabulation
	Paranoid ideation, delusions, hallucinations	
	Incoherent speech	

From Palmateer LM, McCartney JR: *J Gerontol Nurs* 11(2):6-16, 1985.

cause they provide clear standards for judging performance. Teachers also must provide clear feedback on the quality of the learners' performances, help them feel pride and satisfaction in their achievements, and assist as the learner tries to maintain manageable levels of anxiety.[59]

SUMMARY

This chapter deals with assessing motivation and the need for education and clinical evidence of readiness. Knowledge of patterns of health beliefs, behavior and perceived self-efficacy, and the psychosocial impact of illness helps the caregiver to anticipate certain levels of readiness. General principles of motivation, valid in any learning situation, should be used to attain efficient learning.

Assessing motivation requires an understanding of the aims of health teaching as well as skill in gathering and validating information by means of interview, informal conversation, observation, available tools, and health records.

STUDY QUESTIONS

1. It has been said that patients seek help when they are no longer able to cope with their problems at their current level of understanding. If this statement is at least partly true, what are the implications for health care services?
2. List the questions that you would ask to assess need and motivation to learn in each of the following nursing situations?
   a. You are going to catheterize a patient after delivery.
   b. As a public health nurse you are to visit the home of a sick 3-year-old child and must help the mother carry out the physician's orders to force fluids.

c. As a nurse working in a gynecology clinic, you are to teach breast self-examination to groups of women in the waiting room.

d. As a public health nurse you are to teach a 10-year-old boy, who is mentally retarded, blind, and suffering from cerebral palsy, how to feed himself.

3. For each description of patient behavior that follows, indicate possible explanations in terms of the psychosocial adaptation to illness model.

The importance of proper timing and sensitivity to the patient's feelings was made evident in the case of Mike S., a 21-year-old college student who sustained a T10 fracture in a skiing accident. His first admission lasted 3 months; during this time he was apathetic and easily discouraged. He preferred to stay in bed as much as possible, covering himself from head to toe with a sheet. A common statement heard in reference to Mike was, "He certainly has potential but just won't use it. . . ."

A trial of voiding was attempted even though Mike indicated he didn't care if it worked or not. Needless to say, the trial was unsuccessful. . . .

It was true that Mike did have potential for rehabilitation, but he was unable to mobilize this potential because he did not yet have the necessary strength to accept his disabled body. Not only was his bladder in shock, but also his mind and spirit. Mike was discharged to his home to return in 3 months. He left as an angry, depressed young man, unable to see much future in his life as a paraplegic. . . .

On readmission, there was a noticeable change in Mike's attitude toward himself. He had obviously used his 3-month vacation from the hospital in a constructive way. He had developed many plans and ideas to improve his self-care. He was also interested in getting rid of the catheter. . . .*

4. Do you agree or disagree with the following statement? The better nurses understand the patient, the more success they should have in getting him or her to follow their advice in matters related to his or her health? Explain why you agree or disagree.

5. The following statement is from Conte and others:
Some of our patients revealed that when they were first advised to take anti-hypertensive medications, they had doubts as to the accuracy of the diagnosis. Some said they had taken their hypertension seriously only after an unusual or frightening event had occurred as a result of their hypertension or after they learned of its dangers. This suggests that early patient education regarding hypertension could prevent many unnecessary complications.†
Do you agree?

---

*Delehanty L, Stravino V: Achieving bladder control, *Am J Nurs* 70:312-316, 1970.

†Conte A and others: Group work with hypertensive patients, *Am J Nurs* 74:910-912, 1974.

REFERENCES

1. Auerbach SM and others: Anxiety, locus of control, type of preparatory information and adjustment to dental surgery, *J Consult Clin Psychol* 44:809-818, 1976.
2. Bandura A: Self-efficacy mechanism in human agency, *Am Psychol* 37:122-147, 1982.
3. Barsky AJ and others: Silent myocardial ischemia, *JAMA* 264:1132-1135, 1990.
4. Becker MH and others: The health belief model and sick-role behavior, *Health Educ Monogr* 2:409-419, 1974.
5. Becker MH, Janz NK: The health belief model applied to understanding diabetes regimen compliance, *Diabetes Educ* 11:41-47, 1985.
6. Becker MH, Maiman LA: Sociobehavioral determinants of compliance with health and medical care recommendations, *Med Care* 13:10-24, 1975.
7. Becker MH, and others: A new approach to explaining sick-role behavior in low-income populations, *Am J Public Health* 64:205-216, 1974.
8. Broussard EE: Assessment of the adaptive potential of the mother-infant system: the neonatal perception inventories, *Semin Perinatol* 3:91-100, 1979.
9. Crate MA: Nursing functions in adaptation to chronic illness, *Am J Nurs* 65:72-76, 1965.
10. Dunnell K, Cartwright A: *Medicine takers, prescribers and hoarders*, London, 1972, Routledge & Kegal Paul.
11. Fielding R: Patients' beliefs regarding the causes of myocardial infarction: implications for information giving and compliance, *Patient Educ Couns* 9:121-134, 1987.
12. Fitten LJ, Lusky R, Hamann C: Assessing treatment decision-making capacity in elderly nursing home residents, *J Am Geriatr Soc* 38:1097-1104, 1990.
13. Fogel CI, Woods NF: *Health care of women: a nursing perspective*, St Louis, 1981, Mosby–Year Book.
14. Fredette SL: A model for improving cancer patient education, *Cancer Nurs* 13:207-215, 1990.
15. Furstenberg AL, Davis LJ: Lay consultation of older people, *Soc Sci Med* 18:827-837, 1984.
16. Geen RG, Beatty WW, Arkin RM: *Human motivation*, Boston, 1984, Allyn & Bacon.
17. Given CW and others: Development of scales to measure beliefs of diabetic patients, *Res Nurs Health* 6:127-141, 1983.
18. Hans A: Postpartum assessment: the psychological component, *JOGNN* 15:49-51, 1986.
19. Harwood A, editor: *Ethnicity and medical care*, Cambridge, Mass, 1981, Harvard University Press.
20. Horn B: Cultural beliefs and teenage pregnancy, *Nurse Pract* 8(8):38-39, 1983.
21. Houston-Miller N: Questions and answers, *J Cardiac Rehabil* 4:104-106, 1984.
22. Janz NK, Becker MH: The health belief model: a decade later, *Health Educ Q* 11:1-47, 1984.
23. Jones PK, Jones SL, Katz J: Improving follow-up among

hypertensive patients using a health belief model intervention, *Arch Intern Med* 147:1557-1561, 1987.

24. Josten L: Prenatal assessment guide for illuminating possible problems with parenting, *MCN* 6:113-117, 1981.

25. Kasl SV: The health belief model and behavior related to chronic illness, *Health Educ Monogr* 2:433-454, 1974.

26. Klausmeier HJ: *Educational psychology,* ed 5, Philadelphia, 1985, Harper & Row.

27. Kluckhohn FR, Strodbeck FL: *Variations in value orientations,* Evanston, Ill, 1961, Row, Peterson.

28. Lederer HD: How the sick view their world, *J Soc Issues* 8(4):4-15, 1952.

29. Lewis FM, Daltroy LH: How causal explanations influence health behavior: attribution theory. In Glanz K, Lewis FM, Rimer BK, editors: *Health behavior and health education,* San Francisco, 1990, Jossey-Bass.

30. Lowery BJ, DuCette JP: Disease-related learning and disease control in diabetics as a function of locus of control, *Nurs Res* 25:358-362, 1976.

31. Maslow AH: A theory of human motivation, *Psychol Rev* 50:370-396, 1943.

32. Matson RR, Brooks NA: Adjusting to multiple sclerosis: an exploratory study, *Soc Sci Med* 11:245-250, 1977.

33. Mechanic D: *Public expectations and health care,* New York, 1972, John Wiley & Sons.

34. Michielutte R and others: Knowledge of diabetes and glaucoma in a rural North Carolina community, *J Community Health* 9:269-284, 1984.

35. Mishel MH, Murdaugh CL: Family adjustment to heart transplantation: redesigning the dream, *Nurs Res* 36:332-338, 1987.

36. Morisky DE and others: The role of needs assessment in designing a community-based mammography education program for urban women, *Health Educ Res* 4:469-478, 1989.

37. Mullen PD, Hersey JC, Iverson DC: Health behavior models compared, *Soc Sci Med* 24:973-981, 1987.

38. Nathanson GA: Sex roles as variables in preventive health behavior, *J Community Health* 3:142-155, 1977.

39. Norris CM: The work of getting well, *Am J Nurs* 69:2118-2121, 1969.

40. Oakley A: *Women confined: towards a sociology of childbirth,* Oxford, 1980, Martin Robertson.

41. Pill R, Stott NCH: Concepts of illness causation and responsibility: some preliminary data from a sample of working class mothers, *Soc Sci Med* 16:43-53, 1982.

42. Prewitt VR: Health beliefs and AIDS educational materials, *Commun Health* 12(2):65-76, 1989.

43. Robinson D: *The process of becoming ill,* London, 1971, Routledge & Kegan Paul.

44. Rolland JS: Toward a psychosocial typology of chronic and life-threatening illness, *Fam Sys Med* 2:245-261, 1984.

45. Rosenstock IM: The health belief model and preventive health behavior, *Health Educ Monogr* 2:354-386, 1974.

46. Rosenstock IM: Historical origins of the health belief model, *Health Educ Monogr* 2:328-335, 1974.

47. Rosenstock IM, Strecher VJ, Becker MH: Social learning theory and the health belief model, *Health Educ Q* 15:175-183, 1988.

48. Rutledge DN, Davis GT: Breast self-examination compliance and the health belief model, *Oncol Nurs Forum* 15:175-179, 1988.

49. Safer MA and others: Determinants of three stages of delay in seeking care at a medical clinic, *Med Care* 17:11-28, 1979.

50. Slavin RE: *Educational psychology: theory into practice,* ed 2, Englewood Cliffs, NJ, 1986, Prentice-Hall.

51. Spirito A and others: Screening measure to assess knowledge of diabetes in pregnancy, *Diabetes Care* 13:712-718, 1990.

52. Stacey M: Charisma, power and altruism: a discussion of research in a child development centre, *Sociol Health Illness* 2:64-90, 1980.

53. Suchman EA: Stages of illness and medical care, *Health Hum Behav* 6:114-128, 1965.

54. Toner JB, Manuck SB: Health locus of control and health-related information seeking at a hypertension screening, *Soc Sci Med* 13A:823-825, 1979.

55. Vargus JH, Robertson PH: Plug into consumer thinking, *Group Pract J* 33(4):54-60, 1984.

56. Volker DL: Needs assessment and resource identification, *Oncol Nurs Forum* 18:119-123, 1991.

57. Watkins PN and others: Psychological stages in adaptation following burn injury: a method for facilitating psychological recovery of burn victims, *J Burn Care Rehabil* 9:376-384, 1988.

58. Wlodkowski RJ: Making sense out of motivation: a systematic model to consolidate motivational constructs across theories, *Educ Psychol* 16(2):101-110, 1981.

59. Woolfolk AE: *Educational psychology,* ed 4, Englewood Cliffs, NJ, 1990, Prentice-Hall.

60. Young R: Prevention in American II, *Health Med* 3:1-17, 1985.

61. Zola IK: Pathways to the doctor—from person to patient, *Soc Sci Med* 7:677-689, 1973.

CHAPTER 4

Objectives in patient education

The goal of health teaching is to elicit positive behaviors from the patient. The patient and the health team determine the goals, taking into consideration the individual's health, social needs, and capacity to learn. Objectives guide teaching and learning activities. The major purpose of evaluation is to determine if the patient has incorporated the appropriate behaviors. Making knowledgeable decisions about goals and stating them precisely and completely provide clear direction in teaching the patient. Poorly determined goals or an inability to communicate them result in confusion throughout the teaching-learning process. This chapter discusses the determination of goals, rules for the statement of goals, the value of a system that classifies patients' anticipated behaviors, and domains in which patient education goals fall.

BEHAVIORAL OBJECTIVES AS EDUCATIONAL TOOLS

With present knowledge of teaching and learning, we cannot predict all the goals that should or can be met during a particular teaching episode. Because of this uncertainty, some individuals take the position that specification of objectives before instruction is restrictive. This position challenges the teacher's and the learner's ability to predetermine what the learner needs. In addition, a narrow focus of predetermined objectives restricts potentially valuable instruction. Although the degree of validity of this argument is not really known, the weight of present opinion supports the use of objectives. However, it advises against becoming overprescriptive, and teachers must constantly be aware that additional objectives may be needed.

At this time behavioral objectives form the most widely used system of planning in education. Other useful schemes, such as disjointed incrementalism and correction of objectives through feedback, have been adopted. Many providers combine all three of these approaches and use them whenever appropriate. Disjointed incrementalism involves moving toward short-term goals without clear long-range goals. It also involves specifying objectives in terms of moving away from a bad situation. In the feedback model, the teacher may have either a general or specific notion of the learning goals. However, these goals are viewed as fallible tools that are clarified by the outcomes of teaching-learning. Teachers and learners, however, should not allow themselves to rely on excuses to avoid the hard work of determining what needs to be learned.

Other weaknesses of behavioral objectives are as follows: (1) they do not show the complex manner in which ideas are related, and therefore they have no higher level structure; (2) other than hunch or intuition, no procedures exist for justifying the exclusion or inclusion of a given objective, unless that objective relates to an obviously unnecessary task; (3) there is no consistent view of the origin of objectives; (4) they conflict with exploratory learning; and (5) they often communicate intent ambiguously.[20]

Still others object to the notion of negotiated behaviors as the outcome of teaching, believing that patients have a right to information, which they may or may not choose to use to make a behavioral change. Underlying this line of reasoning are the views of those such as Popkewitz,[27] who argues that the forms of knowledge chosen in educational

Nursing diagnosis: Progressive acquisition of maternal role behaviors related to seeking and gaining experience in child care.

Long-term goal: Attainment of the maternal role

Short-term goal: Further acquisition of prenatal maternal role behaviors

The client will:

1. Describe her own philosophy of child care and discipline method.
2. Complete preparation of an area for the infant in the home, including acquisition of initial feeding, clothing, and furniture supplies.

Nursing interventions (directed toward accomplishment of short-term goals):

1. Share knowledge of alternate methods of child care and parenting and discuss advantages and disadvantages with client.
2. Reinforce client's efforts to gain experience in child care, and explore resources where such experience can be gained.
3. Provide opportunity for discussion of types of supplies necessary for infant care such as clothes, furniture, and feeding equipment.

Nursing diagnosis: Beginning maternal acquaintance related to early contact with newborn.

Long-term goal: Maternal attachment

Short-term goal: Continued interaction with newborn

The client will:

1. Use touch with her infant, progressing from fingertips to contact with her whole hand and from the infant's extremities to the infant's trunk.
2. Identify specific characteristics of the newborn that differentiate the infant from other newborns.
3. State that she is comfortable when touching, handling, feeding, and/or bathing the infant.

Nursing interventions (directed toward accomplishment of short-term goals):

1. Provide extended contact with the infant.
2. Use positive reinforcement of client's early attempts at handling and feeding infant.
3. Point out positive feedback behaviors from the infant to the mother.
4. Conduct a modified Brazelton Newborn Assessment to help acquaint the mother with infant's responses to stimuli.
5. Provide opportunities for feeding and bathing the infant, with help available as needed.

FIGURE 4-1. Examples of positive nursing diagnoses with interventions. (From Stolte KM: *MCN* 11:13-15, 1986.)

situations make assumptions about the relationship of people to their institutions and about power and control. Power relations are also present in the manner in which knowledge is codified. The codification also establishes a legitimacy to a social order. Considerable evidence exists of the validity of this line of reasoning in patient education. The goals have tended to be provider goals. Behavior change toward these goals is the dominantly accepted currency of teaching. The knowledge base used is the provider's.

Work on nursing diagnoses provides other classification systems that serve to integrate nursing activity, including learning and teaching. Diagnostic categories such as knowledge deficit and self-care deficit are primarily focused on learning, while others such as ineffective coping and noncompliance frequently require learning. Also, impaired home maintenance management, altered parenting, and self-care deficits often require retraining. Impaired social interactions, altered role performance, decisional conflict, health-seeking behaviors, and ineffective breastfeeding also may require teaching.[7] Stolte is concerned that many nursing diagnoses as presently constituted have a problem or illness orientation.[33] She suggests examples of positive diagnoses with interventions, as in Figure 4-1.

Objectives also reflect philosophic positions and serve as implementation tools. Providers face several questions of philosophy with regard to patient teaching. One issue concerns the amount and type of information that should be shared with patients as well as the degree of independence that should be allowed or should be required of them while participating in health care. Beliefs regarding the release of information may be altered when researchers are better able to describe the effects of giving information to or withholding it from patients and the effects of teaching them independence or dependence. Ideologically, patients are moving toward independent choice. Providers are responding by adjusting care to individual preferences whenever possible.

Who should determine the direction of a patient's training? It is a question that is being asked today and is being resolved by institutional policy statements or by operating procedures that include rules for the instruction of patients. These policies and procedures are followed unless the provider believes that such instruction is not in the patient's best interest.

To promote a unity of purpose, many health agencies have developed and instituted statements of philosophy and goals that provide clear direction. A portion of a statement of philosophy from the nursing department at Boston's Beth Israel Hospital provides the following example:

"The patient's rights include but are not limited to:

- A recognition of his vulnerability when faced with actual or potential illness, unfamiliar and frightening technical procedures, a strange environment, and a multitude of health care workers who use terms that he may not understand.
- The right to have his physical and emotional needs identified by his nurse and validated by him, as his condition permits, as well as his and his family's responses to care.
- The right to have his perception of his condition recognized, respected, and acted on.
- The right to have his family and others who are significant in his life included in decisions related to his care.
- The right to receive current and accurate information in order to maintain a healthy lifestyle and/or cope with his illness, consistent with his ability to absorb such information at any point in time."[8]

When developing a teaching plan, staff should express objectives in written form so that they can be relayed to the learner and to other health workers. Writing the objectives also helps the teacher envision how they might be taught. Frequently, objectives are extended over a period of time, as shown in the box on p. 47.

MAJOR GOALS OF PATIENT EDUCATION

Since its rebirth in the 1960s, patient education has helped patients reach a number of health care goals: individual and family development, rehabilitation, informed consent, compliance or adherence, coping, and self-care. Health care systems use has also been a goal but will not be discussed here. Information about programs with these goals and about compliance and adherence may be found in Chapter 10. The movement toward self-care is described in Chapter 11. Wellness, as a domain,

---

EXAMPLE OF GOALS FOR LEARNING EXTENDED OVER TIME

Main objective: To follow a restricted sodium diet

Week 1	Week 2	Week 3
To name all foods common to the usual eating pattern that have high sodium content	To plan from memory nutritious menus that are within the sodium allotment	To accommodate the new eating pattern in situations such as social functions and being away from home
To agree that a restricted sodium diet may have some merit	To verbalize willingness to follow a restricted sodium diet	To follow the restricted sodium diet without fail
	To prepare foods without using salt	

---

is in the process of developing. Much of the patient education literature falls in the following categories (although these are not entirely mutually exclusive).

Individual and family development

The focus of patient education in this domain is on supporting and enhancing normal development. Actual work concentrates on preparing for birth, parenting infants and young children, and preventing disruptions in normal development created by medical events during the years when children are most dependent. Development in other phases of the life cycle and longitudinal developmental processes used for adapting to certain health conditions (for example, chronic illnesses) are seldom considered in this framework.

Rehabilitation

Rehabilitation implies that the patient is functioning as completely as possible in all spheres of life within the limits imposed by the disease and its treatment after an illness or trauma that cannot be cured. Rehabilitation is both a goal and a treatment approach applicable to many different groups with disabling disorders: cancer, spinal cord injury, stroke, low back pain, chronic obstructive pulmonary disease, postmyocardial infarction, or

heart surgery. Recently, geriatric rehabilitation and assessment units have been developed to avoid placing patients in nursing homes after an acute illness.

Informed consent

Informed consent is primarily known as a legal concept that determines if a patient has knowingly consented to care. It is also an ethical relationship between patient and provider in which the patient acts intentionally, with understanding, and without controlling influences. As a legal doctrine it is rooted in case law but has been codified in 23 states. The focus in law has been on standards of disclosure and causation, with different jurisdictions holding that the standards of adequate consent are what other physicians would disclose or what a reasonable patient would need. Little attention has been directed toward what the consenting individual understands.[2,11]

Individual physicians who are not agents of the state cannot directly be compelled to obtain informed consent. Patients can only sue for damages after there has been a failure to disclose. Informed consent in research has been mandated and monitored by federal controls and regulations. However, no similar institutional controls exist for clinical medicine, and informed consent as a practice of respecting autonomy has never had a sure foothold in medical practice.[11]

Informed consent requires disclosure of material facts about the nature of, the expected benefits of, and the serious risks of or the side effects of (and alternatives to) a therapy. It is frequently not thought of as "education." However, evidence has accumulated that shows patients often have consented without thoroughly understanding. Evidence also reveals a number of clinical situations in which the legal doctrine was not approximated in practice.[28,19]

Faden and Beauchamp see informed consent as requiring disclosure of a core of facts and individualized education in a participatory process that extends over time with the goal being substantially autonomous patient decisions.[11] The American Hospital Association Policy and Statement on the Patient's Choice of Treatment Options indicates that health care institutions should have methods to identify circumstances under which the patient's authority to determine the course of treatment may be constrained. The patient may require recourse to the judgment of others, including the courts.[1] Institutional ethics committees are doing some of this work.

As recently as the 1950s, it was not unusual for physicians to withhold information from patients who were seriously or terminally ill on the grounds that the truth was not always in the best interest of the patient. Physicians claimed that patients did not always want to know the truth, could not always comprehend it, and could be harmed by it. Physicians were skeptical that laypersons could make intelligent choices about the kind of care necessary for the treatment of a specific medical problem. It is clear that truth telling is much more central in medical practice than it was 20 or 30 years ago. However, informed consent is not well conceived in some areas of practice. In rehabilitation, treatment may extend over many months or years with no attempts to reaffirm patient consent.[6] One of the most common medical interventions, prescribing drugs, is frequently conducted without any patient consent at all.[29] A worldwide trend leans toward increasingly stringent requirements in randomized clinical trials. However, studies of physicians' attitudes toward informed consent indicate ambivalence.[34] Health care providers continue to be concerned about problematic situations in which competent patients' choices seem to be irrational (biased toward the present and not to the future)— their values making no sense.[5]

While informed consent is a concept supported by patient education, legal standards influence the hospitals' presentation of this material. Since the legal responsibility for obtaining informed consent belongs to the individual performing the procedure (usually a physician), the courts have consistently limited nursing liability in informed consent law. A recent Connecticut case held that the hospital has no legal duty to obtain the patient's informed consent, only a monitoring responsibility to ensure that consent has been obtained. Fiesta[12] indicates that a nurse who obtains consent for the physician may become part of the informed consent litigation, and if the hospital, by policy, requires nurses to obtain consents, the hospital is incurring liability.

Coping

Coping has been defined as specific cognitive and behavioral acts used by individuals to minimize a perceived threat and its meaning or to solve illness-related adaptive tasks. Relevant outcomes involve the patient's perceived control over illness and feelings of well-being. To facilitate coping, the patient can change external factors, alter meaning, control the emotional reaction to the threat, and solve illness-related adaptive tasks. Natural support systems are useful. Specific problem-focused coping actions might include seeking information or advice about diagnosis and treatment, making social comparisons, carrying out self-care, negotiating expectations with family members and professionals, setting concrete limited goals, rehearsing outcomes, withdrawing, and sharing concerns.

Text continued on p. 54.

Date	Nursing diagnosis	Expected outcome	D/L	C/P	Nursing orders	Int.	Res.
	Potential alteration in health management related to: a. Knowledge deficit: 1) disease process 2) home care management 3) community resources	Health management as evidenced by: a. Ability to verbalize accurate knowledge about disease process b. Ability to demonstrate performance of home care management requirements c. Ability to verbalize available community resources and how to contact them	Dis.		a. Assess readiness to learn, i.e., level of anxiety, pain, verbalized interest, attention span. a. Plan teaching sessions with significant others as appropriate. a. Evaluate effectiveness of teaching based on attainment of expected outcomes. a. Discuss disease process. a. Explain and demonstrate necessary home management skills. 1) wound care 2) inspect for wound infection, temperature, swelling, redness, drainage. If present call M.D. 3) continue with adequate hydration measures 4) knowledge of medications (Pharmacy consult) 5) activity—avoid heavy lifting, straining for 6 weeks 6) incorporate rest periods and gradually increase activity 7) discuss ability to maintain lifestyle with one kidney a. Discuss appropriate community resources available and how the patient may contact them. (List resources.) 1) 2) 3) 4) a. Contact Continuing Care Coordinator to assist with referrals.		

Post-op general—nephrectomy: potential alteration in health management   PS 603-1-22   6/84

FIGURE 4-2. Standardized care plan: post-op general nephrectomy. (From Richter N: *Mich Hosps* 21[2]:25-29, 1985.)

Instructions:

1. Complete INITIAL ASSESSMENT; DATE and INITIAL.
2. Identify patient teaching outcomes (skills or knowledge that the patient needs to demonstrate).
3. Identify all methods and patient teaching materials used. Include classes attended by patient.
4. Note DATE/INITIALS each time the patient/family is taught; along with comments regarding patient's progress when indicated.

PATIENT IDENTIFICATION PLATE

5. Note DATE/INITIAL when outcome is met (when learning has occurred).

Initial assessment	(DATE)	PATIENT READINESS TO LEARN (E.G., ASKING QUESTIONS, INTEREST IN DISCHARGE) BARRIERS (HANDICAPS, ACUITY OF ILLNESS) MOTIVATION
	(INITIALS)	LEARNING NEEDS IDENTIFIED BY PATIENT

	Patient teaching outcomes	Methods, materials (DATE/INITIAL)	TAUGHT (DATE/INITIAL)	Progress and comments	Patient outcome met PATIENT (DATE/INITIAL)	FAMILY (DATE/INITIAL)
Initial plans	States purpose of home total parenteral nutrition (HPN)					
	Identifies components and functions of HPN: • catheter • nutrient fluids • pump to control rate and volume of nutrients					
	States advantages and possible risks associated with HPN					

FIGURE 4-3. Patient teaching flow sheet for home parenteral nutrition (From Konstantinides NN: University of Minnesota Hospitals and Clinics, 1985).

	Patient teaching outcomes	Methods, materials (DATE/ INITIAL)	TAUGHT (DATE/ INITIAL)	Progress and comments	Patient outcome met	
					PATIENT (DATE/ INITIAL)	FAMILY (DATE/ INITIAL)
Hickman/Broviac catheters	Describes anatomical placement of catheter					
	Describes what to expect before, during and after insertion procedure (refer to operative checklist)					
	Demonstrates techniques to prevent infection • proper handwashing • cleaning work space • aseptic technique in working with supplies • storage of supplies at home					
	Demonstrates placement of heparin lock					
	Demonstrates changing the injection cap					
	Demonstrates cleaning skin exitsite					
	Describes actions for catheter complications • signs of infection (local and systemic) • catheter clotting • catheter break/leak • air embolism					

Signature and classification			

FIGURE 4-3, cont'd. For legend see opposite page.   *Continued.*

	Patient teaching outcomes	Methods, materials (DATE/ INITIAL)	TAUGHT (DATE/ INITIAL)	Progress and comments	Patient outcome met	
					PATIENT (DATE/ INITIAL)	**FAMILY** (DATE/ INITIAL)
Parenteral fluids	Reads TPN label for accuracy of composition and checks condition of fluids					
	Connects cassette tubing to bag and primes tubing					
	Adds filter and needle to tubing and connects to catheter					
	Demonstrates use of infusion pump including setting rate and volume to be infused					
	Demonstrates procedure to begin fluid administration					
	Demonstrates procedure to end fluid administration					
	Describes actions for infusion equipment problems: • pump not working • accidental tubing disconnections • leaking filter • pump alarms					
	Demonstrates fat emulsion set-up and infusion process (if applicable)					

FIGURE 4-3, cont'd. For legend see p. 50.

	Patient teaching outcomes	Methods, materials (DATE/ INITIAL)	TAUGHT (DATE/ INITIAL)	Progress and comments	Patient outcome met	
					PATIENT (DATE/ INITIAL)	FAMILY (DATE/ INITIAL)
Home management	States methods for obtaining supplies at home					
	Describes actions to insure safety at home: • uses medical alert card or bracelet • identifies plan for activities—walking, bath or shower, exercise • tapes and clamps catheter					
	Demonstrates actions for self-monitoring at home: • oral temperature • urine test for sugar • body weight					
	Describes symptoms and actions to take for hypoglycemia					
	Describes symptoms and actions to take for hyperglycemia					
	Describes schedule for TPN and daily activities					
	Identifies names and phone numbers of health care providers to contact: • local resources • UMHC resources					

Signature and classification			

FIGURE 4-3, cont'd. For legend see p. 50.

DETERMINATION OF LEARNING OBJECTIVES

Based on assessment of the need to learn and motivation as outlined in Chapter 3, diagnoses and learning objectives are developed with the patient, the family, or both. Protocols, standard care plans, and standards of care that provide guidance for the development of objectives (always within the context of professional judgment) are available today. Examples are shown in Figures 4-2 and 4-3.

An example of a standardized nursing care plan from one medical center may be seen in Figure 4-2.[31] A home health care agency developed standardized nursing care plans partly to document quickly the service provided in a manner that met professional standards, legal guidelines, and third party payer requirements. The plans include the following elements: nursing diagnostic statement (if no nationally accepted statement was available, one was developed); a patient-centered goal indicating the behavior expected of the patient or the

significant other as a result of nursing intervention; a teaching plan with specific objectives; a flow sheet to document teaching and achievement of each objective by the patient or the significant other; a target date for accomplishing each objective to fulfill Medicare's requirement of justifying the initial and ongoing need for services; and nursing orders (prescriptions for care designed to solve a problem by a specified time).[14] Figure 4-3 shows a well-developed set of teaching outcomes incorporated in a flow sheet for home parenteral nutrition.[17] Adequate learning on the part of patient and family is absolutely essential for this therapy. It allows patients to return home rather than remain hospitalized for nutritional support.

Another source of objectives for patient education comes from outcome standards defined for an area of practice. An especially well-done set of standards has been developed for rheumatology nursing practice[26] (Figure 4-4).

Yet another approach to establishing essential

Outcome standard: The individual incorporates pain management techniques into daily life.

Criteria:
1) Verbalizes that pain is characteristic of rheumatic diseases
2) Identifies factors that exacerbate or influence pain response
3) Identifies changes in quality or intensity of pain
4) Establishes realistic pain relief goals
5) Verbalizes that pain often leads to the use of nontraditional and unproven self-treatment methods
6) Identifies pain management strategies
7) Uses appropriate pain management measures

Outcome Standard: The individual incorporates as part of daily activities those measures to manage stiffness.

Criteria:
1) Explains the relationship between stiffness and disease activity, medication, and activities of daily living
2) Verbalizes changes in the intensity and duration of stiffness
3) Describes appropriate methods of decreasing stiffness
4) Describes a schedule of daily activities which takes into account the intensity and duration of stiffness
5) Uses appropriate methods for decreasing stiffness

FIGURE 4-4. Outcome standards for rheumatology nursing. (From American Nurses Association and Arthritis Health Professions Association: *Outcome standards for rheumatology nursing practice,* Kansas City, Mo, 1983, The Association.)

Outcome Standard: The individual achieves self-care independently or with the use of resources.

Criteria:

1) Identifies factors that interfere with the ability to perform self-care activities
2) Identifies alternative methods for meeting self-care needs
3) Initiates alternative methods for meeting self-care needs

Outcome Standard: The individual incorporates as part of daily activities those measures necessary to modify fatigue.

Criteria:

1) Explains the relationship of fatigue to disease activity
2) Differentiates between psychological and physical factors that may cause fatigue
3) Identifies measures to prevent or modify fatigue
4) Uses measures to prevent or modify fatigue

Outcome Standard: The individual attains and maintains optimum functional mobility.

Criteria:

1) Identifies factors which interfere with mobility
2) Describes measures to prevent loss of motion
3) Uses measures to prevent loss of motion
4) Uses appropriate techniques and/or assistive equipment to aid mobility
5) Identifies community resources available to assist in managing mobility
6) Identifies environmental (home, school, work, community) barriers to optimum mobility

Outcome Standard: The individual and family have necessary information about the disease process and the therapy to make self-care management decisions.

Criteria:

1) Describes an appropriate plan for managing personal health care
2) Explains reasons for choices in personal management behaviors
3) Verbalizes sufficient information to meet self-management needs according to a personal value system
4) Identifies personal and community resources that may provide information or assistance

Outcome Standard: The individual achieves a balance between the stress imposed by the rheumatic disease and personal fulfillment.

Criteria:

1) Verbalizes psychologic and physical stress factors
2) Identifies appropriate strategies for coping with personal stress
3) Revises expectations regarding amount and type of activity possible in daily life
4) Identifies available resources
5) Uses available resources

Outcome Standard: The individual achieves a reconciliation between self-concept and the physical and psychologic changes imposed by the rheumatic disease.

Criteria for Individual:

1) Verbalizes an awareness that changes taking place in self-concept are a normal response to rheumatic disease
2) Identifies strategies to cope with altered self-concept

Criteria for family:

1) Verbalizes role changes
2) Identifies strategies to cope with role changes

FIGURE 4-4, cont'd. For legend see opposite page.

Prevention (349 incidents)
1. *Avoids allergens*
   foods
   pollens
   animal danders
   dust
   feathers, stuffings
   fungal spores/molds
   nonspecific combinations of allergens
2. *Avoids irritants and other precipi-*
   tants
   extremes in air temperature, humidity, wind velocity, etc.
   dampness
   fumes (smoke, gas, chemicals, smog)
   exercise
3. *Controls or avoids emotions that trig-*
   ger attack
   fears, anxieties, or stress
   anger, resentment, or jealousy
   excitement
4. *Takes action on exposure to aller-*
   gen/irritant to minimize effects
5. *Takes preventive medicine*
   routine
   anticipatory
6. *Ensures that medications for relief of*
   symptoms are accessible
7. *Uses some form of mind control to*
   prevent attacks
8. *Cooperates in the treatment of upper*
   respiratory infection

Intervention (763 incidents)
9. *Takes ameliorative or corrective ac-*
   tion when attack starts
   stops precipitating activity or leaves
   precipitating situation
   takes medication/uses bronchodilat-
   ing inhaler
   drinks fluids
   clears air passages (coughing, pos-
   tural drainage, etc.)

controls breathing, does breathing
exercises
improves ventilation in room/gets
more air
uses water vapor inhalation (steam or
cool water)
positions body to ease breathing
rests; engages in quiet activities
uses biofeedback
uses relaxation therapy
treats associated symptoms (e.g.,
cold water on swollen eye)
makes conscious effort to concentrate on something else
10. *Practices a variety of intervention*
    strategies, depending on the pro-
    gression/severity of symptoms
    decides whether intervention/help is
    needed and whether it should be
    immediate or can be delayed
    tries another intervening action when
    first action is ineffective
    seeks help from family members or
    other adults when own interven-
    tions don't work
    requests specific therapy from inter-
    mediary, when required
    reports symptoms to adult and relies
    on adult for intervention
    seeks medical help when self-treat-
    ment measures do not work
11. *Develops or requests individually*
    adaptive intervention
12. *Uses medicine correctly*
    recognizes undesirable side-effects
    of medication and reports same
    takes medicines in proper dose, at
    correct intervals, and under pre-
    scribed conditions
13. *Remains calm during attack*
    stays calm; controls emotions (fear,
    anger, anxiety)
    relaxes and allows medicine to work

FIGURE 4-5. Critical self-management competencies for children with asthma. (From
McNabb WL, Wilson-Pessano SR, Jacobs AM: *J Pediatr Psychol* 11:103-117, 1986.)

Compensatory behaviors (199 incidents)

14. *Discusses asthma with peers, makes them understand restrictions, and seeks/accepts peer support*

15. *Accepts primary responsibility for managing own condition*

    reconciles strong personal desire in order to avoid precipitation or exacerbation of symptoms

    reminds adult of treatment schedule

    alerts adult about possibility of attack

    relies on own resources

    (does not know what to do in case of attack)[a]

16. *Exhibits determination to overcome limitations or expand capabilities*

    participates in physical activities according to capabilities

    builds up tolerance to allergens or exercise

    has developed creative alternatives to restrictions posed by asthma

17. *(Denies, resents, hides, or blames self for asthma)*

18. *Accepts/cooperates with regimen even if painful or restrictive*

19. *Avoids using the asthma to manipulate people/get attention*

    avoids conscious precipitation of attack or use of symptoms to manipulate others

    minimizes own problem to help another

20. *Treatment hindered by figure in authority*

    (adult forced the child to do something detrimental to asthma)

    (parent used child's asthma to manipulate child)

    (adult failed to assist child or to comply with protocol/therapy)

    (adult denied the attack)

    (adult fostered child's depending on others for treatment)

21. *(Family problems triggered child's asthmatic attack)*

FIGURE 4-5, cont'd. For legend see opposite page.

objectives for teaching was used by McNabb in developing a typology of the behaviors of children with asthma that are critical in preventing or ameliorating acute episodes and exhibiting the appropriate adjustment to having asthma. These behaviors (Figure 4-5) were identified using the critical incident technique. Children with asthma, their parents, and health professionals provided more than 1300 reports of actual occasions when a child took or failed to take some action that affected the management of his or her condition.[23]

STATEMENT OF OBJECTIVES

Objectives reflect decisions regarding philosophy, the use of research results, learner motivation and need to learn, continuity in learning, sequential arrangement of the behavior to be learned, and priority of learning. Objectives involving what is to be learned must be communicated adequately to the learner and to other workers. Objectives must outline new behaviors that will occur because of changes in the learner's thinking as a result of the educative process.

Each objective must point out a behavior and a content. Statements such as "Develop critical thinking" lack content. Develop critical thinking about what? "Read a chapter of the textbook." What should the student read? Behavior is not defined in the statements "Display a positive attitude," "Babies need protection," "Smoking is a hazard," and "Antibiotics fight infection." What is the learner to do with these generalizations or topics—mem-

---

RELATIONSHIP BETWEEN MAIN OBJECTIVES AND SUBOBJECTIVES

Situation 1: The patient is a person with a newly diagnosed case of diabetes.
Main objective: To administer insulin to oneself without assistance (psychomotor, cognitive, affective)
Subobjectives:
   A. To identify injection sites according to a system of rotation, avoiding tissue where absorption will not take place (cognitive, comprehension)
   B. To use aseptic technique in caring for equipment and giving the injection (For classification, see text.)
   C. To draw a determined amount of solution into a syringe, accurate within 2 units of insulin (psychomotor, mechanism)
   D. To inject the insulin into subcutaneous tissue, avoiding the bloodstream (psychomotor, mechanism; cognitive, comprehension)
   E. To assume responsibility for insulin administration, without fail (affective, valuing)
   F. To take appropriate therapy for complications—mild hypoglycemia, insulin reaction, or skin breakdown (cognitive, comprehension, or application, depending on how different the situation is from that which the patient has encountered before)

Situation 2: A public health nurse is teaching a wife and a daughter how to care for a bedfast elderly father and husband. The patient moves little but has not been incontinent. He has had no skin breakdown to the present but, according to the wife, has been allowed to lie in one position for 4 hours. The main objective is part of the more encompassing objective, to avoid harmful consequences of bed rest.
Main objective: To avoid decubitus ulcer formation (psychomotor, cognitive, affective)
Subobjectives:
   A. To recognize any evidence of tissue breakdown by criteria of color, sensation, and response to massage (cognitive, comprehension; psychomotor, perception)
   B. To reposition the patient at least every 2 hours, so that the body is resting on the same surface only every fourth time (psychomotor, mechanism; cognitive, comprehension)
   C. To keep all linen wrinkle free (psychomotor, mechanism; cognitive, knowledge)
   D. To massage vigorously, at every turning, the skin that has been receiving pressure from body weight (psychomotor, mechanism)
   E. To report to the public health nurse or physician evidence of incontinence or skin breakdown, within 4 hours after it is observed (cognitive, knowledge)

---

orize them, apply them, believe in them? If content or behavior is missing, the objective cannot guide teaching and learning. As shown below, the objectives from the box on p. 47 specify both behavior (indicated by italics) and content (indicated by regular type).

   To name all foods common to the usual eating pattern that have high sodium content
   To agree that a restricted sodium diet may have some merit

To plan from memory nutritious menus that are within the sodium allotment
To verbalize willingness to follow a restricted sodium diet
To prepare foods without using salt
To accommodate the new eating pattern to situations such as social functions and being away from home
To follow the restricted sodium diet without fail
Each of these objectives contains a single be-

havior and a single content. Examples of multiple behaviors and areas of content are as follows:

To *plan* and *serve* nutritious menus that are within the sodium allotment (two behaviors)

To *verbalize* willingness to follow a restricted sodium diet and activity limitations (one behavior and two content areas)

This error in objective writing—specifying several behaviors or areas of content in one objective—is not as serious as failure to define the objectives precisely. If the behaviors vary in level of accomplishment, area of content, or both, they may be taught at different time periods; however, it will be awkward to use the objectives for singular lessons.

An objective may be precisely stated by describing the important conditions surrounding the performance and by specifying the criteria of acceptable performance. These techniques are not useful with all objectives but may greatly clarify some.[21] In an objective previously stated, the learner is required to accommodate his or her sodium allotment to the conditions of attending social functions and being away from home. Another requires planning menus by recalling them from memory.

An acceptable level of functioning is indicated in several of the objectives. The learner is expected to name *all* the foods common to the usual eating pattern that have high sodium content, rather than to name 5, or 10, or some. The goal is for the learner to follow the restricted sodium diet without fail, rather than to follow it sometimes or usually. The minimum acceptable performance may sometimes be defined by a time limit, such as when a mother must learn to avoid chilling her baby by not prolonging his bath. It also may be defined by an acceptable deviation, such as taking a particular medication within a half hour of the designated time or measuring a dosage of medicine for injection within 2 minims of the correct dosage.

A means of communicating learning goals precisely is to define the social and physical settings for the patient as well as the level of stress within which the patient must function. As staff become proficient in formulating objectives, they will no doubt find themselves using other ways of con-

structing specificity. For further discussion of these methods in an excellent self-learning presentation, I suggest that the student read *Preparing Instructional Objectives* by Robert Mager.[21]

Since learning is the ultimate goal and does not always follow from teaching, objectives are designed to present information that the learner must learn rather than information the teacher is to teach. The objectives in learning to follow a restricted sodium diet were correctly stated in terms of the learner. Another possible wording of these objectives may make the following description of learner behavior more explicit:

The patient names all foods common to his or her diet that have high sodium content.

The patient plans from memory nutritious menus that are within the sodium allotment.

The infinitive form used previously to state the objectives merely eliminates repetitious words. The following are examples of objectives, which are not desirable, stated in terms of teacher behavior:

To teach the patient to name all foods common to his or her diet that have high sodium content.

To teach the patient to plan from memory nutritious menus that are within the sodium allotment.

Depending on the words used, a description of behavior may be more or less precise. When behavior is described, it is best to use verbs that have fewer interpretations. Also, there are verbs that denote an internal state such as thinking, believing, or feeling. These should be avoided, since such states cannot be evaluated except as manifested in observable behavior. The following lists give examples of verbs that have relatively broad and relatively specific interpretations, respectively:

Terms with many interpretations[15]

To know (recall, relate, understand, identify?)
To understand (know, relate, identify?)
To be familiar with (know, understand, recognize?)
To realize (discover, appreciate, comprehend?)
To appreciate (realize, know, understand?)
To believe (realize, have faith in?)
To have faith in (believe, hope, trust?)

To be interested in (be aware of, to like?)

To enjoy (relish, love, or be pleased with?)

To value (appreciate, hold in high esteem?)

To feel (receive an impression, be impressed with, respond?)

To think critically (evaluate, apply, synthesize?)

To think (understand, conceive, imagine, reflect, infer, judge?)

To really understand[23]

To fully appreciate[23]

Terms with few interpretations

To identify

To list

To compare and contrast

To predict

To interpret

To recall

To label

To choose

To select

To volunteer

To translate

To apply

To recognize

To state

To classify

To differentiate

To construct

To order

To describe

To demonstrate

It is not possible to list all behavioral terms that may be used in objectives. Rather, think about the broadness or specificity of meaning that the term has and choose that which is specific and denotes observable action. Lists of verbs classified by domain and level of learning within that domain are available.[25]

It is entirely acceptable to state in general terms a main objective describing the overall goal of teaching, as long as components of this main objective are expressed more specifically in subobjectives. Two such examples are shown on p. 58. Of course, the group of subobjectives should represent all components necessary to accomplish the main objective. The main objective may, in turn,

be part of a larger overall goal, such as the goal in Situation 1 for a patient with diabetes to attain independence in daily living. The terms in parentheses are explained in the next section of the chapter.

The terms in main objectives must be general to communicate the breadth of the goal and guide large segments of learning. However, teaching cannot be adequately carried out from main objective alone. The specific content of a lesson derives from careful definition of specific behavior and content, at approximately the level of generalization of the subobjectives for the learning plans in the two situations just presented.

Readers should test their understanding by comparing these objectives with the criteria for precise statement: naming of a single behavior and content, definition of conditions for behavior and criteria of acceptable performance, statement in terms of learning outcomes rather than the process of learning or teaching, description of specific observable behavior, and comprehensiveness of the subobjectives in relation to the main objective.

If the teacher is inexperienced, information about the subject being taught changes, or the abilities of the learners vary, objectives will need to be revised continually. Staff will need to devote time to teaching plan revision and individualization.

A meaningful objective is one that succeeds in communicating the writer's instructional intent to the reader. Testing the clarity of a stated objective involves asking a staff member, a family member, or a patient to indicate behaviors that are expected to occur when the learner reaches the goals. Analysis of evaluation instruments that the staff intends to use or has used may show that the behavior desired is quite different from that which the objective states. This may be brought to the staff's attention by the learner who complains about being expected to know something when it was not part of the instruction or is not useful to him or her. Such a situation requires an analysis to determine the behavior that is desired.

Staff sometimes say they cannot put their objectives into words. These comments may indicate lack of skill with objectives. Since not every person is likely to attain a high level of skill in writing objectives, objectives exchanges have been developed. That is, educators can write to the exchange and obtain sets of objectives for a particular content area in a particular grade level. Obviously, the exchange does more than provide well-written objectives. These sets represent alternative ideas about goals and can instruct the teacher. Such an endeavor would be excellent for every area of patient education. It is likely that staff who can choose from a list of well-stated, potential objectives for a particular patient will be more motivated to teach. The skills required for choosing objectives—recognizing a well-stated objective and matching the patient's situation to the right objectives—are simpler and less time consuming than those required for composing objectives, that is, conceptualizing and expressing goals in precise language. Study questions at the end of this chapter provide practice in spotting errors in writing appropriate patient education objectives.

TAXONOMIES OF EDUCATIONAL OBJECTIVES
Development of the taxonomies

In the late 1940s a group of psychologists and educators became concerned about the need for defining levels of behavior according to complexity and about agreeing on terms to denote these levels. Such a step was vital not only to communication among all those concerned with learning but also to progress in research on the relationship between educating and evaluating. A committee approached the problem by developing taxonomies of behaviors found in objectives used in educational institutions and in the literature. The behaviors were divided into three domains: (1) cognitive, dealing with intellectual abilities, (2) affective, including expression of feelings in the areas of interests, attitudes, values, and appreciations, and (3) psychomotor, dealing with skills commonly known as motor skills. Each domain was to be ordered in taxonomic form of hierarchy; that is, those complex behaviors

at the upper end of the taxonomy (number 5.0 or 6.0) diminished to the simple behaviors at the lower end (numbered 1.0). Effort was made to incorporate the results of personality and learning research into the structure.

At the completion of the cognitive domain taxonomy, the authors believed that they had not succeeded in obtaining complete and sharp distinctions among behaviors.[4] When the taxonomy is used in patient teaching, this weakness is compounded by the fact that the taxonomy was developed from school objectives, which, particularly in the affective domain, seem to differ from some of the behaviors that health learners need to develop. Although the exact classification of behaviors may not always be clear-cut, general classification is sufficient for use of the taxonomy to be beneficial to the health care provider.

An abbreviated adaptation of the completed parts of the taxonomy of the cognitive domain is given on pp. 62 and 63. Proposals for the psychomotor domain (pp. 64, 65, 66), the perceptual domain (pp. 67, 68), and the affective domain (pp. 69, 70) are also presented. More complete descriptions of the behaviors may be found in the original sources. The reader should become familiar with the levels of behavior and be able to classify educational objectives into low, middle, and high levels of each domain. More detail is provided here to broaden the reader's concept of the major categories.

The cognitive and psychomotor domains are ordered on the concept of complexity of behavior, whereas the affective domain represents increasing internalization or commitment to a feeling, thus also requiring more complex behavior at higher levels. Classification into domains represents emphases only, with objectives clearly belonging in one domain rather than another.[20] Classifications of the objectives in the box on p. 58 were indicated in parentheses following the statement of each objective. Multiple entries are listed in order of decreasing emphasis. For example, the objective regarding identifying injection sites is primarily cognitive in that the basic essential behavior is knowledge of good sites for the purpose of injec-

COGNITIVE DOMAIN

1.00 Knowledge

Knowledge, as defined here, involves recall or remembering of information.
1.10 *Knowledge of specifics*
    1.11 Knowledge of terminology
    1.12 Knowledge of specific facts
1.20 *Knowledge of ways and means of dealing with specifics*
    1.21 Knowledge of conventions (characteristic ways of treating and presenting ideas and phenomena)
    1.22 Knowledge of trends and sequences
    1.23 Knowledge of classifications and categories
    1.24 Knowledge of criteria
    1.25 Knowledge of methodology
1.30 *Knowledge of the universals and abstractions in a field*
    1.31 Knowledge of principles and generalizations
    1.32 Knowledge of theories and structures

2.00 Comprehension

This represents the lowest level of understanding. It refers to a type of understanding. The individual knows what is being communicated and can make use of the material or idea being communicated without necessarily relating it to other material or seeing its fullest implications.
2.10 *Translation*
    Comprehension is evidenced by the care and accuracy with which the communication is paraphrased or rendered from one language or form of communication to another. Translation is judged on the basis of faithfulness and accuracy, that is, on the extent to which the material in the original communication is preserved although the form of the communication has been altered.
2.20 *Interpretation*
    The explanation or summarization of a communication. Whereas translation involves an objective part-for-part rendering of a communication, interpretation involves a reordering, rearrangement, or new view of the material.
2.30 *Extrapolation*
    The extension of trends or tendencies beyond the given data to determine implications, consequences, corollaries, effects, and so forth which are in accordance with the conditions described in the original communication.

3.00 Application

The use of abstractions in particular and concrete situations. The abstractions may be in the form of general ideas, rules of procedures, or generalized methods. The abstractions may also be technical principles, ideas, and theories, which must be remembered and applied.

From Bloom BS and others: *Taxonomy of educational objectives: Handbook I: Cognitive domain,* New York, 1977, Longman.

COGNITIVE DOMAIN—cont'd

4.00 Analysis

The breakdown of a communication into its constituent elements or parts, that the relative hierarchy of ideas is made clear or the relations between the ideas expressed are made explicit, or both. Such analyses are intended to clarify the communication, to indicate how the communication is organized and the way in which it manages to convey its effects, as well as to indicate its basis and arrangement.

4.10 *Analysis of elements*
Identification of the elements included in a communication.

4.20 *Analysis of relationships*
Identification of the connections and interactions between elements and parts of a communication.

4.30 *Analysis of organizational principles*
Identification of the organization, systematic arrangement, and structure which hold the communication together. This includes the "explicit" as well as "implicit" structure. It includes the bases, necessary arrangement, and mechanics which make the communication a unit.

5.00 Synthesis

The putting together of elements and parts to form a whole. This involves the process of working with pieces, parts, elements, and so forth, and arranging and combining them in such a way as to constitute a pattern or structure not clearly present before.

5.10 *Production of a unique communication*
The development of a communication in which the writer or speaker attempts to convey ideas, feelings, or experiences or all three to others.

5.20 *Production of a plan, or proposed set of operations*
The development of a plan of work or the proposal of a plan of operations. The plan should satisfy the requirements of a task that may be given to the student or that he may develop for himself.

5.30 *Derivation of a set of abstract relations*
The development of a set of abstract relations either to classify or explain particular data or phenomena, or the deduction of propositions and relations from a set of basic propositions or symbolic representations.

6.00 Evaluation

Judgments about the value of material and methods for given purposes: quantitative and qualitative judgments about the extent to which material and methods satisfy criteria; use of standard of appraisal. The criteria may be determined by the student or given to him.

6.10 *Judgments in terms of internal evidence*
Evaluation of the accuracy of a communication from such evidence as logical accuracy, consistency, and other internal criteria.

6.20 *Judgments in terms of external criteria*
Evaluation of material with reference to selected or remembered criteria.

PSYCHOMOTOR DOMAIN: A TENTATIVE SYSTEM

1.00 Perception

Process of becoming aware of objects, qualities, or relations by way of the sense organs.

1.10 *Sensory stimulation*

Impingement of a stimulus(i) on one or more of the sense organs.

1.11 Auditory

1.12 Visual

1.13 Tactile

1.14 Taste

1.15 Smell

1.16 Kinesthetic

1.20 *Cue selection*

Identification of the cue or cues, associating them with the task to be performed, and grouping them in terms of past experience and knowledge. Cues relevant to the situation are selected as a guide to action; irrelevant cues are ignored or discarded.

1.30 *Translation*

The mental process of determining the meaning of the cues received for action; it involves symbolic translation, that is, having an image or being reminded of something, "having an idea," as a result of cues received; insight; sensory translation; and "feedback."

2.00 Set

A preparatory adjustment or readiness for a particular kind of action or experience.

2.10 *Mental set*

Readiness, in the mental sense, to perform a certain motor act. This involves, as prerequisite, the level of perception already identified. Discrimination, using judgments in making distinctions, is an aspect.

2.20 *Physical set*

Readiness in the sense of having made the anatomic adjustments necessary for a motor act to be performed, including sensory attending and posturing of the body.

2.30 *Emotional set*

Readiness in terms of attitudes favorable to the motor act's taking place.

Modified from Simpson EJ: *The classification of educational objectives in the psychomotor domain.* In *Contributions of behavioral science to instructional technology: the psychomotor domain,* Mt Rainier, Md, 1972, Gryphon Press.

tion. However, a psychomotor element exists; the individual must find the sites through visual and tactile inspection and with a lesser affective component—belief in the value of identifying sites correctly. The objective regarding drawing solution into the syringe is primarily psychomotor, but the individual must understand this task and believe in the importance of accurate measurement.

The group formulating the cognitive and affective taxonomies found that there was much more concern in educational settings with cognitive than with affective matters. Attention to definition of terms and to methods of evaluation was considerably greater for cognitive objectives than for affective objectives. Because of inadequacy in the evaluation of affective objectives, they were used hesitantly in school curricula.

PSYCHOMOTOR DOMAIN: A TENTATIVE SYSTEM—cont'd

3.00 Guided response

The overt behavioral act of an individual under the guidance of the instructor. Prerequisite to performance of the act are readiness to respond and selection of the appropriate response.

3.10 *Imitation*

The execution of an act as a direct response to the perception of another person performing the act.

3.20 *Trial and error*

Trying various responses, usually with some rationale for each response, until an appropriate response is achieved.

4.00 Mechanism

Learned response has become habitual. The learner has achieved a certain confidence and degree of skill. The act is a part of his or her repertoire of possible responses to stimuli and to the demands of situations where the response is an appropriate one. The response may be more complex than at the preceding level; it may involve some patterning of response in carrying out the task.

5.00 Complex overt response

Performance of a motor act that is considered complex because of the movement pattern required. A high degree of skill has been attained, and the act can be carried out with minimum expenditure of time and energy.

5.10 *Resolution of uncertainty*

Performance of a complex act without hesitation.

5.20 *Automatic performance*

Performance of finely coordinated motor skill with a great deal of ease and muscle control.

6.00 Adaptation

Altering motor activities to meet the demands of new problematic situations requiring a physical response.

7.00 Origination

Creating new motor acts or ways of manipulating materials out of understandings, abilities, and skills developed in the psychomotor area.

In the democratic traditions of the Western world the individual's beliefs, attitudes, and values are private matters, with education and indoctrination sometimes very closely related.[18] These same difficulties with justifying objectives, defining behaviors, and knowing how to teach them pertain to patient teaching in the affective domain. For example, is it an invasion of privacy and an unrealistic goal to teach children to value cleanliness when they cannot be expected to maintain this value at home?

Besides establishing definitions that facilitate communication, the taxonomy of educational objectives also clarifies certain teaching decisions. In the cognitive domain, learning at the lowest level—acquiring information—can be achieved by a great

---

PSYCHOMOTOR DOMAIN

1.00 Reflex movements

   1.10 *Segmental reflexes*
   1.20 *Intersegmental reflexes*
   1.30 *Suprasegmental reflexes*

2.00 Basic-fundamental movements

   2.10 *Locomotor movements*
   2.20 *Nonlocomotor movements*
   2.30 *Manipulative movements*

3.00 Perceptual abilities

   3.10 *Kinesthetic discrimination*
   3.20 *Visual discrimination*
   3.30 *Auditory discrimination*
   3.40 *Tactile discrimination*
   3.50 *Coordinated abilities*

4.00 Physical abilities

   4.10 *Endurance*
   4.20 *Strength*
   4.30 *Flexibility*
   4.40 *Agility*

5.00 Skilled movements

   5.10 *Simple adaptive skill*
   5.20 *Compound adaptive skill*
   5.30 *Complex adaptive skill*

6.00 Nondiscursive communication

   6.10 *Expressive movement*
   6.20 *Interpretive movement*

From Harrow AJ: *A taxonomy of the psychomotor domain,* New York, 1972, Longman.

---

variety of learning experiences, including lectures, printed material, and pictures or illustrations. Attainment of the higher categories of the domain requires much more investment of time and energy on the part of the teacher and the learner, with the learner actively working through problems and the teacher helping the learner attain insight into the processes to be learned. It is believed that the same is probably true of the levels of the affective domain[18] and possibly for the psychomotor. Evidence that the individual learner has the ability to reach objectives at higher levels of the domain must be accompanied by a willingness of the learner and the teacher to commit sufficient time and energy to the venture.

Several taxonomies of the psychomotor domain have become available. For example, psychomotor levels have been outlined by Dave.[9] In addition to the Simpson taxonomy,[32] one other is presented in brief form.[16] It provides an additional description of the differences in levels of psychomotor behavior. One taxonomy that focuses on perception, which is basic to all psychomotor functioning, is most useful (see pp. 67, 68). Perception is the act of extracting information from the welter of stimuli impinging on the sense organs. It can be distinguished from the cognitive domain, which refers to judgments made from memory and to mental operations performed in the absence of stimuli. The taxonomy of the perceptual domain is based on a summary of research. It is arranged in a hierarchy of increasing information extraction and is not limited to any single modality of sensory input. Moore notes that the difference between behavior termed "intuitive" and other behavior may lie in the amount of information extracted from the stimulating situation and the degree of its association with previously extracted information.[24]

A word must be said about undeveloped taxonomies that would be most helpful in patient education. Taxonomies of situations are not available. Behavior varies considerably in each situation.[18] This development would be important because patient educators are regularly faced with having to

PROPOSED TAXONOMY OF PERCEPTUAL DOMAIN

I. Sensation

Behavior that demonstrates awareness of the informational aspects of the stimulus energy.

A. Detection and awareness of change. Detection threshold measures in all sensory modes.
   1. Ability to specify the attribute that has changed.
   2. Ability to specify the direction of change.
   3. Ability to specify the degree of change.

II. Figure perception

Behavior that demonstrates awareness of entity.

A. Discrimination of unity; discrimination threshold measures in all sensory modes.
   1. Ability to judge brightness as a property of the stimulus under varying illumination.
   2. Ability to judge distance and location of light and sound.
   3. Ability to judge tactile form qualities such as hardness, sharpness, etc.

B. Sensory figure-ground perceptual organization.
   1. Awareness of the relationships of parts to each other and to the whole.
   2. Awareness of relations between the parts and the background, matrix, or context.

C. Resolution of detail.
   1. Response to detail within the sensory (visual and auditory) world.
      a. Ability to judge size as a property of the stimulus at various distances.
      b. Ability to judge shape as a property of the stimulus regardless of orientation.
      c. Tests of field-dependence.
      d. Tests of spatial orientation.
      e. Other.
   2. Response to detail within the sensory (visual and auditory) field.
      a. Ability to discriminate symmetrical figures.
      b. Ability to discriminate asymmetrical figures.
      c. Ability to perceive rapidly successive bits of information.
      d. "Nonsensory" figure-ground segregation.
      e. Other.

III. Symbol perception

Behavior that demonstrates awareness of figures in the form of denotative signs when associated meanings are not considered.

A. Identification of form or pattern and relation of discrete information into visual, auditory, and tactile forms; recognition thresholds in all sensory modalities.
   1. Ability to distinguish curves from rectangles.
   2. Ability to distinguish triangles from squares.
   3. Ability to identify letters and digits.
   4. Ability to respond appropriately to gross facial expressions.
   5. Ability to distinguish tones in a musical chord.
   6. Ability to abstract a melody line from its variations.
   7. Ability to distinguish color components of a visual spectrum or composition.
   8. Ability to respond appropriately to verbal directions.
   9. Ability to respond appropriately to written directions.
   10. Other.

From Moore MR: *Audio Vis Commun Rev* 18:379-413, 1970.   *Continued.*

PROPOSED TAXONOMY OF PERCEPTUAL DOMAIN—cont'd

III. *Symbol perception*—cont'd
  B. Naming classification of forms and patterns.
    1. Ability to recognize faces and identify people by name.
    2. Ability to identify simplications and schematic drawings.
    3. Ability to name complex objects, pictures, places, melodies, tastes, odors, etc.
    4. Ability to read and comprehend concrete nouns and verbs denoting physical activity.
    5. Ability to indicate similarities and differences between visual, auditory, or tactile forms or their representations and to classify them.
    6. Other.
IV. *Perception of meaning*
  Behavior that demonstrates awareness of the significance commonly associated with forms and patterns and events and the ability to assign personal significance to them; interpretive ability.
  A. Mental manipulation of the identified form or pattern.
    1. Ability to reproduce forms, tunes, or syllables by memory.
    2. Ability to overcome the constancies of brightness, color, size, and shape.
    3. Other.
  B. Ability to attach significance to a symbol and to relate symbols to achieve a significant synthesis.
    1. Understanding of the various parts of speech; comprehension of language.
    2. Ability to make simple associations in all sensory modalities: for example, clouds mean rain, smoke means fire.
    3. Ability to understand verbal imagery, similes, metaphors, analogies, and other figures of speech—connotative meanings.
    4. Other.
  C. Ability to attach significance to a series of events occurring over a period of time.
    1. Insight into cause and effect relationships.
    2. Discovery of new relationships.
    3. Ability to generalize, understand implications, and make simple decisions.
    4. Other.
V. *Perceptive performance*
  Behavior that demonstrates sensitive and accurate observation, ability to make complex decisions where many factors are involved, and ability to change ongoing behavior in response to its effectiveness.
  A. Demonstration of a successful analytical or global approach to problem solving in all areas of endeavor.
  B. Diagnostic ability with respect to mechanical or electrical systems, medical problems, artistic products, etc.
  C. Insight into personal, social, and political situations where awareness of attitudes, needs, desires, moods, intentions, perceptions, and thoughts of other people and oneself is indicated.
  D. Demonstration of artistry and creativity in any medium.
  E. Other.

AFFECTIVE DOMAIN

1.00 Receiving (attending)

1.10 *Awareness*

Awareness is almost a cognitive behavior. But unlike knowledge, the lowest level of the cognitive domain, awareness is not so much concerned with a memory of or ability to recall an item or fact as with the phenomenon that, given an appropriate opportunity, the learner will merely be conscious of something—that he or she will take into account a situation, face or event, object, or stage of affairs.

1.20 *Willingness to receive*

At a minimum level we are describing here the behavior of being willing to tolerate a given stimulus, not to avoid it.

1.30 *Controlled or selected attention*

There is an element of the learner's controlling the attention here, so that the favored stimulus is selected and attended to despite competing and distracting stimuli.

2.00 Responding

2.10 *Acquiescence in responding*

The student makes the response but he or she has not fully accepted the necessity for doing so.

2.20 *Willingness to respond*

There is the implication that the learner is sufficiently committed to exhibiting a behavior so that he or she does so not just because of a fear of punishment, but "on his own" or voluntarily.

2.30 *Satisfaction in response*

Behavior is accomapnied by a feeling of satisfaction, an emotional response, generally of pleasure, zest, or enjoyment.

3.00 Valuing

3.10 *Acceptance of a value*

The learner is sufficiently consistent that others can identify the value and sufficiently committed that he or she is willing to be so identified, but there is more of a readiness here to reevaluate his or her position than would be present at higher levels of valuing.

3.20 *Preference for a value*

Behavior at this level implies not just the acceptance of a value to the point of being willing to be identified with it, but more, a seeking it out and wanting it.

3.30 *Commitment*

Belief at this level involves a high degree of certainty. There is a real motivation to act out the behavior.

4.00 Organization

4.10 *Conceptualization of a value*

At this level the quality of abstraction or conceptualization is added. It permits patients to understand how the value relates to those that they already hold or to new ones that they are learning to hold.

From Krathwohl DR and others: *Taxonomy of educational objectives: Handbook II: affective domain*, New York, 1964, Longman.

Continued.

AFFECTIVE DOMAIN—cont'd

4.00 Organization—cont'd

4.20 *Organization of a value system*

Objectives properly classified here as those that require the learner to bring together a complex of values, possibly disparate values, and to relate them in an ordered fashion with one another. Ideally, the ordered relationship will be one which is harmonious and internally consistent.

5.00 Characterization by a value or value complex

5.10 *Generalized set*

A generalized set is a basic orientation that enables individuals to reduce and order the complex world about them and to act consistently and effectively in it. The generalized set may be thought of as closely related to the idea of an attitude cluster.

5.20 *Characterization*

Here are found those objectives that concern the individual's view of the universe, his or her philosophy of life . . . a value system having as its object the whole of what is known or knowable.

---

predict an individual's behavior from one occasion to another over a period of time. Because no taxonomy exists in this area, individual differences are presently emphasized when comparative statements are made about the problematic performances of many individuals.[13]

A second, useful taxonomy is one of social skills. Social skills are the least well taught component of patient education. However, for patients with chronic illnesses these skills are crucial. The patient with chronic obstructive pulmonary disease may have physiologic difficulties that result from the effects of strong frustrating emotions on the reactive respiratory tract.[10] Voysey speaks of "impression management": the skill of managing social encounters learned by parents of disabled children. She describes the following specific skills: distinguishing true sympathy from mere curiosity; defining some categories of others' actions as insignificant; and predicting others' responses. Other skills in managing the impression follow on the basis of the assessment. Those with rheumatoid arthritis must learn to deal with the uncertainty of

the disease course and develop skills such as pacing activities and walking as if they were not suffering.[35] Persons with ulcerative colitis sometimes use "front men," who know about the patients' situations and work in collusion with them, to explain or justify their unconventional behavior or to conceal their disability. These patients have to learn strategies for scheduling time, using backup people who can take over their activities if they are indisposed.[30]

Use of the taxonomies

The ultimate usefulness of taxonomies of this type depends on the unique instructional procedures of each category. Most of the taxonomies presently available may not be fully developed.

Classifying a group of objectives according to the taxonomy can be helpful in three ways: (1) if an objective is difficult to classify, it may be that the behavior is not stated precisely enough—especially for objectives in the cognitive domain—the one most completely developed; (2) in trying to find the correct classification, the teacher is

EXAMPLES OF HEALTH TEACHING OBJECTIVES ACCORDING TO THE TAXONOMIES OF EDUCATIONAL OBJECTIVES

COGNITIVE DOMAIN

Knowledge — To describe three main purposes of the cough, turn, deep-breathe regimen following surgery

To state why the mother's diet may affect breast-feeding

Comprehension — When changing a surgical dressing, to recognize when something has been contaminated

To translate instructions on a medicine bottle into appropriate action

Application — To apply principles of asepsis to washing a wound with pHisoHex

Given a general knowledge of safety, to plan how to rid a house of safety hazards

Analysis — To identify factors that cause bowel upsets

To distinguish how a quack's argument differs from scientific reasoning

Synthesis — To design an ileostomy bag that suits the patient's needs better than do available commercial ones

To interpret to others the feelings experienced during illness

Evaluation — To assess the health care the patient is receiving in terms of its completeness, the patient's satisfaction with it, and the results obtained

AFFECTIVE DOMAIN

Receiving — To be aware that others are available to help

To tolerate having a retention catheter

Responding — To cooperate with the insertion of a nasogastric tube

To feel some satisfaction in caring for a baby

Valuing — To accept many of the limitations in life imposed by heart disease

To desire positive health rather than mere absence of disease

Organization — To relate to others in a manner consistent with rehabilitation goals

To regularly choose those alternatives of action that are consistent with good parenting

Characterization by a value or value complex — To develop a code of behavior consistent with respect for the health of the patient and others

Continued.

forced to compare the complexity of behavior that is being sought with the learner's present behavior. The teacher then can compare the distance between the two levels with the amount of time, the motivation, and the quality of teaching that is available; (3) if a group of subjectives is at widely variant levels, the teacher may have misjudged the learner's ability or may have stated the behaviors poorly.

The objectives in the learning plan for the patient with newly diagnosed diabetes can be used to illustrate these considerations. "To use aseptic technique in caring for equipment and giving the injection" is difficult to classify. The use of aseptic technique in psychomotor activities is implied, but the objective is not stated precisely enough to determine its cognitive aspect. If the objective read,

---

EXAMPLES OF HEALTH TEACHING OBJECTIVES ACCORDING TO THE TAXONOMIES OF EDUCATIONAL OBJECTIVES—cont'd

PSYCHOMOTOR DOMAIN (SIMPSON)

Perception	To recognize the "feel" of holding a baby with good balance
	To recognize the difference between systolic and diastolic blood pressure sounds
Set	To demonstrate a well-balanced stance with crutches
	To demonstrate correct placement of sphygmomanometer and stethoscope
Guided response	To discover the most efficient method of diapering a baby through trial of various procedures
	To imitate the blood pressure measurement procedure after demonstration
Mechanism	To control the fall of mercury in the sphygmomanometer at 2 to 3 mm Hg per heartbeat
Complex overt response	To pass a tube through the nose into the stomach skillfully with a minimum of discomfort or danger to the patient
	To measure blood pressure within 1 minute, accurate to ± 5 mm Hg mercury, in comparison with an expert
Adaptation	To perform one's own design for turning, moving, and transferring a hemiplegic person, weighing 100 pounds more than oneself, in a home environment
Origination	(Rarely used in patient education)

"To follow the prescribed procedure in maintaining asepsis in caring for equipment and giving the injection," it would imply cognitive level probably at knowledge, whereas "To apply principles of asepsis in administering insulin" specifies the application level of the cognitive domain—a more complex behavior. "To assume responsibility for insulin administration, without fail" is clearly in the middle level of the affective domain, for it requires at least an acceptance on the part of the learner that this regimen is important.[18]

Something must be known about the learners in order to determine the goals. The description of Situation 2 on p. 58 presents little information about the learners. Several factors determine whether the objectives are realistic for these particular learners. What is the relationship between the wife and her daughter? Is the daughter available

to act when help is needed? If the wife is forgetful or overwhelmed by the responsibility of caring for her husband, how much responsibility can she be expected to manage? Are the two physically able to turn the husband? How much do they know about the care of skin, about massage, about turning and positioning, and how motivated are they? Considering the patient's needs, the health care provider must help those in the home reach the objectives in one teaching session.

Given that the learners are capable of reaching the goals planned for them, it should be noted that within each set of objectives for the two situations there is consistency in level; that is, in no instance are there behaviors in the higher levels as described in the taxonomy. Had an objective in the second set read, "To determine a nursing regimen for prevention of decubitus ulcer," this would be at the

ILLUSTRATIVE BEHAVIORAL TERMS FOR STATING SPECIFIC LEARNING OUTCOMES

COGNITIVE DOMAIN	TERMS
Knowledge	Defines, describes, identifies, labels, lists, matches, names, outlines, reproduces, selects, states
Comprehension	Converts, defends, distinguishes, estimates, explains, extends, generalizes, gives examples, infers, paraphrases, predicts, rewrites, summarizes
Application	Changes, computes, demonstrates, discovers, manipulates, modifies, operates, predicts, prepares, produces, relates, shows, solves, uses
Analysis	Breaks down, diagrams, differentiates, discriminates, distinguishes, identifies, illustrates, infers, outlines, points out, relates, selects, separates, subdivides
Synthesis	Categorizes, combines, compiles, composes, creates, devises, designs, explains, generates, modifies, organizes, plans, rearranges, reconstructs, relates, reorganizes, revises, rewrites, summarizes, tells, writes
Evaluation	Appraises, compares, concludes, contracts, criticizes, describes, discriminates, explains, justifies, interprets, relates, summarizes, supports

Modified from Gronlund NL: *Stating behavioral objectives for classroom instruction,* ed 3, New York, 1985, Macmillan.

Continued.

level of synthesis and would be quite incongruous with the rest of that set of objectives.

Various combinations of words can be used to express a given intent. Thus teachers might articulate the objectives differently. For example, consider the alternative ways in which objectives in the case of the bedfast patient in Situation 2 could be stated. "To reposition the patient . . . " could also read, "To turn the patient. . . . " "To recognize any evidence of tissue breakdown . . . " could also read, "To identify. . . ." The content may also be stated differently. "To massage vigorously, at every turning, the skin that has been receiving pressure from body weight" may be stated, "To massage skin areas on which the patient has been lying, at least every 2 hours, or more often if signs and symptoms of breakdown occur."

The content of any main objective may be divided into subobjectives in several ways. One teacher writing the objectives about giving insulin might choose not to consider "using asepsis" in a separate objective but rather to incorporate it along with other safety measures in an objective, "To

administer insulin in a safe manner, using asepsis. . . ." The subobjectives should represent logical groupings. For the psychomotor domain these are primarily tasks such as identifying injection sites, drawing solution into a syringe, or injecting insulin into subcutaneous tissue. For cognitive areas the organizing factor is often a concept such as "tissue breakdown" or "responsibility." To communicate to the learner those things that will be the major topics of his or her effort, each subobjective ought to be of somewhat equal importance.

A situation of imbalance in subobjectives might concentrate on topics such as the angle of insertion, the rate of injection, or the necessity of avoiding the bloodstream, instead of concentrating the single objective of injecting the solution into the tissues. This breakdown would place more emphasis on injection than it actually deserves.

The material on pp. 71 and 72 has been prepared to give the reader an opportunity to relate the taxonomy to behaviors that are being taught. The material on pp. 73 and 74 suggests behavioral terms for stating specific learning outcomes by categories

---

ILLUSTRATIVE BEHAVIORAL TERMS FOR STATING SPECIFIC LEARNING OUTCOMES—cont'd

AFFECTIVE DOMAIN

	TERMS
Receiving	Asks, chooses, describes, follows, gives, holds, identifies, locates, names, points to, selects, sits erect, replies, uses
Responding	Answers, assists, complies, conforms, discusses, greets, helps, labels, performs, practices, presents, reads, recites, reports, selects, tells, writes
Valuing	Completes, describes, differentiates, explains, follows, forms, initiates, invites, joins, justifies, proposes, reads, reports, selects, shares, studies, works
Organization	Adheres, alters, arranges, combines, compares, completes, defends, explains, generalizes, identifies, integrates, modifies, orders, organizes, prepares, relates, synthesizes
Characterization by a value or value complex	Acts, discriminates, displays, influences, listens, modifies, performs, practices, proposes, qualifies, questions, revises, serves, solves, uses, verifies

PSYCHOMOTOR DOMAIN (SIMPSON)

	TERMS
Perception	Chooses, describes, detects, differentiates, distinguishes, identifies, isolates, relates, selects, separates
Set	Begins, displays, explains, moves, proceeds, reacts, responds, shows, starts, volunteers
Guided response	Assembles, builds, calibrates, constructs, dismantles, displays, dissects, fastens, fixes, grinds, heats, manipulates, measures, mends, mixes, organizes, sketches, works
Mechanism	(Same list as for guided response)
Complex overt response	(Same list as for guided response)
Adaptation	Adapts, alters, changes, rearranges, reorganizes, revises, varies
Origination	Arranges, combines, composes, constructs, creates, designs, originates

---

of the cognitive and affective taxonomies of educational objectives.

Use of objectives

Discrepancies in patient and staff objectives are not uncommon. One study found that the goals of physicians treating children with diabetes focused on the long-term threat of diabetic complications, while the goals of the parents concentrated on avoiding the short-term threat (hypoglycemia). Physicians perceived hyperglycemia as significantly more serious than hypoglycemia; achieving normoglycemia involves more risk of hypoglycemic symptoms that can be frightening to families.

The outcome of treatment more closely approximates the parents' goals than the physicians' goals.[22]

There will be certain discrepancies in the patients' and staff's ideas of education as well as other goals that may adversely affect the relationship between the teacher and the learner. In a particular rehabilitation setting, the staff may develop a full list of goals (physical, educational, vocational, and psychologic) that a patient can learn. The patient and family are then interviewed separately, and each is allowed to choose goals. This provides a basis for early identification of conflicts, enhances family-staff-patient interaction through

TABLE 4-1. Sample contract between nurse and client for teaching-learning

Situation: Wife learning to give home care to husband who has had CVA. This is only one element of the contract that would need to be developed with this client.

Elements	Specific contract
What is goal?	To learn to give husband an enema
What does client expect of nurse?	Demonstration of safe procedure adapted to the home and to this patient, with rationale explained and practice supervised
What does client have to offer?	Motivation to learn in order to keep husband at home and in good physical condition
What does nurse expect of client?	Willingness to learn from instruction and practice on her own after initial instruction
What does nurse have to offer?	Expertise in determining when enema is needed, adapting it to individual needs, evaluating its effectiveness, and teaching others how to give the enema
How do we go about working together?	As patient needs his next enema, nurse will explain basis for this decision to wife, plus how to obtain and prepare equipment and give and evaluate enema. Subsequently, wife will begin to make these judgments and do the skills with nurse's help and in 2 weeks will perform independently
Contract to be renegotiated:	At the end of fourth home visit—2 weeks from date of contract initiation or at earlier time if patient's condition or care regarding enema changes or if the nurse or wife believes care is inadequate

negotiation of goals, and encourages the patient and family to be active participants. The goals are later used as bases for follow-up evaluation to discover if the patient is still using those skills at home.[3]

The use of contracts with patients does convert principles basic to learning and the use of objectives into clinical tools. A sample contract may be seen in Table 4-1. Blair reports on the use of contracts in a public health setting. The contract represents a mutual understanding of the reason for the service and indicates problems or areas that will be discussed during the visits. The nurse and patient discuss and clarify the patient's wants and the services that can be provided. It is best to set a limit on the length of time to be expended or on the given number of visits as well as the conditions for renegotiation. Care plans are then based on the contract.

Unfortunately people often do not maintain initial behavior changes. Those factors that cause a patient to adopt a new behavior apparently are not necessarily the same as those required to maintain it. Personal and environmental factors, such as work schedules, social situations, and family conflicts, are problems that require continual confrontations and resolutions. Short-term training influences are usually no match for a multitude of factors that can affect the person's future behavior. Adopting an antihypertension medication regimen, an act that seemingly requires little change in lifestyle, can pose a serious maintenance problem. However, it appears that goal-focused intervention methods and a health care system responsive to individual needs over an extended period of time are of assistance.[36]

SUMMARY

All that is known about producing efficiency in learning is of no use unless the direction that the learning takes is clearly defined. Thus the focus of this chapter has been on determination and communication of desired behavior changes. Taxonomies of educational objectives define and order behaviors in terms of complexity, thereby aiding in communication of goals and decisions regarding teaching and evaluation.

STUDY QUESTIONS

1. The following sentences occur in statements of philosophy and objectives for the nursing services of health agencies. What are their implications for patient teaching in health care provision?
   a. A goal of nursing is to recognize the patient's need for independence.
   b. A goal of nursing is to recognize the patient's desire for self-awareness in relation to the illness.
   c. We recognize the worth and dignity of each individual.
   d. The patient and the family are to participate in setting realistic goals for themselves in the maintenance of health.
2. You are a public health nurse. You are to teach the husband of a woman with Parkinson's disease to care for her indwelling urinary catheter. The husband is highly motivated. In conversing with him, you find that he does not know where the catheter lies after it enters the body, although he does know it drains urine into a container.
   a. Write in correct form the main objectives and the subobjectives.
   b. Designate the priority and sequence of objectives.
   c. Classify the objectives according to the taxonomy of educational objectives and indicate implications of the resulting classification for instruction.
3. Write the objective, "To design an ileostomy bag that suits one's needs better than do available commercial ones," at the knowledge and application levels of the cognitive domain and the valuing level in the affective domain.
4. You have just completed a postpartum study of patients who delivered in your unit. Of the 67 mothers, 56 reported deviations from health in their babies at 10 days of age. What implications does this study have for objectives in the teaching program of the unit?
5. Provide a critique and suggestions for improvement of the following objectives:
   a. The patient will measure her own intake and output and record it as instructed.[34]
   b. When requested, the patient will list in writing, from memory, those foods that are not appropriate on a low-sodium diet.[34]
   c. Each morning the patient will circle, from a list of foods, those that are appropriate on a low-caloric diet.

   d. (1) After discussing the drug handouts with the pharmacist, the patient will know the following information about the medication prescribed:
      (a) The visual identity of each drug
      (b) The name of each drug
      (c) How each drug works with respect to the disease being treated
      (d) Any special instructions regarding administration where appropriate
      (e) Any ancillary information, such as storage or expected side effects, where appropriate
      (f) The common adverse reactions of each drug
      (2) Having learned the above information concerning the medications, the patient will comply intelligently with the medication plan provided him.*
6. Classify the following objectives as (a) patient outcome objectives, (b) teaching outcome objectives, (c) teaching process objectives, (d) learning process objectives, (e) patient education program objectives (for various patients). In addition, critique them.
   (1) Increase the patient's knowledge of illness management.
   (2) Cardiac rehabilitation patients will be able to discuss their diet and modification and its relationship to their convalescence.
   (3) Oncology patients are given the information necessary to maintain normal body functions at a level consistent with the disease and therapy.
   (4) The patient will be able to demonstrate the use of five areas of recording on the voiding record.
   (5) To provide an opportunity for mothers and fathers to share psychologic, emotional, physical, and educational aspects of parenthood.
   (6) The partner of a breast surgery patient will be encouraged to show support to assist the patient toward acceptance and adjustment after surgery.
   (7) Patient describes the relationship between timing and amount of food intake and peak action of insulin.
   (8) To alert the family to the health needs of the patient and to gain their cooperation in enabling the patient to return to a normal way of life after discharge.

REFERENCES

1. American Hospital Association: *Policy and statement: the patient's choice of treatment options,* Chicago, 1985, The Association.
2. Andrews LB: Informed consent statutes and the decision-making process, *J Leg Med* 15:163-217, 1984.

---

*Jinks M, The hospital pharmacist in an interdisciplinary inpatient teaching program, *Am J Hosp Pharm* 31:570, 1974.

 3. Becker MC and others: Goal setting: a joint patient-staff method, *Arch Phys Med Rehabil* 55:87-89, 1974.

 4. Bloom BS, editor: *Taxonomy of educational objectives: the classification of educational goals. Handbook I: Cognitive domain,* New York, 1977, Longman.

 5. Brock DW, Wartman SA: When competent patients make irrational choices, *N Engl J Med* 322:1595-1599, 1990.

 6. Caplan AL: Informed consent and provider-patient relationships in rehabilitation medicine, *Arch Phys Med Rehabil* 69:312-317, 1988.

 7. Carroll-Johnson RM, editor: *Classification of nursing diagnoses;* proceedings of the eighth conference, Philadelphia, 1988, JB Lippincott.

 8. Clifford JC, Horvath KJ, editors: *Advancing professional nursing practice:* innovations at Boston's Beth Israel Hospital, New York, 1990, Springer.

 9. Dave RH Cited in Reilly DE: *Behavioral objectives—evaluation in nursing,* ed 2, New York, 1980, Appleton-Century-Crofts.

10. Dudley DL: *Psychophysiology of respiration in health and disease,* New York, 1969, Appleton-Century-Crofts.

11. Faden RR, Beauchamp TL: *A history and theory of informed consent,* New York, 1986, Oxford University Press.

12. Fiesta J: Informed consent process—whose legal duty? *Nurs Management* 22:17-18, 1991.

13. Frederickson N: Toward a taxonomy of situations, *Am Psychol* 27:114-123, 1972.

14. Gould EJ: Standardized home health nursing care plans: a quality assurance tool, *QRB* 11:334-338, 1985.

15. Gronlund NL: *Stating objectives for classroom instructions,* ed 3, New York, 1985, Macmillan.

16. Harrow AJ: *A taxonomy of the psychomotor domain: a guide for developing behavioral objectives,* New York, 1979, David McKay.

17. Konstantinides NN: Home parenteral nutrition: a viable alternative for patients with cancer, *Oncol Nurs Forum* 12:23-29, 1985.

18. Krathwohl DR, Bloom BS, Masia BB: Taxonomy of educational objectives: the classification of educational goals. *Handbook II: Affective domain,* New York, 1969, David McKay.

19. Lidz CW and others: *Informed consent: a study of decision-making in psychiatry,* New York, 1984, Guilford Press.

20. MacDonald-Ross M: Behavioral objectives—a critical review, *Instruc Sci* 2:1-52, 1973.

21. Mager RF: *Preparing instructional objectives,* Revised ed 2, Belmont, Calif, 1984, David S Lake.

22. Marteau TM and others: Goals of treatment in diabetes: a comparison of doctors and parents of children with diabetes, *J Behav Med* 10:33-48, 1987.

23. McNabb WL, Wilson-Pesano SR, Jacobs AM: Critical self-management competencies for children with asthma, *J Pediatr Psychol* 11:103-117, 1986.

24. Moore MR: The perceptual-motor domain and a proposed taxonomy of perception, *Audio Commun Rev* 18:379-413, 1970.

25. Nuttleman D: Instructional objectives, *Superv Nurse* 8(11):35-44, 1977.

26. Pigg JS, Schroeder PM: Frequently occurring problems of patients with rheumatic diseases, *Nurs Clin North Am* 19:697-708, 1984.

27. Popkewitz TS: *Knowledge, power, and a general curriculum.* In Westbury, I, Purves, AC, editors: Cultural literacy and the idea of general education: eighty-seventh yearbook of the National Society for the Study of Education, Chicago, 1988, University of Chicago Press, pp 69-93.

28. President's Commission for the Study of Ethical Problems in Medicine and Biomedical and Behavioral Research: *Making health care decisions,* Washington, DC, 1982, US Government Printing Office.

29. Quaid KA and others: Informed consent for a prescription drug: impact of disclosed information on patient understanding and medical outcomes, *Pat Educ Counsel* 15:249-259, 1990.

30. Reif L: Beyond medical intervention: strategies for managing life in the face of chronic illness. In Davis MA, Kramer M, Strauss AL, editors: *Nurses in practice: a perspective on work environments,* St Louis, 1975, Mosby–Year Book.

31. Richter N: Patient education: creativity or crunch, *Mich. Hosps* 21(2):25-29, 1985.

32. Simpson EJ: *The classification of educational objectives in the psychomotor domain.* In Contributions of behavioral science to instructional technology: the psychomotor domain, Mt. Rainier, Md, 1972, Gryphon Press.

33. Stolte KM: Nursing diagnosis and the childbearing woman, *Matern Child Nurs J* 11:13-15, 1986.

34. Taylor KM and others: Physician response to informed consent regulations for randomized clinical trials, *Cancer* 60:1415-1422, 1987.

35. Voysey M: Impression management by parents with disabled children, *J Health Soc Behav* 13:80-89, 1972.

36. Wiener CL: The burden of rheumatoid arthritis: tolerating the uncertainty, *Soc Sci Med* 9:97-104, 1975.

CHAPTER 5

Learning

Instructional practices are based on the psychology of learning and on material that has produced results for practitioners in the past. It is true that bright and motivated individuals can learn a great deal without a teacher. However, their efforts to learn can be quite inefficient. Individuals who need to learn health information and skills, even if they are motivated, often do not have sufficient orientation to health matters to attain the goal alone.

It is hoped that after studying this chapter and the following three chapters, the reader will be able to (1) state how findings from learning research are useful in teaching; (2) state the rationale for use of particular methods and techniques in terms of their basis in learning psychology and practicality in a lesson; and (3) evaluate the degree to which a teaching plan is internally consistent. (Do objectives reflect motivation and need to learn? Are content and teaching actions adequate to meet the objectives? Does the evaluation test whether the objectives were met?)

THEORIES OF LEARNING

Learning involves changing to a new state; it is a state that persists. What can be learned? New thinking strategies, new motor skills, and new attitudes are learned in complex patterns that can promote a new performance. General conditions exist (such as reinforcement and transfer) that are applicable to all kinds of learning and learners. Particular conditions that facilitate particular kinds of learning are also present.

Twentieth century learning theories may be classified into two broad categories: *behavioral* and *cognitive*, with Bandura's social cognitive theory containing many key elements of both.[3]

Behavioral learning theory

Behavioral learning theory involves conditioning or reinforcing behaviors. Motivation for behavior change comes from the environment. For example, a person is motivated toward behavior change when he or she is deprived of something or is confronted with a discomforting stimulus. When the response behavior satisfies the need or eliminates the discomfort, the individual is rewarded and the response behavior is reinforced.

Behavior is cued by the stimulus that precedes it, and it is shaped and controlled by the reinforcing stimulus that follows. Most stimuli are environmental events. Changes in responding occur through a learning process called *conditioning*. Most behaviorists recognize two types of conditioning: *classical conditioning* and *operant conditioning*. *Classic conditioning* involves a process of learning in which a stimulus that is initially incapable of evoking a certain response is paired with another stimulus that elicits the response. After associating the two stimuli for a period of time, the formerly neutral stimulus will then elicit the response by itself. For example, a hungry person will begin to salivate when he or she sees food. If a second stimulus, such as the sound of a metronome, is introduced and presented repeatedly along with the food, then if the food is gradually withdrawn, the sound of the metronome alone will elicit salivation. *Classic conditioning* explains why children learn to fear dentists after experiencing pain caused by the dentist.[30]

Operant conditioning, in which a response behavior (operant) produces an effect on the environment (consequent stimuli), is used deliberately as a learning procedure. It is the relationships between behaviors and their consequences that are of interest in operant conditioning, and a number of techniques are used to increase or decrease behavior. Positive reinforcement following a certain behavior increases the probability that the behavior will be repeated under similar conditions. Positive reinforcement is often called a reward. The reward is given following the behavior and is contingent on it. Sometimes the reinforcement is the removal of an aversive agent such as nagging. Removing the aversive agent strengthens the behavior that precedes it. Reinforcers may be food, water, warmth, praise, recognition, grades, or paychecks, and the effects will vary from one individual to another. Extinction is a term that describes the process used to decrease a previously reinforced behavior by ceasing reinforcement. Also, punishment delivered immediately in response to a particular behavior may decrease that behavior; however, the results of punishment are unpredictable. The Premack Principle also is used and theorizes that a particular behavior performed by a person frequently can be used to reinforce a low-frequency behavior. Shaping involves applying reinforcements in accordance with gradually changing criteria. As the performer begins to roughly approximate the target behavior, closer approximations of the final response are needed before reinforcement can be delivered.[53]

In teaching, one must be sure that effective reinforcement is applied to a well-defined behavior so that learners will understand what they did to warrant the reward. As new behaviors are learned, reinforcement is frequent; however, after behaviors are established, reinforcement is given at random to encourage persistence of the behavior.

Cognitive learning theory

In cognitive theory, learning is the development of insights or understandings that provide a potential guide for behavior. New insights lead to a reorganization of the individual's cognitive structure, which is stored internally in visual images and in propositional networks and schemata. Within this framework, learning makes change in behavior possible, although not necessary. Motivation to take action results from a need to make sense of the world and solve problems.

Teachers using this theory would determine the schemata of the learner and would organize content so that it could be assimilated easily into the existing schema. Some learning can be described as an accumulation of new information in memory; however, the basic goal is to direct a longitudinal development of increasingly sophisticated mental models. Each level of learning addresses a larger set of problems. Novices can only relate superficially to the problem area or to the subject matter and must use preexisting schemata to interpret these isolated pieces of data. Experts, on the other hand, quickly identify the problem and know how to approach it, consolidate information in meaningful ways, and monitor and accurately predict the outcome of their performance.[22] In contrast to general learning skills, expertise is increasingly viewed as specific to a particular domain of knowledge or thought.

Social cognitive theory

Social cognitive theory as developed by Albert Bandura[3] is largely a cognitive theory but incorporates principles of behaviorism. According to this theory, humans respond primarily to cognitive representations of the environment rather than the environment itself.

People acquire information, values, attitudes, moral judgments, standards of behavior, and new behaviors through observing others. Infants who are several months old model behavior with competency and continue to do so throughout their lives. Individuals can learn and formulate rules of behavior by observing people, films or videotapes of models, symbolic models (written accounts of a performance), or sets of instructions (compressed accounts of a performance). This coded information serves as a guide for future action. The learner

also gets information about the probable consequences of modeled action. Individuals visualize
themselves executing the correct sequence of actions; therefore cognitive rehearsals and actual performances increase the proficiency of individuals,
give them a sense of efficacy, and reduce the tendency to forget learned behaviors.

In social cognitive theory, behavior is regulated
by perceived effects that often create expectations
for similar outcomes on future occasions. People
will persist for some time in actions that go unre-
warded on the expectation that their efforts will
eventually produce rewarding results. Extrinsic incentives are especially necessary in early stages of
developing competencies (such as playing the
piano) until competency becomes self-rewarding.
The natural social environment is often inconsistent, contradictory, and inattentive. To ensure that
the individual's newly acquired skills generalize
and endure under these less than favorable circumstances, transitional practices must gradually approximate those of the natural social environment.

Much behavior is motivated and regulated by
internal standards and self-evaluative reactions to
the individual's own actions, including self-incen-
tives and self-concepts of efficacy. To function
competently requires skills and perceived self-efficacy. Perceived self-efficacy is a belief in one's
ability to realize a certain level of performance. It
must be distinguished from outcome efficacy,
which judges the likely consequence certain such
behaviors will produce. Judgments of self-efficacy
are based on four principal sources of information:
(1) performance attainments, the strongest of the
sources, involve acting out the desired behavior,
and repeated failures lower self-efficacy; (2) vicarious experiences through observing the performances of others, especially if the model is similar
to the learner in ability, age, sex, and experiences;
(3) verbal persuasion; and (4) perceived physiologic states from which people partly judge their
capability, strength, and vulnerability. For example, cardiac rehabilitation programs are structured
to provide information from these four sources, and
the patient's perceived self-efficacy to perform var-

ious tasks is closely related to whether he or she
will attempt those activities.

TRANSFER OF LEARNING

Transfer of learning, the effect of prior learning
on subsequent learning, is one of the most important products of education, since no learner can
practice for all situations that will arise. It is more
efficient for an individual to learn general information, skills, and ways of thinking and apply them
to a variety of situations instead of learning specifically for each situation. Teaching for transfer is
based on evidence that individuals forget nonsense
material and isolated facts. However, individuals
remember general ideas, attitudes, ways of thinking, and skills that are meaningful to them and that
they have thoroughly learned and applied.

For the transfer of learning to occur, the individual must also recognize that the new situation
is similar to other situations, and he or she must
remember which specific thoughts or behaviors are
appropriate. In behavior learning theory, transfer
has an increased probability for responses occurring in the future because of past performance or
because of the appearance of identical stimuli. In
cognitive learning theory, transfer is not automatic;
when it occurs, it is in the form of generalizations,
concepts, or insights that have been developed in
one situation and are being used in other situations.[58]

Many studies provide evidence that generally
positive transfer increases when overall training
and application conditions coincide. Practice in a
variety of contexts enhances transfer (less like the
original learning). Indeed, extensive, varied practice based on imitating a model and driven by reinforcers can lead to the automatic triggering of a
well-learned behavior in a new context. Other situations call for intentional, mindful abstraction of
something from one context and application to another, deliberately searching for relevant knowledge already acquired.[54] Use of examples aids
transfer, especially if one extracts the rule from the
present example and uses it in new situations.[15]

Intelligence and prior learning influence ease of

transfer. Individuals who have less intelligence and prior learning frequently require instructional support to achieve transfer.[11] Instruction must be planned to ensure that transfer will occur. The process must not simply be left to chance. It is important to remember that what is taught during instruction must be like the situations in which the learning will be used. School learning is sometimes so disconnected from clear goals and real problem situations that the learner does not acquire any cues from it for solving problems in real situations.[15]

Transfer of learning is part of quality of instruction and can be put into context by understanding that learning depends on the following essential factors: learner ability, learner motivation, quality of instruction, and quantity of instruction. Each is necessary to learning but insufficient by itself. To some extent, each can be substituted or traded off. For example, immense quantities of time may be required if motivation, ability, or quality of instruction is insufficient.[60] Pichert has studied the amount of time that patients in a diabetes clinic spent actively involved in teaching-learning situations. He found that almost two thirds of patients' nonwaiting time was spent in assessment and that patients were actively involved in instruction for only 4 to 5 minutes.[46]

MEMORY

Forgetting learned material is one of the banes of our existence. Not using learned material, interference of other learning, loss during reorgani-zation of ideas, or motivated forgetting (which may be subconscious) constitute explanations for not remembering learned materials. Nevertheless, ideas are remembered for a long time, whereas facts are not.

The cognitive process involves the following: (1) selective perception of stimuli from the environment; (2) storage in short-term memory persisting for as long as 20 seconds; (3) encoding (leaves short-term memory and enters long-term memory); (4) storage in a meaningful mode as concepts, propositions, schema, and imagery in long-term memory; (5) retrieval; (6) response generation; (7) performance (patterns of activity that can be observed); and (8) feedback. Instruction can aid each of these steps by providing, for example, differentiation of features facilitating selective perception, verbal instruction or pictures that suggest encoding schemes, or cues that aid retrieval.[21] Retrieval time is slow except for the short-term memory, which holds only about six items. Forgetting is characteristically a progressive loss of precise information about an event rather than the total loss of a stored item and is usually because of the ineffectiveness of search and retrieval processes.

A depiction of the processes and phases of information processing appears in Figure 5-1.

Ways to increase memory retention include fostering intent to learn and to remember, finding meaning in material to be learned, applying newly learned material to a practical situation (practic-

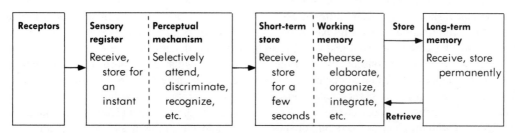

FIGURE 5-1. Processes and phases of information processing. (From Klausmeier HJ: *Educational psychology*, ed 5, New York, 1985, Harper & Row.)

ing), rehearsing remembering, using organizing strategies and visual imagery, and learning over a period of time.

Clinical work has been done on memory loss with aging and on the patient's ability to recall medical advice and informed-consent explanations, particularly involving surgery. When an older person has organic brain syndrome, no known procedures effectively improve memory. But memory loss in the aged is often attributed to a subjective symptom. It may be related to the presence of depression and to stereotypes of aging. Some studies have found that making more demands on the decision-making abilities of elderly patients in nursing homes had the effect of improving health and psychologic well-being. Using interpersonal and gift rewards yielded improvement in short-term memory tests, in nurses' ratings of alertness, and in social adjustment of the group being tested over that of a control group.[32]

Ley has done a series of studies on patient memory of clinical advice and summarizes this work in an excellent article. Neither age nor intelligence showed any consistent relationship with recall, except for one study with patients over 65. Diagnostic statements were best recalled and those concerned with instructions and advice most poorly recalled. These findings seemed to result from perceived "importance" effects. Four methods were found to increase recall: use of shorter words and sentences, explicit categorization, repetition, and use of concrete-specific rather than general-abstract statements (general: "You must lose weight"; specific: "You must lose 7 pounds"). Using these tactics, plus giving instructions and advice and stressing their importance, showed significant differences in the amount of information recalled by patients.[35]

Professionals have been shocked and dismayed at patient recall of informed-consent conversations that generally include explanation of diagnosis, the nature of the illness, proposed surgery, risk of death or complications, benefits, and alternate methods of management with the chances for failure or success. In one study, recall was stimulated at 4 and 6 months postoperatively. Patients could remember fewer than half the items covered, as verified against recordings of the initial conversation.[52] In another study in which recall was checked at 30 minutes and 3 hours postoperatively, patients remembered about three fourths of the material.[50] In another study patients were tested at 4 days postoperatively. The overall retention was 57% but varied widely across topics in the informed-consent interview.[49] These studies were not complete in their description of the initial informed-consent interview; therefore it is difficult to judge whether they provided an optimum treatment to avoid forgetting.

PROBLEM SOLVING

Problem solving is frequently a desired goal in learning situations. It is also an opportunity to apply various learning theories and ideas about levels of learning inherent in taxonomies of educational objectives. Problem tasks are more complex if they have one or more of the following characteristics: (1) incompletely defined alternatives; (2) existence of a number of subproblems; (3) several ways to reach the goal; (4) need for a large number of information sources to solve the problem, or (5) a rapidly changing problem situation.[9] As might be expected with a complex process, problem solving has been broken into a series of steps: (1) identification of the problem; (2) determination of possible actions and their probable results; (3) selection of one action; (4) implementation of it; and (5) evaluation of problem-solving effectiveness.

Learners may need help at any of the stages of problem solving. The teacher may need to help them recognize a problem, for unless they do so, the learners are not likely to act to solve it. Patients often need help in interpreting their feelings of distress so that they can focus on and state a problem. The caregiver often has information needed to solve problems regarding health matters and can be a sounding board and a support as patients think through the problem and arrive at and test solutions.

An individual's ability to solve a problem with little assistance depends on how many of the problem's elements the person already understands. A conceptual framework for linking the problem to the conceptual spaces of the learner helps in dealing with the small short-term memory and may allow retrieval of information already possessed (since the learner did not know that the problem space was related to the present problem).

Until the patient has defined the problem, it cannot be solved. A good definition of the problem may not occur until the problem has been worked on for a while. If a problem is similar to one that the patient has solved in the past, the same strategy can be useful with the new problem. If the problem has a small number of new elements, the patient should be able to adjust that already learned strategy; however, if the number of novel elements is large, it may be necessary to restructure the approach. This is clearly a higher level behavior; each new hypothesis involves a reformulation of the problem by shifting the relationships among the factors. Individuals differ in their repertoires of plans for solutions and in their capabilities for generating new thought patterns.

The following is an example of a nurse helping the patient solve his problem: An elderly man who lives alone has had heart damage and is about to be discharged from the hospital with permanent limitation of activity. He will therefore have a problem in caring for himself as he did before his illness. Although he recognizes the situation as a problem, he needs help in defining its breadth— the extent to which this restriction will affect his daily pattern.

The nurse is a source of information to clarify the meaning of activity restriction. She also knows the amount of energy the patient will expend in different activities and can help him to consider how he can economize it. The patient, with the help of the nurse, concludes that he can meet the restrictions and remain living alone by having his groceries delivered and by allowing a daughter to do his cleaning, washing, and ironing. It is agreed that these new living arrangements will be judged by the amount of energy he must expend, by how tired or how contented he is, and by the physician's opinion about his state of health.

The patient then goes home and tries out the hypothesized solutions, evaluating them as determined. At this stage he again needs the nurse's help, best given in his home, in assessing his subjective feelings of tiredness and the total amount of energy he expends. By visiting the home, the nurse is able to think of new solutions that need to be tried. Of course, the situation in this example may be altered slightly or considerably by such factors as the patient's ability to understand the situation, his emotional readiness to deal with it, a decrease in income, the daughter's moving away, or a change in his health status. This example is not meant to imply that each patient has only a single problem, but such difficulties are often interrelated.

When there are many problems, reaching a solution is not so straightforward. Considerable compromise may be required, as in the plight of an older person with no financial resources and no family but with a fierce desire for independence. Sometimes people are quite incapable of making decisions, either because they cannot reach this level of thinking or because they experience difficulty in advancing through the steps. A man who has had considerable brain damage from a stroke and must be moved from the home is an example of the former condition. The family, nurse, and physician solve the problem for this man because he is incapable of reasoning.

Difficulty in advancing through the steps of problem solving is exemplified by the mother who was distressed because her 2½-year-old daughter was not toilet trained. The mother expressed her disgust with this state of affairs and appeared eager to try solutions. After the nurse and the mother discussed the problem, the mother formulated the following hypothesis: she would consistently praise the child for desired behavior. The mother was never able to test this hypothesis. It became evident that she had such hostile feelings toward the child that she could not control her reactions when, for example, the child had a bowel movement on the kitchen floor. In an emotional situation of this severity the mother might require counseling. In retrospect the statement of the problem had been too limited; the hypothesis was unrealistic. This example shows that emotions are sometimes intertwined with problems that at first may seem to be largely a matter of reasoning.

Motivation plays an important part in problem solving. Families facing stressful events can draw on past experiences to help them solve problems. Individually or collectively, family members can choose a problem-solving possibility according to their perception of the situation. This is true also for individuals who are learning. When a health professional teaches new problem-solving strategies or aids people in further developing those strategies they are already using, the professional and the learner must consider how those particular strategies fit the patient's abilities and life-style.

It is important to provide learners with practice in solving problems; it is also most useful to label the parts of the process they are using and to talk with them about the process as a method. In the following example, parts of the process labeled were later discussed with Mrs. B.

The B. family were basically a "well" family who were experiencing the stresses of normal family development. Separated from her family by a recent move, Mrs. B. first met the community health nurse at an immunization clinic. She eagerly used the nurse's subsequent home visits to increase her understanding of child growth and development and to test out her own ideas about mothering and family life. Johnny, the only child, was 20 months old.

During one home visit the nurse applied the problem-solving method to a developmental question. Mrs. B. had referred to toilet training previously. She picked up the subject again in the following visit.

PROBLEM-SOLVING STEPS
Identification of the problem

MOTHER: I wonder if I should start to do something about toilet training for Johnny.

NURSE: What are some of your ideas about this?

MOTHER: Well, I could let it go for a while, but . . .

NURSE: You're not sure if you want to wait?

MOTHER: Well, no, after all, he's almost 2. I don't want him in diapers until he's 3! We bought him a little potty chair last month. He climbs all over it. (Sighs.)

Determination of possible actions and their probable results

NURSE: What had you thought about doing with the little chair and Johnny?

MOTHER: I could start him on a planned schedule. His B.M.'s are fairly regular. (Discussion follows about schedule, amusements while sitting, possible reactions of child.)

NURSE: You've mentioned two things you might try. First, to let go for a while until Johnny seems more interested; second, to set up a schedule and try to get him into it. There's another idea you might want to consider. Let Johnny get used to sitting on the chair first, and then gradually establish a schedule if he seems ready. (Discussion of probable consequences of this alternative.) All of these are possibilities. Which do you want to check out first?

Selection of one action

MOTHER: Well, maybe he'd be happiest if I first got the idea across to him that he is to *sit* on the potty chair, not climb over it or crawl under it. The schedule could come next. (More discussion as to details of the plan.)

NURSE: You've got some good ideas. Why not try this one idea out? Would you like me to stop by in 2 weeks or so to see how you're doing?

MOTHER: Okay. We might need a little encouragement. Right, Johnny?

NURSE: Don't forget that there's often more than one right way. I'll see you 2 weeks from today. Bye.*[14]

(The steps of action and evaluation of the action took place after this exchange.)

All human tasks can be viewed as procedures, involving individual steps or links and an executive routine that cognitively guides the individual through the task. The previously mentioned example considers a structure for a task that involves

---

*Collins, RD: Problem solving; a tool for patients, too, *Am J Nurs* 68:1483-1485, 1968. (*Author's note:* I have added the headings for these problem-solving steps.)

TABLE 5-1. Stages in arriving at a stable decision

Stage	Key questions
Appraising the challenge	Are the risks serious if I don't change?
Surveying alternatives	Is this (salient) alternative an acceptable means for dealing with the challenge?
	Have I sufficiently surveyed the available alternatives?
Weighing alternatives	Which alternative is best?
	Could the best alternative meet the essential requirements?
Deliberating about commitment	Shall I implement the best alternative and allow others to know?
Adhering despite negative feedback	Are the risks serious if I *don't* change?
	Are the risks serious if I *do* change?

From Janis IL: *The patient as decision maker.* In Gentry WD, editor: *Handbook of behavioral medicine,* New York, 1984, Guilford Press.

primarily cognitive and affective problem solving. Psychomotor skills are series of small tasks that add up to the total skill. It is often useful in designing instruction to analyze the steps of a task and to break them into manageable segments.

To summarize, problem solving involves recognizing and analyzing the problem, recalling or generating a plan for solving the problem, recalling information or gaining new information, producing a solution, verifying the problem-solving processes and solution, and securing feedback and assistance.[30] In addition to assisting learners with steps of the problem-solving process, making use of worked examples of problem solving, and providing initial guidance in applying them, the health professional can improve the learner's knowledge base in the content area of his or her problem. Sometimes, allowing a problem incubation time is helpful. For example, a person must withdraw temporarily from the problem and engage in other activities. Temporary withdrawal allows the person time to forget inappropriate approaches to the problem as well as time to perceive new approaches.

Janis[26] has studied patients as decision makers and has identified five crucial stages that patients must traverse to arrive at a stable decision (Table 5-1). He postulates that if any of the five stages is omitted or carried out perfunctorily, the decision

maker is likely to regret the decision and later to reverse the decision if difficulties arise. Decisional conflict can cause major errors if it is not adequately resolved. Defective coping patterns include defensive avoidance modes in which the individual evades conflict by procrastinating, shifting responsibility to someone else, or using rationalizations to minimize the expected, unfavorable consequences. Hypervigilance is another defective coping measure. The individual searches frantically for a way out of the dilemma by shifting rapidly among alternatives, by impulsively seizing at hastily contrived solutions that seem to promise immediate relief yet overlook the full range of consequences, or by thinking through the problem again and again.

ATTITUDE LEARNING

Attitudes pervade all spheres of learning. During certain periods in health teaching, change of behavior in the affective domain constitutes a major task. Acceptance, an emotional adjustment to illness, is a common task. Attitudes of responsibility are called for in taking health action for oneself and in caring for others. A feeling of courage in illness is recognized frequently as important.

An *attitude* is a learned, emotionally toned predisposition to react in a particular way toward an

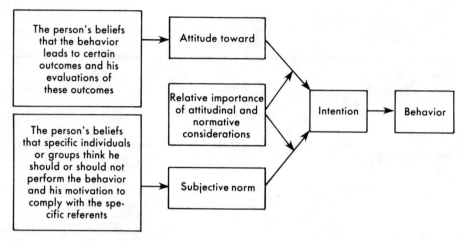

Note: Arrows indicate the direction of influence.

FIGURE 5-2. Factors determining a person's behavior. (From Page MM, editor: The 1979 Nebraska Symposium on Motivation, University of Nebraska, 1980, University of Nebraska Press.)

object, an idea, or a person. *Values,* which are similar but more permanent, are expressions of how individuals believe an object or relationship affects them. Over the years, feelings are gradually developed, become well established, and are reflected in behavior. Often we do not realize that we are acquiring attitudes. Membership in groups, particularly primary ones, seems to influence acquisition of attitudes more than acquisition of concepts or skills. A group's influence on an individual's attitude acquisition is logical, since identification, imitation, and conditioning play an important part in attitude learning.[30] Thus, as an individual is growing up in close contact with the primary group, the family, it seems natural to imitate responsible behavior and be rewarded for it. Imitation evolves into set behavior beliefs or values.

Many studies regarding the relationship between attitudes and behavior do not demonstrate a noticeable correspondence. Product moment correlations are seldom more than 0.30 and often fall near zero. A theory of reasoned action (shown in Figure 5-2) seems to be gaining ground.[17] A per-

son's intention to perform or not perform the behavior is the immediate determinant. Intention is a function of the person's attitude toward the behavior and his or her perception of society's stance on performing the behavior.[18]

Suggestions for teaching attitudes follow directly from knowledge about how they are learned and include employing someone to teach whose attitudes the learner can view and imitate. This model may not be a health professional but possibly another patient with whom the learner can identify and is the reason for establishing colostomy and ileostomy clubs and other such groups. Another way of influencing attitudes is to provide satisfying experiences, so that the person develops a positive response to ideas or feelings associated with the experiences.[30] For example, personnel in a health clinic should try to provide experiences of the sort that help the patient have positive feelings about the clinic.

Kelman believes that significant attitude change always occurs in the context of action. Attitude is not a static psychologic entity but rather an integral part of the action, with each generating the other, constantly tested and reshaped in interaction with relevant others, and characterized by a range of potential action commitments. Latent attitude positions that are already present in the person's range of commitment represent readiness for a shift in attitude, given the proper circumstances. These latent positions may be largely unconscious, or they may be actively entertained by the person but with no opportunity for that person to act. Other competing forces may be keeping the person at the present level. A new event, especially one that is dramatic and compelling and presents new challenging information, may activate the latent position and assist in moving the individual toward a new attitude, especially if the shift is encouraged by relevant authorities.[29]

One of the most formidable problems in changing attitudes is that those reinforced in one part of the individual's life may be extinguished in another. This may be true of health attitudes. For example, the young single mother, who showed signs of developing a responsible attitude toward her infant, lost those feelings when she returned to her peer group, which showed an irresponsibility toward all of life. Understanding also is pertinent to attitude change, particularly when the feeling is not firmly established and not determinative.[31]

The body of research from which role playing is drawn is reliably informative in the area of attitude change. Active participation in role-playing is more effective than passive listening. In role-playing the individual must attempt to duplicate, sincerely and convincingly, a particular attitude held by another person. All techniques of attitude change rely on the assumption that change comes out of conflict, disagreement, inconsistency, or discontent with the existing state of affairs. Group pressure techniques make the individual aware that his or her behavior is in disagreement with the norms of the group. Another technique involves modeling a social behavior that the learner can imitate. Audience participation (group discussion and decision making) helps the learner to overcome feelings of resistance. Persuasion is more successful if the persuader has high credibility based on expertise and trustworthiness.[28] Action is both motivational and informational and plays a vital part in attitude change.[29]

Feelings may reflect the learner's attitudes, or they may be more fleeting expressions of affect. In either case they are constantly present during learning and must be incorporated into the learning process. For example, parent group education is seen as an emotional experience as much as an intellectual one. Therefore expressions of feelings that relate to parent, child, or family living are encouraged.

Those feelings that are close to the surface of consciousness and easily expressed represent an essential part of human existence, even though they are not always recognized as such. Expressing such feelings in a group setting is not usually a part of social communication and can cause some anxiety in group members. However, such exchanges are appropriate in an educational program. A general guideline for every teaching episode might be to assess the learner's feelings about the topic and validate those feelings with him or her. The provider must set up objectives based on learners' feelings and encourage them to express their conscious feelings. The teaching methods outlined in this section are designed to encourage learners to express themselves. Feelings are ever present when the focus of learning is health and illness because the patient's existence is threatened. It is inevitable that staff who have not learned to communicate with patients about feelings will be less successful health teachers.

LEARNING OF PSYCHOMOTOR SKILLS

Anyone recalling the awkwardness of a puppy or child, the unsteadiness of an old man, and relating it to the sure coordination of a skilled artist can observe a variation in motor skills. They can vary with strength, reaction time, speed, balance, precision, and flexibility of tissues. Motor skills are usually composed of an ordered sequence of movement that must be learned. Separate parts of a motor act can be learned and practiced separately as part-skills.

To perform a particular skill, a person must possess a neuromuscular system that is capable of performing the skill and must have an ability to form a mental image of the act. A mental image is created when the learner watches a demonstration that shows the skill as well as points out relevant cues for a successful performance. Relevant cues often involve muscular cues of balance and pull. The typist uses such cues to sense where the fingers are; the horn player uses them to feel the correct lip placement. Cues may also be seen or heard. When learning to walk with crutches, a person must see the floor or objects that might get in the way, hear people approach from behind, and feel whether he or she is balanced. The cues must be obvious to the beginner and often are not noticed much in advance of the action. The person experienced in doing the motor skill can use many cues rather than just the obvious ones. He or she is not confused by irrelevant cues, attending to them with less conscious concentration. Also, the person experienced in motor skills reacts faster and can take advantage of cues far in advance of action. The goal is a smooth, coordinated sequence of action with a minimum expenditure of energy.

The learner practices to develop a proficient performance. The mental image is a guide. At first, however, the teacher may need to guide the person's body so that he or she experiences the physical sensations that accompany correct motions. For example, a nurse might guide a child's hands as he or she learns to drink from a cup. It is best for the learner to practice in a situation that provides cues similar to those provided where the skill will be used. For example, the colostomy patient is taught in a setup that simulates a bathroom at home. During the crucial early stages of practice—a time when bad habits can be formed—information about the patient's progress, or lack of it, is important. Learners often need help in judging their own performances, even though they can often judge someone else's. Eventually, students get messages from their own physical sensations and can decide if their objectives have been accomplished.

Research has not been able to determine the length and frequency of practice sessions needed for various motor skills. It is generally recommended that practice periods be short and infrequent enough to avoid fatigue. Fatigue can cause a decrease in function, with resulting frustration. If the practice period is not long enough to allow the muscles to loosen, the learner will not complete a whole performance. If intervals between practices are too long, the learner may forget.

Cognitive processes are necessary to perceive the nature of the task and to recognize similarities between the present task and previous experiences. The learner must also identify, select, and practice important cues in order for response to occur. Cognitions may also be used to store permanently evaluative feedback as well as causal reasons for a performance outcome. Strategy uses information to direct decisions for purposeful behavior; it is often difficult to observe strategy directly. However, it may be inferred from the pattern of decisions the provider observes in a problem solver. Incorrect cognition or inefficient strategy can retard learning and lower performance quality. Once the cognitions and strategies are adequate, and once the movements can be accomplished, the next most important determinant of adequate learning is "time on task," that is, the amount of time the learner practices.

Once a motor skill has been learned, it can be quickly recaptured even after an interval of many years. It is not possible to make such a definite statement about intellectual learning.

The three phases to skill learning include the cognitive phase, the organizing phase, and the perfecting phase. The cognitive phase is usually of short duration. The learner does not practice much but learns the nature of the skill by observing someone who models the skill and by listening to instructions. The more obvious cues are selected and their distinguishing qualities noted. Feedback is elementary, and errors are many. Speed and coordination are low, and responses are not stable. The organizing phase puts the emphasis on motor function, and some skills become automatic. The perfecting phase involves continuing improvement over a long period of time. Larger behavior units replace the single and intermediate units of the earlier phases.[30]

Training programs to reestablish functions disrupted by nerve damage are developed on the basis of specialized assessments of physiologic readiness. Those patients with varying kinds of damage to the neuromuscular systems may need bladder, voluntary muscle, and speech reeducation.

ADULT LEARNING

All aspects of adult learning are important for application in patient education. This section focuses on adult developmental tasks and on natural patterns of learning in people who are not usually involved in formal school programs. Data from a national sample showed that almost 80% of the population 18 years and over perceived themselves as continuing learners, yet only 3% were engaged in courses or school-like activities. Seventy-six percent had planned one or more self-initiated learning projects in the year before data were collected. The projects had a minimum duration of 7 hours and a mean of 155 hours. Each person averaged 3.3 projects. Many of these adults preferred models of learning in which they were the planner or in which they used an instructional assistant who was personally accessible.

A "shopping center" access to multidisciplinary teams of learning consultants and information brokers was suggested by Penland as a way to package learning assistance for this particular population.[44]

Mezirow[38] has built on the work of Jurgen Habermas to develop an overall conception of the tasks of adult learning. He defines *adult education* as any organized and sustained effort to facilitate learning, especially in a way that enhances the adult's capacity to function as a self-directed learner. Adult learning activity is seen as focused in three domains: (1) technical-work, which deals with the ways the learner controls the environment and uses the traditional hypothetical-deductive theories of learning, (2) interactive or communicative domain, in which education focuses on helping

learners interpret the ways they interact, and (3) emancipatory-self-knowledge domain, which can yield dramatic personal and social change by creating awareness of the way ideologies have created or contributed to our dependency on power resembling a monarchy—meanings that come from uncritically assimilated half-truths of conventional wisdom and power relationships assumed to be fixed.

The emancipatory self-knowledge domain is the most distinctly adult. The challenges of adulthood are seen as involving a process of traveling through an uncertain number of changes that transform the individual to conform with society's perspective of the psychocultural norm. The adult's new experience is assimilated into the standing psychocultural assumptions and transformed by his or her past experience. This process may involve a series of transformations, although a disorienting dilemma is clearly a factor in motivating such a transformation. Although the learner does not return to an old perspective once a transformation occurs, the passage involves difficult negotiation and compromise, stalling, and backsliding. Self-deception and failure are common. The crucial difference between the emancipatory self-knowledge process and that of primary socialization (child) is that adults are capable of being critically reflective. Assistance with perspective change involves helping people to see the problem and providing access to alternate meaning perspectives to help people interpreting their reality. Adult learners then can examine their assumptions critically by using stories and pictures that pose hypothetical dilemmas with conflicting rules and assumptions in the areas of critical concern.

Indeed, support groups often involve adults who come together in response to the same life dilemma. These groups foster critical reflection. They help the participants gain and apply insights to their own lives. One can study the outcomes of this kind of education by interviewing and by comparing movement in the problem awareness, the expectations, and the goals.[38] Health situations frequently cause individuals to feel disoriented and precipitate self-reflection. Most people operate with both personal and cultural myths that order, explain, predict, and place value on the events and circumstances life presents. The myths also provide instructions that guide behavior. In developing a new perspective, the learner must identify conflicting myths, examine their sources, and create new, more suitable myths.[18]

Knowles, who has written widely about andragogy, or the study of teaching adults, sets forth conditions that are necessary for adult learning: (1) an atmosphere that promotes collaboration, mutual trust, respect, and mutual support; and (2) the idea that learners must participate in diagnosing their own needs, formulating their learning objectives, designing and carrying out learning plans, and evaluating their learning. Learning contracts are an effective way to help participants structure their learning.[31]

LEARNING IN CHILDREN

The field of growth and development is a complex one that includes study of individuals at all ages, including children. Ability to learn depends on maturation, and a great deal of maturation occurs in childhood. Readiness to learn in childhood changes considerably, beginning with visual, auditory, and motion stimulation of infants. The primary dimension of children's development is the degree of differentiation they make between the self and other. The child moves toward a clearer distinction between the internal and the external self. The general principles and comments about learning outlined in previous sections of this chapter are applicable to children within their readiness level.

Intellectual development moves from concrete to abstract. Children can use language to represent objects or experiences and can solve problems by direct manipulation of physical objects during the preschool years. Young children are egocentric and interested only in what affects them. They want explanations for everything but are not concerned with supplying reasons for their questions. If children have a background of direct nonverbal experience during the elementary school years, they can verbally manipulate relationships between ideas without having the objects present. As they grow toward adolescence and then adulthood, they gradually come to understand and manipulate relationships between abstractions without any reference to the concrete. Eventually, they can formulate and test hypotheses based on the possible combinations of several ideas.

Children must develop motor skills and feelings as well as grow intellectually. Developing trust in the first 2 years is crucial. At that point children become more autonomous, learning to walk, run, jump, and feed themselves. Between the ages of 3½ and 7, children develop imagination and learn to take the initiative. During the early school years they become industrious, turning their attention to the outside world. As adolescents they develop their identities.[55]

Knowledge of growth and development suggests that teachers should determine realistic objectives and explain them in a way that the child can understand. Allowing children to handle equipment, such as a breathing mask, seems to encourage acceptance of the treatment. This is especially true during the years when direct nonverbal experience is important. Because children under 5 years of age experience egocentricity and fear of injury, they need to know how procedures will affect them. For example, it may be explained to children that during a chest x-ray examination they will just have to stand still, to hold their breath for a few seconds, and not to worry because they will not feel anything.

Research has consistently reported limited periods of behavioral upset followed by rapid recovery after discharge from the hospital. (Children between 6 months and 4 years are the most vulnerable.) Young children, in particular, consider illness to be self-caused and punitive.[56] It has been suggested that if a child is less than 4 years of age, explanation of anatomy and physiology is not useful because the child does not have the necessary understanding and is prone to develop undesirable fantasies. Separation anxiety in this age group is a primary problem. Therefore teaching should stress that the same provider needs to care for the child, and it should encourage the parents to help.

For children over 7 years old, more sophisticated language and drawings can be used. Children of school age also benefit from tours of hospital playrooms and wards and from discussion in which they can learn about their illness, its origins, and proposed plans of treatment. Because school-aged children have a more mature concept of causality, they have the capacity to understand that neither illness nor treatment is imposed on them because of their own misdeeds. These children are able to cooperate with treatment because they can think before they act. Since they can express their feelings in words and have a greater grasp of time sequences, they can better tolerate a separation from their parents.[59]

Children's health attitudes and behaviors show a critical period of change around the time they enter the third grade. Third graders are able to decide whether to report illness or injury. They have developed cognitive abilities, and they have learned the social rules that govern illness and when to seek care. By the sixth grade these abilities are refined.[42]

Adolescents must master the ability to think in abstractions and to imagine the possibilities that are inherent in a variety of situations. Many adolescents need help in thinking through behavioral alternatives. They may need guidance through steps of problem solving and planning. Role playing in peer groups can help illustrate appropriate norms of behavior. It can also translate abstract information into stories that are easier to remember.

A study done across age ranges in chronically ill children illustrates the point. Children under 7 years of age believed that illness was caused by human action. They believed that illness was often caused by their wrongdoing. Germs were usually listed as a cause of illness by 7- to 10-year-olds. Children under 9 years of age were not able to give multiple explanations for disease and their interaction, such as infection and the body's lack of immunity. At 5 to 6 years the child's comprehen-

sion regarding medical procedures and the roles played by medical personnel is determined by the consequences to the child. Consequences might involve punishing the child for being bad. At 7 to 10 years the child could accurately infer the intention of medical procedures and knew that the treatment was intended to help him or her get well. However, children were limited in their ability to infer empathy. Children older than 10 years could infer intention as well as empathy. This study found that egocentric or magical thinking was retained by children during times of high stress. It is not wise to force a child into a higher level of comprehension than his or her emotional needs require. Sometimes, well-informed children cannot cope well with illness. However, improvement in family interactional patterns seems to help those who are coping poorly.

The relevance of this information for teaching is severalfold. The child's maturity level determines his or her ability to absorb information. Therefore knowing a child's maturity level can help determine the objectives and teaching strategies for that child.

A second example is the accommodation the teacher needs to make in explanations when diseases such as epilepsy or cancer do not provide concrete perceptual referents. Appropriate referents can be provided using drawings and analogies. Cancer is explained with drawings showing particular kinds of cells—garbageman cells, police cells, outlaw cells (cancer cells). Treatment is presented as a way to supplement the body's own police and medical forces.[62]

Illness and hospitalization can deprive children of activities central to their growth. Therefore it is necessary to think in terms of substitute experiences that might be provided to protect the child's growth potential.[59] It is also important to relieve the child's anxiety caused by fear of the unknown. Anxiety may be attributed to normal developmental crises, illness, or hospitalization.

Chronically ill children become increasingly able to understand their illnesses as they develop intellectually. Cognitive development brings with it the ability to grasp the meaning of a poor prognosis or of functional limitations. Such understanding may take an emotional toll on the youngster. In a study of children with diabetes, those with more advanced disease concepts were more worried about their diabetes. A child with a good understanding of his or her illness may need less of the clinician's attention from an educational standpoint, but he or she may need more emotional support. The child may need an opportunity to discuss psychosocial issues or to rehearse ways of dealing with future possibilities. An introduction to other persons with diabetes including positive adult models may help the child a great deal.[2]

Adolescents frequently display particular thought patterns involving an imaginary audience or a personal fable, consistent with a stage of intense preoccupation with themselves. They believe that if everyone is watching them and thinking about them, thanks to the imaginary audience, they must be something special, unique, or different. Teenagers with chronic illness may stop taking medications because they believe they are special and different and can manage without the medications. Believing that they are immune to the natural laws that other people must obey can also cause them not to use contraceptives. Unprotected intercourse is not viewed as a risk by the adolescent.[16] Pestrak believes that many adolescents are functioning at a cognitive level that renders them unable to practice most forms of birth control effectively. The effective practice of birth control requires that individuals accept their sexuality and acknowledge that they are sexually active, anticipate the present, and view potential future sexual encounters realistically.[45]

Pridham has presented a useful tool (Table 5-2) describing how features of development are pertinent in helping children deal with procedures.[48]

APPLICATION OF LEARNING THEORIES

All of the theories described in the early part of this chapter have been used in health situations. In this section a number of clinical examples of learning theory application are provided.

TABLE 5-2. Features of development that are pertinent to helping children deal with procedures

	Birth to 2 years	2 to 7 years	7 to 12 years	Adolescence
How the child thinks and problem-solves	Sensory-motor experience develops schema (well-defined and repeated sequences of actions and perceptions). Memory is obvious by 3-4 months and is demonstrated in 2nd year by child's imitations of parents' activities. Between about 18 and 24 months, use of symbols for thought-reasoning-	Preoperational stage (thinking is dominated by the child's perceptions rather than logic). Verbally communicated information is increasingly important in learning; exploratory manipulation of objects also helps the child to learn. Child watches, listens, asks questions (why? how?). Child can (a) label (classify) familiar things; perception is often limited to a single, salient feature, making it difficult for child to see things in a context	Concrete operational phase. Child learns from observing/interacting with peers as well as from own experiences. Can use symbols to organize thoughts and represent experience. Features of thinking include increasing capacity to (a) understand viewpoints of others; (b) see the relative nature of things (e.g., this hurts a little; that hurts a lot); (c) use deductive logic in respect to tangible (concrete) experiences (if this, then that); (d) classify things in terms of several characteristics, implying that the child can	Stage of formal operations. At this point, there is use of reason and logical thinking and interest in theoretically possible problems and questions. The adolescent can engage in self-reflection and think about own thinking and can learn from verbally presented ideas and arguments.

	or differentiate unessential from essential properties of an experience; (b) use memory to reconstruct past events; (c) use imagination to deal with events, people, objects; (d) about age 4, begin to infer outcomes; (e) define objects/events in terms of their use/function. Thinking relies on the child's own point of view (egocentricity), since children do not have the capacity to identify a point of view other than their own. As the child gets older, he or she begins to be able to think in terms of quantities (e.g., to recognize variation in quantity; to use numbers to count). Attention is increasingly selective as the child's schema or perceptual sets become more refined.	view things in context, for example, "The shot hurt, but it will make me feel better;" (e) evaluate painful intrusive actions in terms of logical function rather than in terms of punishment; and (f) understand unseen body mechanics/functions. Child can make use of sensory as well as procedural information.	
	communication appears.		Uncertainty about selves as persons (especially early and middle adolescence); concern about whether or not body, thoughts, and feelings are "normal."
Major fears and worries	After about 6 months: separation from parents; unfamiliar people/experiences/places, especially when not accompanied by parent.	Separation from parents; harm to body, including fears of castration after about age 3; punishment for wrongdoing.	Body injury; disability (loss of body functions); loss of control; loss of status.

Continued.

From Pridham KF, Adelson F, Hansen MF: *J Pediatr Nurs* 2:13-22, 1987.

TABLE 5-2. Features of development that are pertinent to helping children deal with procedures—cont'd

	Birth to 2 years	2 to 7 years	7 to 12 years	Adolescence
Understanding cause and effect	By about 3 months, may associate an action with a result. In second year: magical thinking: belief that what is wished for happens.	Beliefs: (a) everything happens by intention; (b) imminent justice—misbehavior is followed by punishment; (c) belief that events that in fact are associated only by happenstance are connected.	Child 6-8: conclusions are based on perceptions. Child 9-12: applies logical operations (deductive thinking) to concrete (immediately experienced) circumstances. Prior to about 9 years, children are likely to view their illness as a consequence of transgressions of rules. (Rules exist in their own right and misdeeds have their own inherent punishment.) Prior to about 9 years, children are likely to believe that illness is caused by germs whose presence is sufficient for illness. At about 9 years, children begin to understand that (a) an illness may have multiple causes; (b) the body's response to an agent or a combination of agents may vary; and (c) host factors interact with agent(s) to cause illness.	Can use formal rules of logic and evidence to assess cause and effect.
Concept of time	By about 3 months, shows anticipation for feedings. Can wait as a consequence of perceiving clues of a familiar and desired activity.	Organized around familiar/routine activities of daily living. By about age 4, has concept of time and day and knows days of week.	Has a concept of the past and future as well as of the present. Can understand time intervals between events and can tell time by a clock. Sense of time is thus independent of perceptual data, e.g., activities of daily living.	Can synthesize the past, present, and future in thinking.
Intentions, goals, and plans	By about 4 months, may show signs of intention/a sense of making an effort to get a result. In second year, child can make a choice of two options.	About age 4, begins to plan and anticipate actions in the near future; has objectives for activities.	Plans more elaborate projects that involve others to a greater extent.	By midadolescence (about age 15), makes future plans for self. Can think in terms of tasks as well as responsibilities in relation to them.

spoon. The caregiver prompts the child by touching him or her on the wrist, the elbow, and the shoulder and then removes all support. Chaining is a technique used to teach behaviors that normally occur in a fixed sequence, such as washing, toileting, dressing. The caregiver teaches the tasks backwards, teaching the last step first and then backing up in each training session. Often, all three techniques (shaping, fading, chaining) are used together.

Staff may do the beginning teaching with a family member or with the person who is taking over. This person may be taught to carry out the process with staff providing only consultative services. The route that is taken depends on the ability of the lay person to interpret behavior and consistently give the correct response. The route taken may also depend on how well the learner accepts the lay person and on the length of time the two will be together.

A particularly useful example concerns an individual with chronic schizophrenia and uncontrolled hypertension who would not take the medication. Through role playing, this patient's brother was instructed in simple behavioral strategies such as the use of reinforcement and extinction and the use of a detailed monitoring record of the patient's intake of medication. Letters and phone calls from the physician were also used as reinforcers. As a result of the program, the number of hospital days and unscheduled outpatient visits for this individual decreased significantly, producing a considerable cost savings.[47]

Throughout the training period, counts are made of the desired and undesired behaviors and compared with the baseline counts. For this comparison it is useful to make charts of desired behavior and of undesired behavior. The training session number is the abscissa and frequency of behavior is the ordinate. (See reference 4 for example.) The success of the program is evaluated. It may be necessary to make modifications, including switching techniques. Shaping proved to be ineffective for Stevie, the little boy mentioned in the box. Fading was found to be more effective, possibly because

reinforcement is delayed less in this technique. It is possible to misjudge a person's readiness level or the reinforcer of the behavior. Sometimes a new source of anxiety in the patient may disturb the learning process and require a revision of the plan. Staff have an important role in the evaluation of progress. They not only check on the success of the learning process, but they also make sure that the parents see the progress. Progress may be slow.[4]

In another example using behavior modification Berni and others[7] developed a care plan for Billy (see pp. 100, 101).

The theory and techniques of operant conditioning can be used to shape new behaviors, to increase low rates of behavior, to reinstate behavior once exhibited but no longer present, or to eliminate avoidance behavior. Operant conditioning has been used to guide learning of self-help skills in retarded persons and to accelerate them in normal children. These skills include spoon feeding, drinking from a cup, dressing, play skills, ambulation, speech, and toilet using. The operant conditioning technique has been used to extinguish such undesirable behaviors in children as throwing food, undressing, tantrums, and vomiting.

Parents have been taught to use behavior modification with their children. Parents can be taught how to modify any class of overt child behaviors. Behavioral management skills that parents frequently need to learn include (1) obtaining the child's attention before issuing a request; (2) issuing one request at a time; (3) waiting after each request for 8 to 15 seconds without talking; (4) helping the child; (5) assuming a threatening or cajoling expression until the requested action is completed; (6) issuing discipline when the child is noncompliant after the first repetition of the request; (7) praising the child's compliance; and (8) issuing time out.[51]

Three approaches can be used in training parents: educational groups, individual consultations, and controlled learning environments. In the controlled learning environment, parents wear earphones and professionals, who are observing through one-way mirrors, direct the behavior of the parents by trans-

PLAN FOR BILLY'S CARE*

WEEK 1

Overall goal: To teach the patient appropriate behavior in preparation for discharge by discontinuing attention to his excessively "sick" behavior and by reinforcing "well" behavior.

1. *Goal:* To reinforce ambulation and independence.

Inappropriate behavior by patient: Refusing to walk, wanting to be carried, and wanting to use wheelchair

Appropriate behavior by patient: Walking.

Negative reinforcers or removal of positive reinforcers: Removing the wheelchair; reducing nurses' social contact, talking, and playing with Billy

Positive reinforcers: Nurses smiling and joking with Billy within his physical capabilities

2. *Goal:* To teach verbal communication and extinguish pointing, grunting, and whining

Inappropriate behavior: Grunting, pointing, whining, and not talking

Appropriate behavior: Talking

Negative reinforcers or removal of positive reinforcers: Nurses refusing to comply with Billy's nonverbal requests after explaining the program to him; reducing nurses' social contact, talking, and playing with him

Positive reinforcers: Complimenting his efforts to talk; smiling, talking, and playing with Billy when he talks

3. *Goal:* To reinforce "well" behavior by deemphasizing bad health and emphasizing positive factors

Negative reinforcers: Deemphasizing questions and remarks about his health status, not commenting in front of Billy about his condition, refraining from pointing out his blue nailbeds whenever this occurs

Positive reinforcers: Pointing out improvement in his activity, praising him for involvement in the occupational therapy program, praising him when he eats or drinks fluids well

WEEK 2

Overall goal: To make Billy's daily living experience as happy as possible by providing a feeling of security for him and by teaching him "well" behavior within his physical capabilities

1. Omit ambulation as a goal for the present
2. *Goal:* Verbal communication

Negative reinforcers: (add) Requesting verbal responses before complying with Billy's requests when he is not talking as he should, going about necessary tasks in silence

Positive reinforcers: (add) Taking time to read to Billy

3. *Goal:* To reinforce "well" behavior
4. *Goal:* To maintain adequate fluid intake

Negative reinforcers: Responding neutrally when Billy refuses the prescribed fluids

Positive reinforcers: Placing a plastic translucent cylinder at Billy's bedside, filling it with colored water equal to the amount that Billy drinks, and complimenting Billy as the level of water rises

Modified from Berni R, Dressler J, Baster JC: *Am J Nurs* 71:2180-2183, 1971.
*Billy is a 5-year-old who has ataxia telangiectasia.

PLAN FOR BILLY'S CARE—cont'd

WEEK 3
Overall goal:
To make Billy feel worthwhile and needed, with "a place in life," in addition to the goals of the first and second weeks

1. *Goal:* Wheelchair ambulation

Positive reinforcers: Arranging for portable oxygen tank, and praising patient when he goes to the activity room

2. *Goal:* To establish verbal communication
3. *Goal:* To reinforce "well" behavior

Negative reinforcers: Reacting neutrally to signs of health fluctuation

4. *Goal:* To maintain prescribed fluid intake (500 ml)
5. *Goal:* To maintain good nutrition

Negative reinforcers: Ignoring his refusal to eat

Positive reinforcers: Commenting when he eats well, giving him attention and choice at the time his menu is made out, making sure that he is served small portions, scheduling meals after pulmonary therapy, and praising him for what he does eat when he has a poor day

---

mitting messages into the earphones. (This approach can also be used in the home.) The training program may involve general or specific steps for a particular behavior change. Programmed instruction texts are often used to present basic behavioral principles and applications. Instructional techniques include modeling after demonstration by the professional or an informed parent. Videotape feedback for analysis and correction of procedures is also useful.[40]

Behavioral self-management programs follow a specific structure, such as the following example in weight reduction[41]:

1. Self-screening for commitment, time, and energy
2. Definition of the problem in behavioral terms, such as eating less or exercising more

3. Self-observation through record keeping on special forms, to obtain factual information about the internal and external signals that trigger problem behaviors and the resulting consequences
4. Analyzing the problem from the records; asking whether certain thoughts or feelings trigger the behavior
5. Setting reasonable goals with small steps; if the patient feels deprived or overwhelmed, the immediate goals are too high
6. Adopting tactics for change:
   a. Managing the external environment so that negative signals are eliminated (store food in opaque containers) or new positive ones are created (pedometers to measure the distance of walking exercise)

b. Changing self-perceptions as well as thoughts—private monologues that are signals that trigger behaviors

c. Developing social support

d. Using self-rewards

7. Evaluating progress by comparing behavior with the baseline

Many behaviors require continued self-monitoring, which helps maintain motivation and reveals areas that need work. Behavioral self-management programs have been developed for assertiveness, fears and phobias, insomnia, female sexual responsiveness, and drinking behavior.[41] Self-management programs aimed at weight loss may be more effective than behavior modification programs carried out by therapists. Studies examining the effectiveness of programs initiated in therapy show an average of small weight reductions with no further reductions after the formal treatment. Weight lost during treatment may be explained as changes in eating behaviors caused primarily by therapist contact. The patient stops using the techniques after the treatment ends.[18]

Operant conditioning is considerably relevant in helping many patients achieve learning goals. Recently, its focus has become more cognitive, since all behavior is cognitively mediated and affected by expectancies. Guidance in operant conditioning research and practice can be obtained from psychologists who have depth of preparation in learning theory and interpretation of behavior. A major concern about the use of operant conditioning has

---

(A) The health educator (advisor) must explain the concepts of reinforcement and contingency to the client.

(B) The health educator (advisor) should review and discuss each item on the HBCS with the client as follows:

HBCS Item #1

Assist the client in determining a specific priority behavior that he or she would like to change. For the best possible results the health educator should encourage the client to initially choose a behavior that is likely to be readily altered by the HBCS. This will allow the client to become familiar with the HBCS guidelines and demonstrate his/her ability to successfully use these guidelines. As the client gains confidence that compliance with the HBCS guidelines can bring about desired behavior change, he/she will be more likely to apply the same guidelines to behaviors which are more resistant to change.

HBCS Item #2

Help the client set a goal utilizing a basic formula to develop a goal—to/action verb/desired results/time frame/resources required the following goal could be formulated as it relates to exercise. To increase exercise behavior by swimming 20 minutes a day, four days per week at 60 to 80% maximum heart rate, for six consecutive weeks at the local YMCA.

HBCS Item #3

The HBCS provides the client with the opportunity to choose and formally commit to changing a specified behavior over time via the contingency contract provided here. At this point the health educator should review the concept of contingency with the client and subsequently have the said client sign the contract. The reward (employer based or Better Health Certificate) which the client will receive contingent upon reaching his/her behavioral goal should also be specified.

FIGURE 5-4. Health behavior change schedule training steps. (From Cole GE, Friedman GM, Bagwell M: *AAOHN J* 34:132-137, 1986.)

HBCS Item #4

Have the client identify and list the obstacles (deterrents) which he/she expects to encounter in the process of reaching his/her behavioral goal. The purpose of this step is to increase the client's awareness regarding possible difficulties in reaching his/her goals so he/she can make plans to overcome these perceived difficulties. Explain to the client that you realize it is impossible to visualize all the potential problems he/she will encounter, but that it is important to realize that difficulties will inevitably arise.

HBCS Item #5

Help the client to plan ways to overcome difficulties (deterrents) listed on item #4 of HBCS. Explain to the client that even though difficulties inevitably will arise, as discussed under item #4, these difficulties can be overcome via planning, dedication, perseverance, etc.

HBCS Item #6

Help the client determine and list the steps (small, realistic, achievable approximations of the behavioral goals) he/she will need to take to reach the behavioral goal listed in item #2 of the HBCS. At this point the health educator (advisor) must serve as a resource for health information, by responding to the clients' requests for information by subsequently providing educational resource materials.

HBCS Item #7

At this point the health educators (advisor) should help the client choose the appropriate reinforcers (rewards) which can be self-administered contingent upon the successful completion of the steps specified in item #6 of the HBCS. In helping the client carry out this process it will be necessary to explain the "Premack Principle" and if so desired to administer a Reinforcement Survey Schedule which will produce a pool of relevant reinforcers (rewards).

HBCS Item #8

Encourage the client to keep a daily log of failures, successes, and ongoing progress towards, and the completion of specified shaping steps and the terminal behavioral goal. The health educator can facilitate this process by providing the client with a formal behavior change log on which the client can record appropriate information regarding day-to-day progress. At this point it is also important to set a future date and time when the client can report in person on any progress he/she has made. Furthermore, the client should also be reminded that an external reward will be presented to him/her contingent upon successfully completing the behavior change goal.
(C) Congratulate the client for taking his/ her first step towards a longer, more productive, happier, healthier life.

FIGURE 5-4, cont'd. For legend see opposite page.

Continued.

Client _____ Health Advisor _____

Organization _____

Health behavior change schedule (HBCS)

Record the health related behavior (priority behavior) that you would like to change and plan a systematic behavior change program as outlined below.

1) Priority behavior (i.e., smoking, overeating, excessive drinking).

_____

2) Set a specific goal. Include a target date for your goal.

_____

3) Complete the following goal contract and include the reward(s) which is/are contingent upon successfully achieving your goal.

I agree to _____ , on or before _____ .

(WRITE IN YOUR BEHAVIORAL GOAL) (DATE TO BE ACHIEVED)

If I am able to reach my goal in the specified time period, I will receive

_____ .

(REWARD)

_____

(YOUR SIGNATURE)

_____ _____

(HEALTH ADVISOR SIGNATURE) (DATE)

4) List and briefly describe the obstacles (deterrents) you expect to encounter as you attempt to reach your goal.

_____

5) List and briefly describe what steps you will take to overcome the obstacles (deterrents) cited in item 3.

_____

6) Determine and list the steps (small, realistic, achievable goals) you will need to take to reach the goal you listed in item #2. Include a target date for each step.

Step 1: _____ Date _____

Step 2: _____ Date _____

Step 3: _____ Date _____

Step 4: _____ Date _____

Step 5: _____ Date _____

7) Develop a list of rewards—that are inexpensive and unrelated to food or alcohol—which you can treat yourself to upon completing each step listed in item #5.

a) Step 1/reward 1 _____

b) Step 2/reward 2 _____

c) Step 3/reward 3 _____

d) Step 4/reward 4 _____

e) Step 5/reward 5 _____

8) Evaluate your progress by keeping a daily log of your failures, successes and ongoing progress toward your goal listed in item #2. When you reach your specified goal (see item #2) report your success to your health advisor who will make arrangements for you to receive the external reward listed in item #3 of the HBCS.

FIGURE 5-4, cont'd. For legend see p. 102.

been that it may merely change surface behavior without understanding or altering its basic psychologic and physiologic origin. Thus treating pain, vomiting, or anxiety by operant conditioning requires excellent judgment regarding possible causes of the behavior.

Some aspects of chronic pain may also be conceptualized in learning terms. For example, behavior occurring after presentation of a presumed noxious stimulus may be accounted for and modified by principles of learning, whatever the original cause of pain. The problem's becoming chronic provides evidence that it has not been entirely resolved by medical approaches; therefore the opportunities for learning pain behavior patterns by operant mechanisms are increased.

Use of behavioral change techniques in work settings has increased as employers have become interested in promoting good health habits and preventing disease. In a work-site weight control program, a self-motivational program of financial incentives was used and implemented through payroll deduction. Return of incentive dollars to employees depended on progress toward weight goals.[19] A private for-profit health promotion and disease prevention corporation has developed the Health Behavior Change Schedule and Training Steps, reproduced in Figure 5-4.[13]

Applications of cognitive learning theory in health situations have focused on the interaction of cognitive and biologic learning theory in areas such as progressive muscle relaxation and guided imagery and on characteristic or inherent inclinations toward disease.

Relaxation and imagery

The relaxation response is characterized by changes in the sympathetic nervous system causing a decrease in heart rate, blood pressure, respiratory rate, and reported levels of anxiety. A number of reports in the literature describe teaching patients relaxation techniques preoperatively so that patients can use them postoperatively for pain relief. It is believed that increased anxiety and muscle tension can cause increased pain. Although it is common in these studies for patients to report less distress, changes in analgesic intake may or may not be found.[25,33] Patients with cancer who are undergoing chemotherapy and have the goal of decreasing anxiety and side effects have also used relaxation techniques. Some adverse effects, such as withdrawal, insomnia, or hallucinations, have been reported.[12]

A teaching plan for relaxation therapy may be found in Table 5-3. A relaxation script is on p. 109. The four elements necessary to establish a successful relaxation technique are quiet environment, decreased muscle tonus, a mental device, and a passive attitude. Since regular practice (20 minutes, twice a day) is required to learn and maintain this skill, tape recordings of relaxation messages can be useful.[12] The patient is taught to tense and then relax different muscle groups while focusing on the differing sensations. With practice the patient learns to relax without the aid of the therapist or the audio tape.

A closely related technique is systematic desensitization. In this procedure the therapist and the patient create a graduated series or hierarchy of anxiety-producing scenes. The scenes for a patient about to undergo an endoscopic examination might be (1) sitting in a hospital room and thinking about the procedure; (2) being wheeled into the examining room; (3) seeing the doctor and nurse approaching; (4) opening mouth and having local anesthetic swabbed on the throat; and (5) having a tube held in place and feeling like gagging, but being unable to. The patient imagines each scene while under relaxation. When he or she reports anxiety, the scene is withdrawn and the patient practices the relaxation techniques until he or she is again relaxed. Therapy continues with the patient proceeding as far up the hierarchy in each session as possible without experiencing anxiety. Another form of the desensitizing procedure involves actually walking the patient through the procedure rather than using imagined situations. With short hospital stays it may be difficult to complete desensitization before the patient undergoes the medical procedure.[63]

TABLE 5-3. Relaxation therapy patient teaching plan

Objectives	Content	Teaching actions	Outcome criteria
1. Patient will describe what stress is	Stress is the response of the body to change. Small amounts of stress can be helpful in adjusting to change. Large amounts of stress for long periods of time cause wear and tear on the body	Discuss with patient	Patient will describe what stress is and state some examples of stressful situations
2. Patient will describe what relaxation is	Relaxation is a learned behavior. Relaxation can be achieved by various techniques, e.g., meditation, progressive muscle relaxation. Relaxation can produce changes in the body that are opposite of the stress response	Discuss with patient	Patient will describe what relaxation is and its relationship to stress
3. Patient will discuss uses of relaxation	Relaxation is used by some persons to decrease anxiety associated with stressful situations such as treatments, procedures, and pain	Have patient discuss any uses of relaxation that he has knowledge of or experience with	Patient will state some uses of relaxation
4. Patient will identify areas of tension	Signs of tension include tightness, pain. Common areas of tension are face, forehead, neck, and shoulders	Have patient tense arm by clenching his fist, have him describe how it feels. Then have him relax arm and describe difference	Patient will discuss signs of tension and identify common areas of tension
5. Patient will identify relaxing images and mental device	Thinking of pleasant memories or images can enhance relaxation by distracting attention away from stressful situations. Some persons think of pleasant scenes such as lying on a beach or in a field. It is helpful to identify a key work or phrase that can help recall relaxing images (mental device)	Have patient discuss pleasant images. Instructor can provide some guidance with ideas, but he or she may want patient to identify his own images. Encourage patient to elaborate on images, describe details. Ask patient to associate a single word or phrase with each relaxing image	Patient will identify at least one relaxing image and one mental device

From Cobb SC: *Cancer Nurs* 7:157-161, 1984.

TABLE 5-3. Relaxation therapy patient teaching plan—cont'd

Objectives	Content	Teaching actions	Outcome criteria
6. Patient will describe the four elements of relaxation	The four key elements needed in a relaxation technique are: 1. A quiet environment—free of noise, distractions, and interruptions (as much as possible) 2. Decreased muscle tonus—since it is not possible to be tense and relaxed at the same time, learning to relax muscles makes general relaxation easier 3. A mental device—a sound, word or phrase repeated silently or audibly, assists in recalling relaxing images, encourages mental relaxation 4. Passive attitude—let thoughts pass in and out of mind freely. Do not worry about how well you are relaxing	Discuss with patient, provide handout of four key elements	Patient will describe the four key elements of relaxation
7. Patient will demonstrate progressive muscle relaxation	Instruct patient to: 1. Sit quietly in a comfortable position—sitting or semireclining position with all extremities supported is recommended. Lying down is not suggested due to tendency to fall asleep in this position (sleep is not the goal, although if it happens it is okay) 2. Leave eyes open for several minutes, then gradually close and keep closed 3. After several minutes with eyes closed, begin progressive tensing and relaxing of all muscles from feet up	Ensure that room is as private and quiet as possible. Written instructions will facilitate patient practice	Patient will be able to demonstrate progressive muscle relaxation from the feet up

Continued.

TABLE 5-3. Relaxation therapy patient teaching plan—cont'd

Objectives	Content	Teaching actions	Outcome criteria
	The following are some practice techniques to help you do this: a. Legs—tense and relax foot, knee, thigh, then entire leg b. Trunk—pull in abdomen, arch back slightly, relax abdomen, back, legs; bend shoulders back, relax; elevate shoulders, relax. Relax entire trunk c. Arms—bend each hand back and then relax, bend each elbow and relax. Tense and relax entire arm d. Neck—bend head back, bend chin toward chest—bend head right, then left. Relax e. Mouth—clench teeth, relax; frown, relax; smile, relax f. Eye region—wrinkle forehead—frown, relax. Close eyelids tightly—relax Once body feels relaxed, keep muscles relaxed	Instructor may do exercises with patient—provides a role model and helps decrease self-consciousness Instructor may coach patient; e.g., by saying "tense . . . now relax"	
8. Patient will demonstrate rhythmic breathing	Breathe through your nose slowly. Become aware of your breathing. As you breathe out, say mental device to yourself. Breathe easily and naturally. Continue for 10-20 minutes. When finished, sit quietly for several minutes with eyes closed, then with eyes opened. Do not stand up for a few minutes	Instructor demonstrates, then has patient do technique	Patient will show signs of successful relaxation: breathing slows down, face appears relaxed with lips apart, feet move from being parallel to one another to turning apart
9. Patient will describe practice schedule	Technique should be practiced once or twice daily. Excessive use is to be avoided	Have patient keep a log of practice sessions—include when, where, feelings, and sensations	Patients will identify times and places for practice

RELAXATION SCRIPT

Find a comfortable chair and make whatever minor adjustments you need to be as comfortable and unrestricted as possible and let your mind just wander throughout your body. Check your body and get comfortable, relaxed. Loosen any tight clothing. Choose a comfortable position for your body. Make whatever minor adjustments you need to make. Allow yourself to be in the most comfortable position. Then let your attention focus on the very top of your head, on your scalp and forehead, smoothing out all the muscles of your scalp and forehead. Let them go, relax them. Smooth those muscles out and let your scalp rest very comfortably on top of your head. Let that relaxation move over your eyebrows, eyelids, even relaxing your eyes behind your closed eyelids, letting your eyes rest quite comfortably. Continue to let the relaxation flow over your cheeks, lips, and chin, letting your whole face become quite comfortably heavy and relaxed. Allow the muscles that hold up your jaw to relax; just let them go.

Let go of any tension in your tongue. Let your tongue rest very comfortably, puddled in your mouth. Relax your throat and your vocal cords.

Let the relaxation continue to flow down the back of your head. Let go of all the muscles along your neck and down your shoulders. Smooth out all the muscles of your neck and shoulders. Think of any tension here as a tiny knotted rope that you untie and let hang loose and limp. Smooth them out and just let them hang loose, limp, and relaxed. Relax your shoulders and all the neck and let that relaxation flow down into your arms, relaxing all the muscles of your upper arm down to your elbows and your forearm, smoothing out those muscles and letting them go. Let go of

the muscles around your wrists and hands, all the way down to your fingertips. Let your arms become comfortably heavy and relaxed. As your arms become more and more heavy and relaxed, let the blood flow more comfortably into your fingertips. When you let go of the tension in your arms and shoulders, the blood flows more easily into your fingertips. This is a sign of relaxation.

As you continue to relax your head and face, your neck and shoulders and arms, let your attention move to your upper back and smooth out all the muscles along your shoulders and upper back. Continue to relax all the way along your spine, down your middle back, smoothing out all the muscles down into your lower back. Continue to let go all the way down into your waist and buttocks. Feel that relaxation.

Allow the relaxation to come around the side of your chest. Let go of all the muscles between every rib, smoothing them out and letting go of any tension. With every breath, allow your chest to become more and more relaxed. Observe your breathing with every breath. As you inhale air, allow your stomach to blow up like a balloon. As you exhale, let your stomach fall back into your spine. Allow your breathing to be smooth, normal, rhythmic. Allow yourself to let go with every breath. Continue to let go, with your abdomen feeling the wave of warmth and relaxation.

Let go of all the muscles around your hips and pelvis, letting your whole pelvic area relax and smooth out. Let that relaxation flow down to your thighs, knees, your shins, calves, letting your legs become comfortably heavy and relaxed. Let go of your ankles, heels, feet—even the soles of your feet and toes. As your legs become comfortably heavy, blood flows again more easily to the toes, and your feet become comfortably warm.

Feel your body from the very top of your head, all the way down to the ends of your toes. Your body is relaxed, peacefully calm, and very quiet inside. Allow your body to relax even more. As you continue to exhale, let your body just float on down through the chair, comfortably heavy and relaxed. Continue to remain awake and alert as you feel yourself relax more deeply. Relaxation allows your whole body to have a very deep rest while you are awake and alert. Relaxation is different from tiredness. While tiredness is a drain of energy produced by too much tension in the system, relaxation allows you to conserve the energy that was formerly used up by tension through deep relaxation, such as you are experiencing now. The body can get a very deep rest and you can feel refreshed and rejuvenated.

As you practice these techniques of deep progressive relaxation, you become more and more capable and effective at relaxing more quickly and more efficiently. You are learning new skills. With increased skills you will learn to use the words calm, very quiet, or relaxed, which will allow you to achieve the same quality of deep relaxation that you are experiencing now. With practice, the depth of the relaxation can also be increased. Again, allow yourself to be alert, conscious, and awake, very relaxed and quiet inside. When you are ready, allow the muscles around your eyes to be less heavy. Move your arms and body little by little. When you are ready, become aware of the room and the environment around you and let your eyes open. Feel your relaxation. When you are ready, just let your eyes open and become aware of the room.

From Guzzetta CE, Dossey BM: *Cardiovascular nursing: body-mind tapestry,* St Louis, 1984, Mosby–Year Book.

EXAMPLE OF GUIDED IMAGERY

NURSE: Bill, how are you feeling about your cardiac catheterization?

BILL: I'm scared. I keep having these ideas about it being awful. All I've ever seen really is stuff on television. It looks scary.

NURSE: I would like to share some positive ideas with you, as well as a few skills that you can use during your procedure to help you. Would you be interested?

BILL: You bet. Can we do it now?

NURSE: Let me ask you a few questions. What is the most perfect, quiet, magic place that comes to your mind which makes you relax and feel good?

BILL: That's easy. My brother and I have some property in southern Colorado. On it is a pond where beavers live and play. Also that pond has big rainbow trout in it. Boy, I'd sure like to go fishing up there soon. Maybe I will as soon as I get over this.

NURSE: Let me guide you with some basic relaxation skills that you can use during your cardiac catheterization. Then I'll use the same information you just gave me about the beaver pond. Okay?

BILL: I'm ready. [Bill was on his bed lying at a 30-degree angle.]

NURSE: Bill, with your eyes closed and your body relaxed and lying still, travel forward 24 hours. It is 7:00 a.m. the morning of your cardiac catheterization. You awake feeling refreshed, relaxed, and confident about your cardiac catheterization that will occur in a few hours. Use these first few alert, awake moments to feel the relaxation from the top of your head to the tip of your toes. [At this point a general, head-to-toe relaxation induction is used.]

Since you feel relaxed, it is now time to get on the stretcher and head to the cardiac catheterization laboratory. You look forward to this day. You will know information soon that will help you in your continued recovery. As you ride down the hall, use this time to focus on breathing in and out and feeling very relaxed. Feel yourself entering the door behind the x-ray department. The cardiac catheterization room is on your left. As you enter the room on the stretcher, you are greeted by two nurses whom you know, and you are delighted. As you move onto the cardiac catheterization table, feel the security of that table as the nurses place a strap over your legs and arms to help you maintain this position. Continue to use this time to concentrate on your breathing and to achieve a deeper state of relaxation.

You hear your cardiologist entering now. He greets you and makes you feel comfortable by his confidence and caring. The procedure is now beginning. Your physician is numbing your skin in your groin area for your comfort during the procedure. Use this time for positive images. Whenever the physician wants you to participate in the procedure by coughing or bearing down as though you were having a bowel movement, you will be able to come back quickly. But until that time, go to your special place.

At this point, feeling confident and relaxed, allow yourself to go to southern Colorado. You haven't been there in a while. Ah, it feels so good. Smell the mountain air, the pine trees so fresh and strong. Look at the different trees—the aspens as their leaves quake in the sun, the magical tall blue spruces with their unmistakable color. Look at the little chipmunks and squirrels playing. Feel yourself with fishing pole in hand with your wonderful black and white no. 4 Rooster Tails and other lures. You are walking down that path which leads to the beaver pond.

Today seems special. This path is exciting. You hear twigs and leaves snap and crunch as you step on them. You feel a balance while you walk. This walk is relaxed, and you have nothing to do today except watch the beavers play and maybe catch some trout.

As you get to the edge of the pond, there are the beavers playing. They look at you; two are in the water, and one is on a log. They are closer to you than they have

From Guzzetta CE, Dossey BM: *Cardiovascular nursing: body-mind tapestry,* St Louis, 1984, Mosby–Year Book.

EXAMPLE OF GUIDED IMAGERY—cont'd

ever been. As they look at you, they say hello and watch you for a while. Neither you nor the beavers are afraid. They continue to play, flapping their tails, diving off logs, showing their long teeth and black soft eyes. You start to fish for the first time in a long while. Feel the excitement of that first cast. It seems perfect. On the first cast, you get a bite, but the trout is just playing with your Rooster Tail. The pond water is clear, and as you pull your line in, you can see two trout following it. Feel that sense of going with the flow. If you catch a trout, fine; and if you don't catch one that also is fine.

As you continue your fishing, you hear your physician tell you that everything is going fine. He asks you to cough, and you do so. Then continue your image; again bring it into full, clear focus, adding more detail—the colors, the smells, the environment, what you are doing, and what the beavers are doing. [A period of quietness is allowed for 5 minutes. The patient continues to image in an alert relaxed state with his eyes closed.]

The next thing you hear is your physician telling you that your procedure is over and it went very well. He briefly tells you that he has found what it is that you both need to know. And he tells you he will give you the details of what was found in the afternoon.

You feel relieved that the procedure went well. Now you are back in your bed with a sandbag on your groin. It weighs 5 pounds and will stay on there 8 hours. Your head is at a 30-degree angle. Feel yourself successfully using the urinal in this position. Give yourself a pat on the back for staying calm and relaxed and being able to image that special pond.

Begin to feel the muscles around your eyes become less heavy. Begin to lighten your arms and legs, and start to move slowly and gently. And when you are ready, just open your eyes and look around.

BILL: You're not going to believe this: I caught two trout during that exercise. I had my doubts when we started, but you know, I've had those kinds of thoughts before; I just never knew I was imaging. I'll sure try that tomorrow. Thanks.

NURSE: Try to do these exercises a few more times on your own, and I'll do it with you one more time before I leave today.

Imagery is a concentrated focusing on images formed in the mind. These are imagined stimuli. Imagery is an extension of everyday thought processes like daydreaming. Distraction, on the other hand, involves focusing on existing stimuli, such as a wall decoration, or bodily sensations, such as breathing. Both techniques, along with others, were used to help children with cancer control pain during intrusive procedures such as bone marrow aspiration. These techniques allow the child to gain control of the situation and participate actively in the treatment.[24] Relaxation is one of the first steps in effectively being able to image. A script for guided imagery may be found on pp. 110, 111.[23]

Self-statement modification procedures target the patient's maladaptive cognitions as the source of emotional turmoil and seek to alter these cognitions. Stress inoculation training is one such procedure. The goal in stress inoculation is to modify the patient's view of the stress through examination of his or her self-talk. Patients are taught new ways to talk to themselves. Anxiety is the patient's cue to rethink the situation and self-talk differently.[63] In cognitive modeling, models verbalize their thoughts as they solve problems and form judgments. Mastery models perform calmly and faultlessly. Coping models begin fearfully but gradually overcome their difficulties. They give voice to their problem solving and determined coping efforts. Coping models are especially used in self-help groups. In teaching cognitive self-regulating skills, modeled self-talk includes a variety of guides such as analysis of task requirements, symbolic rehearsal of a plan of action, self-instructions for performance, coping self-talk to counteract disruptive thought patterns, and self-praise for attainments.[3]

Biofeedback is a process that gives information about bodily processes and provides a way for individuals to modify those processes. For example, information about the individual's brain waves or blood pressure is displayed on a recording instrument. While watching the display, the individual is encouraged to try to make a change, for example, in blood pressure. Biofeedback from the muscles of the forehead and neck is used to relieve tension headaches.

Attributions

Attributions are a form of cognitive interpretation about why something happened. A persuasive theory with mounting and affirming evidence suggests that people tend to attribute the cause of serious illness to their emotional state, their health behaviors, confidence in their ability to control the outcome of the problem, or the ability to contend with uncertainty regarding their condition. This may explain why attributions predict morbidity in some serious illness.[1] Most patients report an attribution. Those reporting a causal explanation have a more positive physical or emotional outcome than patients who fail to report.[57] Obviously, health professionals are interested in helping patients and significant others build adaptive attributions.

Some examples may be helpful. Bar-On reports a study of male patients less than 60 years old who had had their first myocardial infarction. Their attributions about the cause and outcome of the infarction formed five clusters: (1) some of the patients attributed the myocardial infarction to fate,

luck, or the pressures of life; (2) some denied the problem and said that the infarction was a matter of chance, that they would continue to do what they had been been doing; (3) some wanted to control the future by building their bodies and following their physicians' advice; (4) some believed that their anger had caused the attack and that with the help of physician and family, they would be able to cope; and (5) some believed that their bodies were vulnerable because of inherited tendencies, smoking, or bad habits; however, they believed that medication would help. Those with the fourth pattern of attribution were more likely to recover and return to work.[5]

Likewise, a study of parents who cared for their adult children with schizophrenia discovered four patterns of attribution for the cause of the illness and for appropriate caretaking: (1) schizophrenia was caused by chemical imbalance, and care should be oriented to monitoring and limiting the ill member's intake of chemicals; (2) the adult children could be persuaded to respond to reason; (3) symptoms were largely out of the individual's control but could be reduced if he or she avoided certain environments that exacerbated symptoms; and (4) since the symptoms were the patient's way of coping with the confusion, the appropriate model of care was gentle support.[10]

Finally, an interesting treatment for hypochondriasis approaches the disorder as sensory amplification of normal bodily sensations or symptoms of trivial disorders. The resulting alarm heightens arousal and self-scrutiny, which further amplifies the sensations. The cognitive-educational treatment approach teaches patients to focus on relaxing and on benign sensations, provides information about the somatic manifestations of stress, and asks patients to explore which emotional states exacerbate their symptoms. An educational approach is more acceptable to these patients than is therapy.[6]

In a number of clinical situations, several behavioral and cognitive techniques are used. For example, coping strategies for pain tolerance might include distraction, self-relaxation, imagery, calming self-instruction on how to prepare for and han-

TABLE 5-4. Proposed protocol for training pill swallowing

Child doesn't swallow pills	
Due to skills deficit	**Due to behavioral noncompliance**

1. *Relaxation*
  a. Use quiet, relaxed environment.
  b. Teach relaxation breathing (i.e., tell child to take deep breaths and exhale slowly while making a hissing noise, may also repeat word such as "relax" or "calm" to himself).
2. *Modeling*
  a. Begin with candy that can be easily swallowed.
  b. Model swallowing and demonstrate how to cope with a failure (i.e., "I didn't do very well, but that's OK, I'll try it again").
3. *Practice*
  a. Have child place candy in mouth and allow it to dissolve to the desired size, then swallow.
  b. Child may be encouraged to take water and tilt head back to swallow candy.
  c. Encourage child gradually to swallow the candy sooner after it is placed in the mouth (i.e., before it shrinks).
4. *Reinforcement*
  a. Provide agreed-upon reward (e.g., hugs, praise, or trinkets) immediately after the child swallows the candy.
  b. Immediately after the child swallows two consecutive candies (in mouth less than 15 sec) of same size, provide agreed-upon reward (e.g., favorite food, money, short game).
5. *Repeat*
  a. After two successful trials & reward, move to slightly larger size candy and repeat steps 2-4. Repeat until approximate size of medication to be swallowed is reached.
6. *General considerations*
  a. Do not try to trick or shame child into swallowing pills.
  b. Allow child to progress at his/her own pace.
  c. Make sure child knows difference between practice candy and real medicine.
	1. *Reinforcement*
	Parents should immediately and liberally reward child for promptly taking oral medications at scheduled times. Praise in front of significant family members and the reason for the reinforcement should be included.
	2. *Extinction*
	The child's complaints, whining, and attempts to delay medications should be ignored by parents. Children should be told why they are receiving the medications, but this should not be repeated each time medications are scheduled.
	3. *Time out*
	The child should be placed in a nondangerous, nonreinforcing environment for a minimum of 10 minutes by parents, for refusal to take scheduled medications. The child should be required to be quiet for the last 5 minutes of this period, even if more than 10 minutes elapse. The above contingencies should be explained to the child and one warning be given prior to use of time out. Immediately after time out is concluded, the child should again be told to take his/her medication. If he/she refuses, time out should be repeated until compliance is obtained.
	4. *General considerations*
	  a. This program will only work if the child's caretakers are calm and above all *consistently stick with the program*.
	  a. Any behavior of the child that allows delay or circumvents delivery of medication (e.g., running away, hiding, physical resistance) will become more frequent. Therefore, these behaviors must be met with time out.
	  c. Use procedure 1 in behavioral noncompliance protocol to maintain compliance.

If both behavioral noncompliance and skills deficits are present, both parts of the protocol should be used.

From Funk MJ, Mullins LL, Olson RA: *Child Health Care* 13:20-23, 1984.

dle painful sensation, cognitive reappraisal of aversive events, and self-affirmation of capabilities.[3] Other clinical examples follow:

- Adherence to an exercise regimen involves shaping, behavioral contracting, and cognitive strategies such as goal setting and coping thoughts. Fading during formal exercise sessions, formal reinforcements, and asking patients to self-monitor daily pedometer readings also are useful regimens.[37]
- For 3- to 6-year-old children undergoing cardiac catheterization, behavioral rehearsal involves a tour, doll play, and coloring books that demonstrate distraction strategies for coping with the catheterization. First the doll is restrained on the catheterization table, then the child is so restrained to practice responses for coping with distress. The child's favorite records are played during the catheterization. The nurse specialist informs the child of progress, and he or she is given a bravery badge at completion of the procedure. When compared with a control group, rehearsed patients cried significantly less, showed less gross body movement during the catheterization, and had less anxiety after the procedure.[39]
- For patients undergoing chemotherapy for cancer, conditioned nausea and vomiting were caused by repeated association of the pharmacologic side effects with environmental stimuli, so that sights, smells, taste sensations, and even thoughts associated with the chemotherapy process elicited anxiety, nausea, and vomiting. Progressive muscle relaxation training with biofeedback was used, as was systematic desensitization, and attentional diversion.[8]
- Table 5-4 shows a protocol for training a 9-year-old boy in pill swallowing, with treatment for skills deficit and for behavioral noncompliance.[20]
- Leventhal sees compliance within a self-regulation model in which patients generate their own representations of health threats. They consider information supplied by the media, friends, and health practitioners, as well as their own body symptoms and sensations. On the basis of these representations, they plan and act. Practitioners rarely elicit these models from patients. However, in the future they must do so and must fit their interventions into those models. Of course, they will need to alter incorrect goals and teach skills needed to reach the patients' defined goals. Only in this way will long-term compliance be attained.[34]

Availability of these behavioral and cognitive techniques greatly expands the repertoire of skills that can be taught to patients and expands the approaches to understanding patient education interventions.

SUMMARY

Since fulfillment of particular objectives is the purpose for educational efforts, the teacher draws on a core of knowledge about learning to guide the change, including growth, development, and memory. For cognitive behaviors, it is important to establish a bridge of meaning between old and new understandings. Attitude learning requires opportunity for imitation of a model; motor skills benefit from practice with feedback. Operant conditioning involving discriminate use of behavior reinforcers has already been shown to be significant in health care.

Klausmeier defines the following basic conditions of learning: (1) organizing and sequencing of learning tasks, (2) focusing learner attention on the learning tasks and the means of attaining them, (3) aiding learners in setting goals, (4) supplying models, (5) guiding learners' activities verbally, (6) managing practice effectively, (7) providing for individual differences, (8) evaluating learners' performance and providing feedback, (9) providing for retention, and (10) providing for transfer.[41]

STUDY QUESTIONS

1. Pelco[43] describes an approach to teaching a 4-year-old child how to take a capsule, using behavioral learning principles. Label the behavioral approaches being used.

Teaching action	Behavioral approach

a. The child refused to accept any capsules.

b. Therapist showed child how to swallow by putting capsule between fingers, placing on back of tongue, taking a sip of juice, tilting head, and swallowing.

c. Explain to child that she could earn pennies to buy toys displayed in the room, by doing what therapist asked.

d. When child refused to swallow, therapist placed his hand over the child's and guided it through the steps, until she successfully swallowed capsule.

e. Pennies and praise were given even if physical guidance was used and child swallowed smaller capsule.

These steps were followed until the child could consistently swallow prescription-sized capsules. The parent was trained how to maintain routine capsule acceptance postintervention.

2. Following are sequential responses of patients who had suffered myocardial infarctions. Indicate possible rationale for the behavior, in terms of theory about motivation and learning.

A first response to this illness was anxiety and a frantic search for a "cause" of the illness, as a way to control the disease by excluding this activity.

Some patients had an urgent need for rigid definition by the physicians about the correct way and extent of exerting themselves during convalescence and later—a kind of bargaining for control of the symptoms.

Some patients wished to remain confused about their understanding of the illness.

Other patients sought to identify with others whom they knew had suffered a coronary occlusion. This helped to decrease the ambiguity they experienced in the early stages of the illness because, by following the pattern of the convalescence of their colleagues, they were able to structure some expectations for their own future.[36]

3. An assumption on which parent group education can be based is that parents learn best when they are free to create their own response to a situation. At no time does the leader pressure toward group consensus or conformity. What possibly conflicting learning principles are involved in the decision to function according to this assumption?

4. Some findings suggest a relationship between feelings of guilt on the part of parents of disabled children and the adequacy of their knowledge.
   a. What could explain this relationship?
   b. How would you use this information?

5. In one study of postoperative recall of an informed-consent discussion,[52] the following points were made. Critique their logic, based on your knowledge of patient learning.
   a. "There were repeated instances in each conversation in which the patient was asked if he understood the explanations, and questions were answered as they arose. We believe, therefore, that all patients completely understood the information imparted."
   b. "The patients studied had been educated by their previous experience with their disease; all had chronic heart disease and had been hospitalized many times for diagnostic and therapeutic procedures."

REFERENCES

1. Affleck G and others: Attributional processes in rheumatoid arthritis patients, *Arthritis Rheum* 30:927-931, 1987.
2. Allen DA and others: Concerns of children with a chronic illness: a cognitive-developmental study of juvenile diabetes, *Child Care Health Dev* 10:211-218, 1984.
3. Bandura A: *Foundations of thought and action: a social cognitive theory,* Englewood Cliffs, NJ, 1986, Prentice-Hall.
4. Barnard K: Teaching the retarded child is a family affair, *Am J Nurs* 68:305-311, 1968.
5. Bar-On D, Cristal N: Causal attributions of patients, their spouses and physicians, and the rehabilitation of the patients after their first myocardial infarction, *J Cardiopulm Rehabil* 7:285-298, 1987.
6. Barsky AJ, Geringer E, Wool CA: A cognitive-educational treatment for hypochondriasis, *Gen Hosp Psychiatry* 10:322-327, 1988.
7. Berni R and others: Reinforcing behavior, *Am J Nurs* 71:2180-2183, 1971.
8. Burish TG and others: Behavioral relaxation techniques in reducing the distress of cancer chemotherapy patients, *Oncol Nurs Forum* 10:32-35, 1983.
9. Campbell DJ: Task complexity: a review and analysis, *Acad Manag Rev* 13:40-52, 1988.
10. Chesla CA: Parents' illness models of schizophrenia, *Arch Psychiatr Nurs* 3:218-225, 1989.
11. Clark RE, Vogel A: Transfer of training principles for instructional design, *Educ Commun Tech J* 33:113-123, 1985.
12. Cobb SC: Teaching relaxation techniques to cancer patients, *Cancer Nurs* 7:157-161, 1984.

13. Cole GE, Friedman GM, Bagwell M: A worksite behavioral health education program based on operant conditioning, *AAOHN J* 34:132-137, 1986.

14. Collins RD: Problem solving: a tool for patients, too, *Am J Nurs* 68:1483-1485, 1968.

15. Cormier SM, Hagman JD, editors: *Transfer of learning,* New York, 1987, Academic Press.

16. Elkind D: Teenage thinking: implications for health care, *Pediatr Nurs* 10:383-385, 1984.

17. Fishbein M: *A theory of reasoned action: some applications and implications.* In Page MM, editor: *Nebraska symposium on motivation,* Lincoln, 1980, University of Nebraska Press.

18. Foreyt JP, Goodrick GK, Gotto AM: Limitations of behavioral treatment of obesity: a review and analysis, *J Behav Med* 4:159-174, 1981.

19. Forster JL and others: A work-site weight control program using financial incentives collective through payroll deduction, *J Occup Med* 27:804-808, 1985.

20. Funk MJ, Mullins LL, Olson RA: Teaching children to swallow pills: a case study, *Child Health Care* 13:20-23, 1984.

21. Gagne RM: *The conditions of learning,* ed 3, New York, 1977, Holt, Rinehart & Winston.

22. Glaser R, Bassok M: Learning theory and the study of instruction, *Annu Rev Psychol* 40:631-666, 1989.

23. Guzzetta CE, Dossey BM: *Cardiovascular nursing,* St Louis, 1984, Mosby–Year Book.

24. Hockenberry MJ, Bologna-Vaughn S: Preparation for intrusive procedures using noninvasive techniques in children with cancer: state of the art vs. new trends, *Cancer Nurs* 8:97-102, 1985.

25. Horowitz BF, Fitzpatrick JJ, Flaherty GG: Relaxation techniques for pain relief after open heart surgery, *Dimens Crit Care Nurs* 3:364-371, 1984.

26. Janis IL: *The patient as decision maker.* In Gentry WD, editor: *Handbook of behavioral medicine,* New York, 1984, Guilford Press.

27. Janz NK, Becker MH, Hartman PE: Contingency contracting to enhance patient compliance: a review, *Patient Educ Couns* 5:164-178, 1984.

28. Kelman HC: Attitudes are alive and well and gainfully employed in the sphere of action, *Am Psychol* 29:310-324, 1974.

29. Kelman HC: The role of action in attitude change. In Page MM, editor: *Nebraska symposium on motivation,* Lincoln, 1980, University of Nebraska Press.

30. Klausmeier HJ: *Educational psychology,* ed 5, New York, 1985, Harper & Row.

31. Knowles MS: *Andragogy in action,* San Francisco, 1984, Jossey-Bass.

32. Langer EJ and others: Environmental determinants of memory improvement in late adulthood, *J Pers Soc Psychol* 37:2003-2013, 1979.

33. Lawlis GF and others: Reduction of postoperative pain parameters by presurgical relaxation instructions for spinal pain patients, *Spine* 10:649-651, 1985.

34. Leventhal H, Zimmerman R, Gutmann M: Compliance: a self-regulation perspective. In Gentry WD, editor: *Handbook of behavioral medicine,* New York, 1984, Guilford Press.

35. Ley P: Memory for medical information, *Br J Soc Clin Psychol* 18:245-255, 1979.

36. Martin HL: The significance of discussion with patients about their diagnosis and its implications, *Br J Med Psychol* 40:233-242, 1967.

37. Martin JE, Dubbert PM: Behavioral management strategies for improving health and fitness, *J Cardiac Rehabil* 4:200-208, 1984.

38. Mezirow J: A critical theory of adult learning and education, *Adult Educ* 32:3-24, 1981.

39. Naylor D, Coates TJ, Kan J: Reducing distress in pediatric cardiac catheterization, *Am J Dis Child* 138:726-729, 1984.

40. O'Dell S: Training parents in behavior modification: a review, *Psychol Bull* 81:418-433, 1974.

41. Ormiston L: Self-management strategies. In Squyres W, editor: *Patient education: an inquiry into the state of the art,* New York, 1980, Springer.

42. Palmer BB, Lewis CE: Development of health attitudes and behaviors, *J Sch Health* 46:401-402, 1976.

43. Pelco LE and others: Behavioral management of oral medication administration difficulties among children: a review of literature with case illustrations, *J Dev Behav Pediatr* 8:90-96, 1987.

44. Penland P: Self-initiated learning, *Adult Educ* 29:170-179, 1979.

45. Pestrak VA, Martin D: Cognitive development and aspects of adolescent sexuality, *Adolescence* 20:981-987, 1985.

46. Pichert JW, Hanson SL, Pechmann CA: A system for assessing use of patients' time, *Eval Health Prof* 8:39-54, 1985.

47. Pinto RP, Sirota AD, Brown WA: Behavioral instruction for a patient's relative to increase antihypertensive compliance, *Psychosomatics* 26:677-679, 1985.

48. Pridham KF, Adelson F, Hansen MF: Helping children deal with procedures in a clinic setting: a developmental approach, *J Pediatr Nurs* 2:13-22, 1987.

49. Priluck IA, Robertson DM, Buettner H: What patients recall of the preoperative discussion after retinal detachment surgery, *Am J Ophthalmol* 87:620-623, 1979.

50. Reading AE: Psychological preparation for surgery: patient recall of information, *J Psychosom Res* 25:57-62, 1981.

51. Rickert VI and others: Training parents to become better behavior managers, *Behav Modif* 12:475-496, 1988.

52. Robinson G, Merav A: Informed consent: recall by patients tested postoperatively, *Ann Thorac Surg* 22:209-212, 1976.

53. Rosser RA, Nicholson GI: *Educational psychology,* Boston, 1984, Little, Brown.

54. Salomon G, Perkins DN: Rocky roads to transfer: rethinking mechanisms of a neglected phenomenon, *Educ Psychol* 24:113-142, 1989.

55. Smart MS, Smart RC: *Children: development and relationships,* ed 4, New York, 1982, Macmillan.

56. Thompson RH: *Psychosocial research on pediatric hospitalization and health care,* Springfield, Ill, 1985, Charles C Thomas.

57. Turnquist DC, Harvey JH, Andersen BL: Attributions and adjustment to life-threatening illness, *Br J Clin Psychol* 27:55-65, 1988.

58. Vojtecky MA: An adaptation of Bigge's classification of learning theories to health education and an analysis of theory underlying recent health education programs, *Health Educ Q* 10:247-262, 1984.

59. Waechter EH: *Nursing care of children,* ed 10, Philadelphia, 1985, JB Lippincott.

60. Walberg HJ: Instructional theories and research evidence. In Wang MC, Walberg HJ, editors: *Adapting instruction to individual differences,* Berkeley, Calif, 1985, McCutchon Publishing.

61. Whitney LR, Barnard KE: Implications of operant learning theory for nursing care of the retarded child, *Ment Retard* 4:26-29, 1966.

62. Whitt JK, Dykstra W, Taylow CA: Children's conceptions of illness and cognitive development, *Clin Pediatr* 18:317-339, 1979.

63. Williams CL, Kendall PC: Psychological aspects of patient education for stressful medical procedures, *Health Educ Q* 12:135-150, 1985.

CHAPTER 6

Teaching: theory and interpersonal techniques

While caregivers have been teaching, they also have been assessing the patients' needs to learn, they have been motivating the patients, and they have been defining objectives for the patients. Now they try to produce behavior change, including change in thoughts, in feelings, and in the meaning of experience that will eventually yield observable behavior change. The common notion that teaching just gives information to a class disregards other essential facets of the task. This limited perspective does not take into account the variety of teaching methods and techniques available or the kinds of behavior changes possible.

BEHAVIORALLY ORIENTED TECHNIQUES

Because the need for patient education is so great and the resources often seem so limited, it is easy to fall into a pattern of simply providing general information to patients and referring to this service as education. The patients' focus is not on learning all there is to know about a treatment or a disease. They are interested in using the information to manage their own health situations. Chronic illnesses necessitate active patient participation in development, implementation, and follow-up of treatment goals. Reaching the goals requires support and reinforcement. The ability to deliver this kind of patient education may require changes in the methods and structures health care institutions use to relate to patients. Examples of new delivery systems that support patient education may be found in Chapter 10. Analysis of the many research studies that support the systems may be found in Appendix E.

Two examples of behaviorally focused teaching techniques may be helpful. When campers with diabetes learned about a new food and participated in preparing it, they were more likely to select it for a snack at a later time as compared with a group that received a traditional lecture or discussion on trying new foods or a control group given a general nutrition class.[39] A behavioral focus may be developed for cognitive learning as well. For example, it would be valuable to women who are at risk of bearing a child with muscular dystrophy or who have a neural tube defect. Instruction to assist patients in making a decision about childbearing used structured scenarios such as having a handicapped child (see example in box) or not bearing another child. The women "tried out" the outcomes of each scenario as if that decision had been made. They could also have used imagery-based decision making to imagine the feelings and bodily sensations that would ensue.

Such active learning focuses on the behavior of making a decision. Reviews of research on patient education for those with chronic disease show that (1) any education is better than none, and (2) behaviorally oriented patient education is 150% to 300% more effective than didactic programs. The critical features accounting for the success of behaviorally oriented education include emphasis on certain aspects of the process. For example, emphasis is placed on self-care behaviors (rather than on the disease process), use of mechanisms to alter the self-care environment (such as reminder systems), regular contact with the same health care provider, and incentives.[40]

STRUCTURED SCENARIO

Imagine that . . .
Your child would always require the same care as an
   infant. How do you feel that you would respond to
   the situation? Which statement most closely reflects
   your feelings?
_____ I could manage.
_____ I don't know whether I could manage.
_____ I couldn't manage.
_____ Other, explain briefly.[2]

From Arnold JR, Winsor EJT, McDowell RL, Jr: *Clin Pediatr*
25:345-348, 1986.

INSTRUCTIONAL FORMS

A number of learning tools are available: printed
material in books and pamphlets, programmed instruction, pictures and other visual aids (including
television and motion pictures), certain situations
and environments, and individuals and groups. Depending on the learner and the material, these tools
more or less provide self-instruction for the learner.
Although individuals learn many things without a
teacher, most need a teacher part of the time. Today
the teacher is less a dispenser of information—
factual material—than a programmer and designer
of many kinds of learning experiences. They reach
toward particular goals and use a combination of
tools, including their relationship with the learner.
Teachers who are less knowledgeable and skilled
in teaching tend to be rigid in their responses. Often
responses are limited to giving the learner information the teacher thinks is needed. Skilled teachers are more flexible in that they can alter their
teaching according to the learner's responses and
are capable of using many techniques and tools in
appropriate ways. These behaviors fall on a continuum. It is important to determine where present
teaching behaviors fall.

The reader will recall from the last chapter that
the theory of instruction concerned with taking best
advantage of the learning process is not fully developed. Instructional psychology is a linking science between scientific knowledge about human
behavior and knowledge gained from educational
practice. It has been best developed for behavioral
learning theory, with a technology of instruction in
programmed instruction and operant conditioning
techniques. These techniques have led to impressive accomplishments, particularly in circum-
scribed situations and with relatively specifiable
and less complex aspects of human behavior. Currently cognitive psychology is the dominant theoretic force in instructional psychology[23] and is developing a technology of instruction.

In the meantime it would be useful to have an
overview of the differences and common elements
of instructional forms that have grown up in practice. After contemplating learning in terms of its
broad classes: direct experience through reinforcement, observation of a model, and symbolic systems, including natural language, it is necessary to
examine the instructional side of the situation. Reinforcement has the limitation of being ambiguous
because it does not indicate the critical alternatives
the learner faces in making a decision. It presents
only the consequences of the former performances.
Teachers can make the situation less ambiguous by
immediately reinforcing the learner's positive behavior or by making clear the feature of the stimulus that is to be attended. Language is an instructional device par excellence. A word indicates not
only a perceived referent but also the excluded set
of alternatives. The major limitation of language
in instruction is not only that it demands literacy
but that instruction in it is limited to rearranging,
ordering, and differentiating knowledge or information that the learner already has available from
other sources, such as modeling or personal experience. Modeling is graphic but does not always
reveal reasons for action.

According to one point of view, all of these
instructional forms that seem to have widely different topographies can lead some learners to the
same end performance and, to some extent, convey
the same information. All of them increase the
amount of information conveyed (information den-

TABLE 6-1. Summary of instructional methods

Instructor-centered	Interactive	Individualized
Lecture	**Class discussion**	**Programmed instruction**
Students are passive Efficient for lower learning levels and large classes	Class size must be small May be time-consuming Encourages student involvement	Most effective at lower learning levels Very structured Students work at own pace Students receive extensive feedback
Questioning	**Discussion groups**	**Modularized instruction**
Monitors student learning Encourages student involvement May cause anxiety for some	Class size should be small Students participate Effective for high cognitive and affective learning levels	Can be time-consuming Very flexible formats Students work at own pace
Demonstration	**Peer teaching**	**Independent projects**
Illustrates an application of a skill or concept Students are passive	Requires careful planning and monitoring Utilizes differences in student expertise Encourages student involvement	Most appropriate at higher learning levels Can be time-consuming Students are actively involved in learning
	Group projects	**Computerized instruction**
	Requires careful planning, including evaluation techniques Useful at higher learning levels Encourages active student participation	May involve considerable instructor-time or expense Can be very flexible Students work at own pace Students may be involved in varying activities

Experiential learning methods

Field or clinical	Laboratory	Role playing	Stimulations and games	Drill
Occurs in natural setting during performance Students are actively involved Management and evaluation may be difficult	Requires careful planning and evaluation Students actively involved in a realistic setting	Effective in affective and psychomotor domains Provides "safe" experiences Active student participation	Provide practice of specific skills Produces anxiety for some students Active student participation	Most appropriate at lower learning levels Provides active practice May not be motivating for some students

From Weston C, Cranton PA: *J Higher Educ* 57(3):259-288, 1986.

TABLE 6-2. Matching domain and level of learning to appropriate methods

Domain and level	Method
Cognitive domain	
Knowledge	Lecture, programmed instruction, drill and practice
Comprehension	Lecture, modularized instruction, programmed instruction
Application	Discussion, simulations and games, computer-assisted instruction, modularized instruction, field experience, laboratory
Analysis	Discussion, independent/group projects, simulations, field experience, role-playing, laboratory
Synthesis	Independent/group projects, field experience, role-playing, laboratory
Evaluation	Independent/group projects, field experience, laboratory
Affective domain	
Receiving	Lecture, discussion, modularized instruction, field experience
Responding	Discussion, simulations, modularized instruction, role-playing, field experience
Valuing	Discussion, independent/group projects, simulations, role-playing, field experience
Organization	Discussion, independent/group projects, field experience
Characterization by a value	Independent projects, field experience
Psychomotor domain	
Perception	Demonstration (lecture), drill and practice
Set	Demonstration (lecture), drill and practice
Guided response	Peer teaching, games, role-playing, field experience, drill and practice
Mechanism	Games, role-playing, field experience, drill and practice
Complex overt response	Games, field experience
Adaptation	Independent projects, games, field experience
Origination	Independent projects, games, field experience

From Weston C, Cranton PA: *J Higher Educ* 57(3):259-288, 1986.

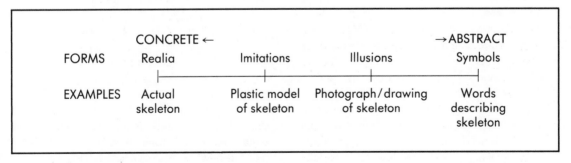

FIGURE 6-1. Form of instructional materials: the abstract-concrete continuum. (From Weston C, Cranton PA: *J Higher Educ* 57:259-288, 1986.)

sity), from reinforcement, to modeling, to language.[47] Obviously, research is not complete. Although this chapter will point out reasons for choosing one approach or form rather than another, it is important to remember that various instructional forms overlap in their degrees of effectiveness.

Instructional materials have three basic components: (1) a delivery system, which is the physical form of the materials and hardware used to present stimuli to the learner, such as handouts, slides, computer-assisted instruction, or a person; (2) a content or message; and (3) a form or condition of abstractness. Figure 6-1 shows an example of the abstract-concrete continuum.[56]

Methods are also instructor centered, interactive, individualized, or experiential (Table 6-1) and can be matched with domains and levels of learning (Table 6-2).[56]

A 1983 survey of health promotion programs in Michigan hospitals reported on the percentage of educational programs using each of the following instructional techniques: written materials, 87%; audio-visual materials, 78%; discussion groups, 67%; demonstrations, 64%; one-to-one discussion-counseling, 57%; and role playing–modeling, 27%.[48]

CHOOSING THE CONTENT TO TEACH

Teachers make decisions about the content of lessons by determining what a patient needs to know from the established body of knowledge. It is rare to have research verifying content. Most research deals with the process of teaching. Either it avoids consideration of content or standardizes it. Several studies of persons undergoing threatening procedures (gastroendoscopy, removal of children's orthopedic casts) have found that people who are told about typical physical sensations showed less distress than did those told only about the procedure or those not given any preparatory information. The messages are directed toward the patient's five senses. Using information gathered from former patients, those undergoing treatment are told what they will feel, see, hear, taste, or smell during the procedure. However, they are not advised about the level of intensity because that varies among individuals. Note that the sensation content describes the event from the patient's point of view, whereas the less effective description about how and where a procedure will be done represents the provider's point of view.[33]

TEACHER-LEARNER RELATIONSHIP

Studies of provider-patient relationships have frequently raised questions about quality of interactions. In one such study physicians spent little time informing their patients, overestimated the time they had spent, and underestimated patients' desires for information.[55] In addition, quality of interpersonal skills has been found to influence patient outcomes. Most studies show a significant, positive relationship between interpersonal skills and patient satisfaction with the visit, a modest but fairly consistent relationship between patient satisfaction and adherence,[4] and potential for significantly reduced malpractice litigation.[46] Other studies have found physicians inaccurate in predicting patient satisfaction.[42] Many patients prefer highly affective as well as highly informative interaction styles.[46] Patients want providers to reassure them, support them, and acknowledge their feelings. Patients would also like an opportunity to respond to information the provider has given them.[41] Interventions providing patients with information and skills that enable them to ask questions of and negotiate with their providers have been greatly effective.[26,52]

Teacher-learner relationships require commitment. The individual or group of learners must receive teaching until the goals are reached, until instruction is no longer profitable, or until the learner withdraws. This does not mean that clinicians take on the responsibility for solving the problems. However, clinicians set goals in learning to address particular problems. Clients need to understand how the teacher-learner relationship can assist them, how long it will last, and when they can have uninterrupted sessions with the practitioner.

This commitment is made as part of a profes-

is limited but critical in teaching the client how to alter maladaptive cognitive processes and environmental contingencies.

Several points can be made about these models.

1. Problems between helpers and recipients can arise when each is operating on a different model. Indeed, the wrong models may be in place in a number of areas.
2. Some data support the hypothesis that models in which people are held responsible for solutions are more likely to increase their competence.
3. Some authors (Brickman and others) indicate a preference for the compensatory model, noting that it is the only one that justifies the act of helping (since the recipient is not responsible for problems) but still leaves patients with a sense of control over their lives (since they need the help to find a solution).
4. Many questions remain. Are some helping models better than others or only acceptable for some patients? Has there been historic evolution of dominant models applied to different populations? For example, the compensatory model in childbearing situations is now emerging over the previously predominant medical model.

The compensatory model is probably most congruent with the teaching approach advocated here—one with mutual participation by client and practitioner.

ORAL TEACHING

Since teaching is communicating, which is accomplished in large part by language, the teacher must be skilled in the use of language. Clinicians need special knowledge of language because of two conditions inherent in health teaching: medical terminology is foreign to much of the public, and individuals with considerable health needs often have poorly developed language skills that result in low levels of understanding. The next chapter focuses in detail on the kinds of words and sentences that are difficult for many patients to understand.

The use of written information would no doubt improve patients' retention of information. The use of another device, called "advanced organizers," produced significant increases in recall. In this study the advanced organizers were category names to organize the material. The material used in the experiment consisted of the following statements:

1. You have a chest infection.
2. And your larynx is slightly inflamed.
3. But I think your heart is all right.
4. We will do some heart tests to make sure.
5. We will need to take a blood sample.
6. And you will have to have your chest x-rayed.
7. Your cough will disappear in the next two days.
8. You will feel better in a week or so.
9. And you will recover completely.
10. We will give you an injection of penicillin.
11. And some tablets to take.
12. I'll give you an inhaler to use.
13. You must avoid cold draughts.
14. You must stay indoors in fog.
15. And you must take two hours' rest each afternoon.*

The advanced organizers were used as follows:
I am going to tell you:

what is wrong with you;

what tests we are going to carry out;

what I think will happen to you;

what treatment you will need; and

what you must do to help yourself.

First, what is wrong with you . . . (statements 1-3)

Secondly, what tests we are going to carry out . . . (statements 4-6)

Thirdly, what I think will happen to you . . . (statements 7-9)

Fourthly, what the treatments will be . . . (statements 10-12)

Finally, what you must do to help yourself . . . (statements 13-15)*

---

*From Ley P and others: A method of increasing patients' recall of information presented by doctors, *Psychol Med* 3:217-220, 1973.

Notice that the category names are not medical terms; rather, they are categories meaningful to patients.

One physician used a taped final interview with his patients as a means of improving understanding and retention. On the average, patients listened to the tapes 3.5 times. Most patients had spouses or relatives who also listened. Nearly all the patients felt that they were helped by this tool.[9]

Analogies are frequently used in teaching, presumably to give meaning to health ideas by relating them to information that is commonly known. For example, a film on diabetes explains the body's use of food as similar to the use of fuel by a car engine. The normal mechanism of blood glucose triggering release of insulin can be compared with a thermostat regulating a furnace to maintain an even temperature. The tissue of a colostomy stoma may be described as the same type as that inside the mouth, since the mouth is the beginning of the alimentary canal. It has been suggested that this explanation will help to remove the mystery and fear of what the stoma looks like before the patient has seen it.[31] A cardiac monitor may be explained to patient and family as being "like having a cardiogram all the time," since the patient is likely to have had that experience.

Analogies seem to be useful in bridging the gap to new experiences; however, they can be interpreted incorrectly and lead to incorrect action. Besides independently thinking through the strengths and weaknesses of a particular analogy, providers should try it out on patients and ask what they think it means. Sometimes caregivers' thought patterns are so different from their patients' that it is difficult to predict patient interpretations.

Because of their backgrounds, health professionals may tend to overuse verbal instruction. They often value independence and symbolic learning. They may therefore choose a verbal means of instruction to motivate a person, when joining the patient in the health action would be more effective. Expressing the idea in words can serve to maintain a professional distance from patients and at the same time create a student-teacher role hierarchy and a status gap between helper and patient. It may, however, fail as a teaching technique if used exclusively.

In earlier chapters the patient–health professional relationship (especially involving the physician) is described as under attack for some of its basic assumptions. One such critique explains that withholding information from the patient is a means of maintaining patterns of dominance and subordination in the society, with physicians serving as the agents of the larger society. Patient education can extend this dominance-submission relationship or it can encourage patients not to accept without question the orders and advice of professionals acting as social control agents.

Other critiques that do not interpret the relationship difficulties as part of a broader social strategy have simply pointed out the distortion of patient intent by health professionals in their use of language. Analysis by Cousins of several patients who were labeled as denying their health problems found that these patients were really acting rationally in exploring other options and opinions regarding their problems.[13] The term "denial" seemed to be applied from the narrow perspective of a physician who believed the patient was not strictly complying with medical advice. The focus was not on the patient's effort to cope with the health problem by using numerous resources.

It is not unusual to find patient satisfaction strongly related to ratings of physician courtesy, information giving, and listening.[12] For example, one study found that patient noncompliance with medications was significantly related to the patient's dissatisfaction with physician communication. A subgroup of the population studied (patients with functional headaches—a disorder) had clear and elaborate definitions of their symptoms and were dissatisfied with physician communication. Another dissatisfied group were those who remained worried about the possibility of serious illness and had not been reassured by the physician. What appeared to be most important was the patient's expectation of what the contact with the physician would yield.[21]

The following relevant question arises: Do professionals have the skills necessary for patient instruction? One study of house officers found their skills in facilitating patients' understanding of their illnesses and of providing explanations of the illnesses were underdeveloped and a source of discomfort for the doctors.[18]

The idea of a contract between patient and professional, introduced in Chapter 4, serves as a way of clarifying expectations for the interaction it motivates and structures. Those persons who cannot commit themselves to action because of denial, confusion, or grief, or who cannot make decisions about their treatment because of medical emergencies, are not able to contract. Characteristics and examples of good patient contracts may be seen in Table 6-3.[30] Note that these characteristics reflect the instructional principles of clear feedback, pos-

TABLE 6-3. Good patient contracts: characteristics and examples

Characteristics of a good patient contract	Questions health professionals can ask to help patient set an achievable goal	Sample contract: Mr. Dixon, 47, is an obese businessman, who had a heart attack 4 months ago. His goals:	Sample contract: Ms. Waverly, 56, is a plump woman with angina pectoris, who finds she snacks constantly. Her goals:
Realistic	Does goal seem possible? Have you ever had regular exercise? Sound reasonable at this time?	Walk the dog.	Lose weight.
Measurable	How often can you do this? What will show you have done this?	Walk the dog *around the lake for 30 minutes*.	*Lose 5 pounds*
Positive	What goals are you working *toward*? What are you going to do for yourself? What strengths can you build on?	*I will* do the following exercise . . .	*I will* lose weight by a. Eating three meals b. Sitting down to eat c. An evening snack of an apple or other fruit
Time-dated	When can you start this? What will you do in the next 2 weeks?	Walk the dog each night *before supper for the next 2 weeks*.	Lose 5 pounds by *the end of the month, which is my birthday*.
Written	Could I write down your ideas? Would you write down these goals we are discussing?	Will walk dog 30 minutes around a lake before supper—2 weeks.	I'll lose 5 pounds by my birthday. 1. Eat three meals a day 2. Sit down 3. Fruit snack at bedtime
Rewardable	If you make this effort, what reward could you give yourself?	New walking shoes if I accomplish my goal.	A long-distance telephone call to my sister.
Evaluated	How can I help you evaluate your goals? Can you share your goals with anyone?	I'll come back in to see you to report progress in 2 weeks.	I'll ask my sister to work on these goals with me. I will send you a postcard the first of next month with my results.

From Herje PA: *Nurse Educ* 5:30-34, 1980.

itive expectations and rewards, and commitment within the professional-patient relationship.

Of course, many opportunities exist for the improvement of the professional-patient relationship. Teaching is not only a direct source of benefit to patients from skills and information learned but could be an important vehicle for improved relationships between professionals and patients.

DEMONSTRATION AND PRACTICE

Demonstration involves an acting out for learners—showing them. It includes showing an intellectual skill or an attitude as well as showing the correct performance of a motor skill. It may also involve setting up conditions for patients to demonstrate to themselves that they can accomplish something. For example, working on a treadmill can persuade a cardiac patient that he or she can exercise. The interpersonal techniques discussed in the previous section are prime ways to demonstrate ideas, solve problems, or develop positive attitudes. The learner has to practice to learn these techniques. Learners can practice by working through exercises and by functioning in mock or real situations that require use of the skill or attitude.

Demonstration is a performance of procedures or psychomotor skills, which, combined with practice, is the method most suited to attaining skills. Skills are not learned separately from attitudes and factual knowledge; demonstration and practice sessions are usually combined with giving information and with discussion sessions in order to clarify the patients' concepts and feelings.

The purpose of the demonstration is to give the learner a clear mental image of how the skill is performed. Therefore assurance that the demonstration is adequately seen is of prime importance. If the motions are limited, as they are in giving an injection, probably no more than a few people can see clearly enough. Presentations of a prime view by television or motion picture may be necessary if the groups are large. In some instances an over-the-shoulder view of the demonstrator provides the learner with a clear idea of the way he or she must perform the action. When the demonstrator is removing fluids from a vial and giving an injection, the mirror image that the viewer receives by *facing* the demonstrator is not entirely realistic.

The mental image must be accurate; therefore the demonstration has to be practiced and critically examined before it is presented. The learner, who is not knowledgeable about the skill, will have difficulty distinguishing irrelevant and incorrect actions from those that are relevant and correct. A demonstration that shows a baby being bathed in a tub without the nurse's testing the temperature in any way provides an incorrect model, even though the temperature may have been checked before the demonstration began. Another irrelevant action might be taking the baby's temperature before the bath, which, without an explanation, would imply that this always should be done. The teacher must expect that learners will mimic the demonstration down to the tiniest detail; therefore the demonstration must be so accurate that the learner will be able to perform without error.

Equipment must be tested before the demonstration. It is disruptive to be demonstrating the transfer of a patient from wheelchair to bed and discover that a lock on the wheelchair is broken. This is not to say that a lesson can or should be absolutely error free. An occasional mistake can be useful to show how the teacher goes about correcting it. This may occur when the nurse is ready to dry the baby and finds that the towel was left on the other side of the room. Continual errors, however, can be confusing to the learner.

It is important to *show* the entire procedure that the learner will be expected to perform. I remember a film demonstrating a baby bath, in which the way to cleanse the baby's genitals was talked about but never shown. In addition, the verbal instructions dealt only with the cleansing of female genitals. Imagine a new young mother who has been told that "it is very important to wash in these folds." This teaching gives neither information about why "it is very important" nor an adequate notion of how to go about the task.

Learners need practice to develop motor skills; therefore the teaching plan must incorporate a time for patients to practice. When equipment is sufficient and the group is small enough, practice may begin with the learner's redemonstrating the skill immediately after the teacher finishes. Additional practice should take place in a setting similar to that in which the skill will be performed. The teacher must supervise enough to provide feedback for a correct performance and to stimulate motivation if necessary.

To compensate for failing senses, such as failing vision in patients with diabetes, patients often have to learn how to use special aids for doing tasks. Not only are the materials (tools) different, but also the mode of demonstration has to be altered to compensate for the failing sense. It is reported that persons with diabetes often have difficulty in correctly assessing their visual loss and may in addition have neuropathy, which can affect the equipment that should be chosen. When the patient has slight visual impairment, the use of brighter lighting, a white background, and glass rather than plastic syringes can help. The patient can use a longer syringe with bolder markings and wider spaces between calibrations or a magnifying device. Other aids for needle insertion into the bottle are available. The patient can detect when the insulin bottle is empty by taking a marble out of a dish with each dose or by injecting air into the vial and listening for the bubbles. Inserting the needle from the skin surface gives better control. Also available is a scale with braille markings. A number of other tools and procedures are described in books on rehabilitation to use with persons who have visual and other handicaps.

SUMMARY

In general, this chapter focuses on broad categories of instructional forms and, in particular, on interpersonal interaction between learners, the teacher, and other learners. The chapter also broadly outlines direct experience in educational and real world settings, as well as discusses the use of language.

Chapter 7 focuses on the teaching tools to use independently or within a teacher-learner relationship. Chapter 8 discusses instructional alignment—a powerful idea outlined in previous chapters that appraises the extent to which instructional assessment and processes match the intended outcomes.[11] Most instruction suffers in the quality of instructional alignment; however, a fine tuning will likely yield vastly superior learning outcomes.[11]

STUDY QUESTIONS

1. "Teaching the Patient About Open Heart Surgery" is the title of an article in the October 1965 issue of the *American Journal of Nursing*. In explaining to the patient, the nurse uses phrases (quoted in part) such as ". . . you have a defective aortic valve"; "the narrowing is due to calcium deposits . . . left behind by infections such as rheumatic fever"; ". . . lack of atmospheric pressure creates a negative pressure, or a pulling force that keeps the lungs always expanded"; "the chest tubes are connected to a closed system called an underwater seal system"; and others. The nurse compares the two pleura to Saran Wrap in explaining that the outside of the lung and the lining of the chest wall slide over each other with perfect ease.[54]
   a. What level of education would a patient probably need to have to understand explanations in this terminology?
   b. Why is the analogy between pleura and Saran Wrap likely to be confusing? Is the comparison of a leaky heart valve to a warped door less confusing?
2. You are teaching a group of parents of mentally retarded individuals about their children's sexuality. It is clear that they need information and that they also need to face and make decisions in the sexual realm of their children's behavior. What general group teaching approaches would you use?
3. When patients were asked if they had been catheterized, most did not know what it meant. How would you alter the question?
4. One study[6] has shown that patients are more satisfied with their physicians when they are given and retain more information about their illnesses. When an experimental group of patients was asked to restate what they had been told, followed by physician feedback, retention of the information was 83.5% compared with 60.8% in a control group in which this teaching was not used. Patient satisfaction also was higher in the experimental group. List three principles used in this experimental treatment.
5. For burn rehabilitation, the patient's and the family's competence in carrying out exercise programs, proper skin care, and the prescribed wearing of pressure splints is essential for the control of scarring and contractures. A survey of occupational therapy departments in hospitals with burn

units found reports of the use of the following types of educational materials: verbal instructions, 97%; handwritten instructions, 64%; pamphlets or booklets, 49%; typed instructions, 49%; pictures of scarring, 45%; slides, 15%; and movies, 4%. Content to be taught includes proper wearing of splints, active exercise program, contact person for emergencies, positioning techniques, mechanism of scarring, wearing of pressure garments, passive exercise program, emotional aspects of skin care, and wearing of support stockings.[34] Is this a good match between content and teaching materials?

6. Read Glendon M: Teaching Harry what we'd thought he knew, *Nursing 85* 15(7):44-45, 1985,[24] and identify the patient problems and the kind of teaching interventions used.

7. In training asthmatic children to use their nebulizers correctly, the following steps were carried out in this order: (1) learners were given the rationale behind each nebulizer technique, (2) the trainer modeled the technique and then the subject tried to perform the behavior correctly, (3) the trainer provided feedback and reinforcement. When learners had difficulty with a particular behavior, the trainer broke the overall technique down into small sequenced steps.[38] Does this represent optimum use of learning principles? How could the procedure be improved to stimulate and support learning?

REFERENCES

1. Abarbanel J, Zinner E, McDowell RL Jr: Parent-infant support groups in a pediatric practice, *Clin Pediatr* 25:345-348, 1986.
2. Arnold JR, Winsor EJT: The use of structured scenarios in genetic counseling, *Clin Genet* 25:485-490, 1984.
3. Auerbach AB: *Parents learn through discussion*, New York, 1980, John Wiley.
4. Bartlett EE and others: The effects of physician communication skills on patient satisfaction, recall, and adherence, *J Chron Dis* 37:755-764, 1984.
5. Beckie T: A supportive-educative telephone program: impact on knowledge and anxiety after coronary artery bypass graft surgery, *Heart Lung* 18:46-55, 1989.
6. Bertakis KD: The communication of information from physician to patient: a method for increasing patient retention and satisfaction, *J Fam Pract* 5:217-222, 1977.
7. Brickman P and others: Models of helping and coping, *Am Psychol* 37:368-384, 1982.
8. Brown DG, Glazer H, Higgins M: Group intervention: a psychosocial and educational approach to open heart surgery patients and their families, *Soc Work Health Care* 9:47-59, 1983.
9. Butt HR: A method for better physician-patient communication, *Ann Intern Med* 86:478-480, 1977.
10. Christianson C: Support groups for infertile patients, *JOGNN* 15:293-296, 1986.
11. Cohen SA: Instructional alignment: searching for a magic bullet, *Educ Researcher* 16(11):16-20, 1987.
12. Comstock LM and others: Physician behaviors that correlate with patient satisfaction, *J Med Educ* 57:105-112, 1982.
13. Cousins N: Denial, *JAMA* 248:210-212, 1982.
14. Crowe L, Billingsley JI: The rowdy reactors: maintaining a support group for teenagers with diabetes, *Diab Educator* 16:39-43, 1990.
15. Cwikel JM, Israel BA: Examining mechanisms of social support and social networks: a review of health-related intervention studies, *Pub Health Rev* 15:159-193, 1987.
16. DeBasio N, Rodenhausen N: The group experience: meeting the psychological needs of patients with ventricular tachycardia, *Heart Lung* 13:597-602, 1984.
17. Duer JD: Group dissemination of breast self-examination training technology, *Patient Educ Couns* 6:160-164, 1984.
18. Duffy DL, Hamerman D, Cohen MA: Communication skills of house officers, *Ann Intern Med* 93:354-357, 1980.
19. Feldman M: Cluster visits, *Am J Nurs* 74:1485-1488, 1974.
20. Field T and others: Effects of ultrasound feedback on pregnancy anxiety, fetal activity, and neonatal outcome, *Obstet Gynecol* 66:525-528, 1985.
21. Fitzpatrick RM, Hopkins A: Patients' satisfaction with communication in neurological outpatient clinics, *J Psychosom Res* 25:329-334, 1981.
22. Follick MJ and others: Quality of life post-myocardial infarction: effects of a transtelephonic coronary intervention system, *Health Psychol* 7:169-182, 1988.
23. Glaser R: Instructional psychology: past, present, and future, *Am Psychol* 37:292-305, 1982.
24. Glendon M: Teaching Harry what we'd thought he knew, *Nursing* 15(7):44-46, 1985.
25. Greene VL, Monahan DJ: The effect of a professionally guided caregiver support and education group on institutionalization of care receivers, *Gerontologist* 27:716-721, 1987.
26. Greenfield S, Kaplan S, Ware JE Jr: Expanding patient involvement in care, *Ann Intern Med* 102:520-528, 1985.
27. Hahn K: Therapeutic storytelling: helping children learn and cope, *Pediatr Nurs* 13:175-178, 1987.
28. Heffron WA and others: Group discussions with the parents of leukemic children, *Pediatrics* 52:831-840, 1973.
29. Heins HC Jr, Nance W, Ferguson JE: Social support in improving perinatal outcome: the resource mothers program, *Obstet Gynecol* 70:263-266, 1987.
30. Herje PA: Hows and whys of patient contracting, *Nurs Educ* 5:30-34, 1980.
31. Hollingsworth CE, Sokol B: Predischarge family conference, *JAMA* 239:740-741, 1978.
32. Jacobs MK, Goodman G: Psychology and self-help groups, *Am Psychol* 44:536-545, 1989.
33. Johnson JE and others: Easing children's fright during health care procedures, *Matern Child Nurs J* 1:206-210, 1976.
34. Kaplan SH: Patient education techniques used at burn centers, *Am J Occup Ther* 39:655-658, 1985.

35. Kulik JA, Mahler HIM: Effects of preoperative roommate assignment on preoperative anxiety and recovery from coronary bypass surgery, *Health Psychol* 6:525-543, 1987.

36. Ley P and others: A method of increasing patients' recall of information presented by doctors, *Psychol Med* 3:217-220, 1973.

37. Main K: The power-load-margin formula of Howard Y. McClusky as the basis for a model of teaching, *Adult Educ* 30:19-33, 1979.

38. Marion RJ, Creer TL, Burns K: Training asthmatic children to use their nebulizer correctly, *J Asthma* 20:183-188, 1983.

39. Maryniuk MD, Kauwell GPA, Thomas RG: A test of instructional approaches designed to influence food selection, *Diabetes Educ* 12:34-36, 1986.

40. Mazzuca SA and others: The diabetes education study: a controlled trial of the effects of diabetes patient education, *Diabetes Care* 9:1-10, 1986.

41. Mendez A, Shymansky JA: Verbal behaviors and patterns exhibited by physicians during genetic counseling sessions, *Patient Educ Coun* 6:165-168, 1984.

42. Merkel WT: Physician perception of patient satisfaction, *Med Care* 22:453-459, 1984.

43. Moore DT: Discovering the pedagogy of experience, *Harvard Educ Rev* 51:286-300, 1981.

44. Moss N: Hospital units as social contexts: effects of maternal behavior, *Soc Sci Med* 19:515-522, 1984.

45. Neale DC: Specifications for small group activities in instructional design, *Instruc Sci* 13:15-35, 1984.

46. O'Hair HD, Behnke RR, Kind PE: Age-related patient preferences for physician communication styles, *Educ Gerontol* 9:147-158, 1983.

47. Olson DR: On a theory of instruction: why different forms of instruction result in similar knowledge, *Interchange* 3:9-24, 1972.

48. Pack BE and others: A review of hospital-based health promotion programs in Michigan nongovernmental hospitals, *Patient Educ Couns* 7:345-358, 1985.

49. Peplau HE: Professional closeness, *Nurs Forum* 8:342-360, 1969.

50. Ramsey AM, Siroky AS: The use of puppets to teach school-age children with asthma, *Pediatr Nurs* 14:187-190, 1988.

51. Reiff MI, Essock-Vitale SM: Hospital influences on early infant-feeding practices, *Pediatrics* 76:872-879, 1985.

52. Roter DL: Patient question asking in physician-patient interaction, *Health Psychol* 3:395-409, 1985.

53. Tarver J, Turner AJ: Teaching behavior modification to patients' families, *Am J Nurs* 74:282-283, 1974.

54. Vavaro FF: Teaching the patient about open heart surgery, *Am J Nurs* 65:111-115, 1965.

55. Waitzkin H: Information giving in medical care, *J Health Soc Behav* 26:81-101, 1985.

56. Weston C, Cranton PA: Selecting instructional strategies, *J Higher Educ* 57:259-288, 1986.

57. Winslow EH, Macvaugh H, III: Coronary artery surgery, *Nurs Clin North Am* 11:371-383, 1976.

CHAPTER 7

Teaching tools: printed and nonprinted materials

Chapter 7 presents technical material about print and audiovisual teaching tools. The information in this chapter shows how to choose, how to develop, and how to decide when to use such tools. Some tools may be self-instructional; however, all are used within the process of teaching, as outlined in this book.

PRINTED AND COMPUTER MATERIALS

When written materials are used as teaching tools, vocabulary and sentence length aren't the only elements that must be considered. Factors such as format, headings, illustrations, line width, type size, and style of writing affect readability but are not incorporated into the readability formulas. The reasoning process the reader must use to understand the material must also be taken into consideration. A difference of opinion may exist about the validity of the information. Therefore the teacher must decide whether the material expresses a point of view he or she wishes to teach. Finally, to be useful the written material must play a part in meeting one of the learning objectives. The provider must decide if the material meets a specific objective before the material is given to the learner to read.

Printed teaching material can be described as a frozen language that is selective in its description of reality (which is both a strength and a weakness). It encourages limited feedback but is constantly available. Print partially relaxes time requirements and is more efficient than oral language (except for those who have not learned to read efficiently) because readers can control the speed at which they

read and comprehend. Certain kinds of thinking seem to demand written expression, and writing requires a sequential presentation. For example, a complex sequence of thoughts that incorporates definitions, qualifications, and logical constraints is expressed best in writing. It can be formulated with care and often without a strict time limit. Most people who have learned to read well generally prefer to acquire information by reading. Reading is ideal for understanding complex concepts and relationships. If the learning objective primarily requires skill in dealing with persons or things, then demonstrations, concrete experience with the activity, and oral coaching and guidance would be more effective than print media.[9]

The various media that can be used for learning possess cognitively relevant characteristics in their technologies, symbol systems, and processing capabilities. Computers are distinguished by their extensive processing capabilities rather than by their access to a particularly unique set of symbol systems (they use words and pictures). In television the symbols can depict action; however, the symbols are transient.[26]

Although some students can learn a particular task regardless of the medium, others need the advantage of a particular medium's characteristics. For example, experts who learn from text, skim rapidly, using trigger words to read selectively and nonsequentially. When memory limits are reached, they stop and summarize the material they have learned. Such processing strategies cannot be used with audiotapes or lectures. Novices take advantage of the text's stability to slow the rate of information processing; as a result they are able to review the material. Pictures that illustrate information central to the text help the reader. If the material is too difficult for the reader; however, he or she must expend a great deal of effort trying to decode the text and possibly increasing the risk of learning failure.[26] This chapter focuses on how to construct tools so that they are most useful to various learners.

Predicting reading comprehension

Although learning by reading is economical in use of teacher time, some people cannot read well enough to use any print material. For many others the materials available are written at a higher level than they can comprehend. Interestingly, this kind of information has been available for years; yet materials still are written at levels that are mismatched (almost always higher) with the skills of the people who use them.

For example, Glanz and Rudd found that the readability levels of 38 print cholesterol education materials averaged grade 11.[20] Content analysis of these materials also suggested a need to better address other heart disease risk factors, portion size, and use of brand name food recommendations. Analysis of 74 English language, patient-education pamphlets developed by the American College of Obstetricians and Gynecologists found that 61 of these pamphlets were written at reading levels of 11th grade or higher. The mean literacy level in the United States is at or below the eighth grade level. A number of sexually active populations, who could benefit from instruction in conception and antepartal care, read at even lower levels.[55]

Other examples include Mathews, Thornton, and McLean's study that analyzed patient education materials for persons with chronic obstructive pulmonary disease and found that the readability level averaged grade 11.8.[30] When technical vocabulary, such as "acute," "aerosol," "allergen," "alveoli," "arrhythmias," "asthma," "bronchial," and "capillaries," was removed, the reading level was reduced to grade 9.9. Printed instructions that come with health care products are also important

to monitor. One study found that eight of fourteen printed instructions for condom use required a high school graduate reading level and none required less than a tenth grade reading level.[40] Table 7-1 presents reading levels of materials from various fields, as measured by SMOG, FOG, and Fry readability formulas.[46]

The presumption that individuals read at the level of their completed formal education is frequently not correct. A recent study found that actual reading levels measured by the Wide Range Achievement test were an average of three grade levels lower than were the reported reading levels indicated by the grade completed.[46]

To match the learner to the material, teachers must know something about the factors that determine readability and must be able to measure it. When the reading level of material is beyond the skill of the learner, comprehension is decreased, recall is sketchy and inaccurate, and motivation for further instruction from printed sources is reduced.

Examples of materials written at high levels and revised to read at much lower levels can be found on pp. 144, 145, and 146.[12,13,16]

Readability can be predicted in three ways: (1) by the Cloze method in which every fifth word in a reading passage is removed, and the reader is asked to fill in the words based on the meaning of other words in the passage; (2) by the predictability of certain words in reading passages; and (3) by formulas based on the length of words and sentences. The formulas themselves are often validated against reading tests. The patient's comprehension can be measured directly with a comprehension test covering the material in the passage.

Various readability formulas may be useful for different kinds of text. For example, the Fry Readability Formula, shown on p. 147, and the graph in Figure 7-1 determines the level of materials from grades 1 through college; however, these are not useful with passages of fewer than 300 words. The FOG Formula, found on p. 148, uses number of sentences and number of polysyllabic words and is useful for grade 4 through college. The Flesch Formula, found in the box on p. 149, uses average

TABLE 7-1. Reading levels of patient education materials

Title of publication	Source	SMOG	FOG	Fry	Avg.
Diabetes					
1. Dining Out Made Simple	Becton-Dickinson (B-D)	10	10.2	8	9.4
2. Fast Food Guide	B-D	8	8.5	6	7.5
3. How to Take Insulin	B-D	8	7.9	4	6.6
4. How to Give a Combination of NPH U100 & Regular U100 Insulin	Yale–New Haven Hospital (YNHH)	9	9.6	11	9.9
5. How to Give Your Insulin	YNHH	8	7.0	8	7.7
6. If You Were in an Accident	Medic Alert	13	14.2	15	14.1
7. Mixing Insulins	B-D	11	13.6	11	11.9
8. Vacation, Travel, and Diabetes	B-D	10	12.3	11	11.5
9. You & Diabetes . . . & Dia-Beta (glyburide)	Hoechst-Roussel	12	14.5	14	13.5
"Diabetes" average-grade levels		9.9	10.9	9.8	10.2
Urinary tract					
15. Acute Cystitis in the Female	Parke-Davis	13	15.3	14	14.1
16. Intermittent Self Catheterization	YNHH	10.	10.7	7	9.2
17. Understanding Acute Urinary Tract Infections	Parke-Davis	13	16.6	12	13.9
"Urinary Tract" average grade levels		12.0	14.2	11.0	12.5
Exercise					
18. A Home Exercise Program	McNeil	9	9.4	7	8.5
19. Exercises for Low Back Pain	McNeil	9	8.8	7	8.3
20. Exercises for the Painful Neck and Shoulder	McNeil	10	9.4	7	8.8
"Exercise" average grade levels		9.3	9.2	7.0	8.5

Contraception

10.	A Guide to the Methods of Contraception	Ortho	15	16.9	14	15.3
11.	After Your Doctor Prescribes the Pill	Ortho	13	14.8	14	13.9
12.	Koro-flex Arching Spring Diaphragm . . .	Holland-Rantos	12	13.0	10	11.7
13.	Questions & Answers About Your Diaphragm/Diaphragm Instructions for the Partner	Ortho	11	12.2	8	10.4
14.	Today Vaginal Contraceptive Sponges	VLI	15	17.2	12	14.7
	"Contraception" average grade levels		13.2	14.8	11.6	13.2

Miscellaneous

21.	Are You Really Serious About Losing Weight	Pennwalt	13	15.2	13	13.7
22.	Cancer—What to Know—What to Do About It	National Cancer Institute	11	11.0	11	11.0
23.	Diverticular Disease	Searle	15	17.3	14	15.4
24.	Heart Attacks—Your Questions Answered	Merck, Sharp & Dohme	11	13.0	10	11.7
25.	Transderm-Nitro How to Use	CIBA	11	12.6	10	11.2
26.	Migraine Information for Patients	Organon	11	11.1	9	10.4
27.	Stress	Blue Cross/Blue Shield	11	13.5	10	11.5
28.	Strike Back at Stroke	American Heart Association	8	7.6	6	7.2
	"Misc." average grade levels		11.4	12.7	10.4	11.5
	AVERAGE READABILITY LEVELS		11.2	12.4	10.0	11.2

From Streiff LD: *Image* 18:48-52, 1986.

TWO EXAMPLES OF READING MATERIALS FOR PATIENTS: ORIGINAL AND REVISED VERSIONS

Example 1: Consent to Operation

Original (25th grade level)

I consent to the performance of operations and procedures in addition to or different from those now contemplated, whether or not arising from presently unforeseen conditions, which the above-named doctor or his associates or assistants may consider necessary or advisable in the course of the operation.

Revised (6th grade level)

I agree to other operations or treatments. My doctors may learn more in surgery. They may think I need other treatments. My doctors will decide in surgery. I agree to let them do the things they think are needed.

Example 2: Patient Education Material

Original (16th grade level)

Angina pectoris is a symptom and not actually a disease. The term refers to a pain in the chest, usually under the sternum (breastbone), which is brought on chiefly by exercise or emotional upsets in a person who has a heart problem. The pain is usually relieved by rest alone, but goes away more quickly with the use of a medicine which helps to bring more blood to the heart muscle.

Revised (7th grade level)

Angina is a feeling. It is not really a disease. The word means a pain in the chest. The pain is felt under the breastbone. A person who has heart trouble may feel this. Exercise or getting upset can cause the pain. The pain usually goes away with rest. It goes away faster if you take medicine. The medicine helps to bring more blood to the heart.

From Davis TC and others: *J Fam Pract* 31:533-538, 1990.

---

sentence length and word length and is useful for grades 5 through college. The SMOG Formula, found on pp. 150 and 151, counts the number of sentences and the number of words with three or more syllables and is useful for grades 5 through college. Meade and Smith have compared readability formulas done on the same health education materials and have found that the Flesch, FOG, and Fry formulas correlate highly with each other.[31]

Of the more than 30 formulas assessing readability,[17] Fry has developed a new one that can assess passages of 40 to 300 words.[18] Fry's formulas use a dictionary that gives grade levels for 43,000 words. Also, several software packages can calculate readability formulas. The user selects several random samples (representative of the text) of 100 words, types the text into the computer, and receives the calculated readability score.[32]

It is not difficult to see intuitively that the readability formulas show only partially the reasons why materials are easy or difficult to understand. Preliminary work is being done in extending the notion of readability to include the structure, texture, and information density of text.[3] Structure is the skeletal outline of the text. The three broad categories of prose structures are: narrative (tells a story), expository (communicates knowledge), and persuasive. Within these are three underlying structures: subordinating, coordinating, and sequential presentation of ideas. Texture is the amount of in-

Text continued on p. 154.

Sample A.

Sample A.

The sample below is a typical patient information handout, written at the reading level of a high school graduate or higher, that would be given to patients whose reading ability appears to be at that level. Sample B below is the same handout, rewritten at a fifth grade level of reading ability, and more appropriate for those patients with less developed reading skills.

STREP THROAT

The physician will treat your strep throat by first ordering a throat culture to make sure you have the streptococcus organism and, if you do, then prescribing medicine. You could receive either a penicillin injection or have to take oral antibiotic medicine for a prescribed length of time. It is essential that you take all the medicine your physician has ordered because if you don't, the infection could continue. When you have finished the oral antibiotic, you may have to come back and see the doctor and have another throat culture. Ask your doctor if you need to return and then call a week in advance for an appointment.

Here are some things you can do. It is important to rest and get sufficient sleep; naps are recommended. Try to drink plenty of water and juice. For example, drink at least five glasses of water and two glasses of juice every day; more if possible. If your throat is painful or you develop a fever, take one or two Tylenol not any more frequently than every four hours. A simple solution of salt water may help the soreness in your throat. Put ¼ teaspoon of salt in one cup of warm water and gargle gently with this as often as needed.

Do not return to work or school until your fever is gone and you have improved. In any case, you must wait at least 24 hours after you have had your shot to return to work or school and, if you are taking oral medication, you must wait at least 48 hours after beginning your pills to go back. This is so you will no longer be contagious when you return.

Follow these instructions and you should be feeling better soon. If you don't improve in a couple of days, however, call the office and ask to speak to the nurse.

Sample B.

The sample patient handout below contains the same information as Sample A above but is written at a fifth grade level of reading ability for those patients with weaker reading skills. Note the simpler vocabulary and sentence structure, the use of questions to focus reader attention on specific points, and the use of bold type to highlight important information.

SORE THROAT CAUSED BY STREPTOCOCCUS

HOW WILL THE DOCTOR TAKE CARE OF MY STREP THROAT?

1. The doctor will order medicine for me. I may have to get a shot (penicillin). I may have to take ___ pills (antibiotic) every day, for ___ days.
2. It is very important that I take all my pills. Even when my sore throat goes away, I must finish taking my pills. If I do not take all my pills, I could get sick again.
3. I may have to come back to see the doctor again. When all my pills are gone, I might need a test (throat culture). If so, I will come back on ___

HOW CAN I HELP MYSELF GET BETTER?

1. I need to sleep more. Naps are important to get more sleep.
2. I need to drink lots of water and juice. Try to drink 5 glasses of water and 2 glasses of juice a day.
3. TYLENOL medicine can be taken, if I feel hot or have a sore throat. Only take one or two pills of TYLENOL at one time. Do not take TYLENOL any more often than every four hours.
4. I can gargle with warm salt water to help my sore throat. Put a small amount of salt in a spoon and add to a cup of warm water. Gargle gently with the warm salt water as often as it helps.
5. I will not go back to work or school until ___. If I feel hot or sick, I will stay home and rest. If my sore throat does not go away in ___ days, I will call the nurse at ___ (telephone number).

WHEN I HAVE A BAD SORE THROAT, IF I SEE A DOCTOR AND TAKE ALL MY PILLS AND REST AND DRINK LOTS OF WATER, THEN I WILL SOON FEEL BETTER.

From Dixon E, Park R: *Nurs Outlook* 38:278-281, 1990.

SAMPLE MATERIAL

WRITTEN AT THE THIRTEENTH GRADE LEVEL

The heart usually receives electrical signals from the sinoatrial node, an area in the top right chamber. In ventricular tachycardia the signals that orchestrate the rhythm originate in the ventricle, located below the atrium. This area of origin results in an erratic beat or rhythm. The erratic beat disables the ventricles from contracting, thus blood is unable to be pumped out adequately. Inadequate blood supply affects all body parts since oxygen and nutrients are located in the blood. When the brain does not receive adequate blood supply, symptoms that include fainting, dizziness, and unconsciousness can occur. Stroke and death are also potential results.

With the knowledge that ventricular tachycardia is an erratic and potentially fatal rhythm that can occur at unpredictable times, physicians usually prescribe medications to control or prevent that rhythm. When medications are unable to keep the erratic beat dormant, the heart may require defibrillation. Defibrillation resets the electrical circuit, allowing the sinoatrial node to once again dominate.

REWRITTEN ON THE SIXTH GRADE LEVEL

Electrical signals from the heart's pacemaker keep the heart beating in a normal way. The pacemaker is called the S-A node and is found in the top part of the heart. Signals can also come from the bottom part of the heart. If they come from the bottom part, an irregular or rapid beat results. Several rapid and irregular beats are called V Tach. V Tach means the heart is not able to pump blood. When this happens, the body is not able to get the blood it needs. Blood carries oxygen and food to the body. One of the body parts that needs blood most is the brain. When the brain does not get blood, it can make a person feel faint or dizzy. It can also cause a stroke or death.

Doctors order medicines to try to control or stop this irregular or rapid beat. The medicines usually control this type of beat. Sometimes they do not work. The heart may then need to be shocked. The shock is given by a machine called a defibrillator. The shock usually helps the heart to reset its signals. It then beats in a regular way. All parts of the body can then get the supply of blood they need.

From Evanoski CAM: *J Cardiovasc Nurs* 4(2):1-6, 1990.

DIRECTIONS FOR USING THE READABILITY GRAPH

1. Select three one-hundred-word passages from near the beginning, middle and end of the book. Skip all proper nouns.
2. Count the total number of sentences in each hundred-word passage (estimating to nearest tenth of a sentence). Average these three numbers.
3. Count the total number of syllables in each hundred-word sample. There is a syllable for each vowel sound; for example: cat (1), blackbird (2), continental (4). Don't be fooled by word size; for example: polio (3), through (1). Endings such as -y, -ed, -el, or -le usually make a syllable, for example: ready (2), bottle (2). I find it convenient to count every syllable over one in each word and add 100. Average the total number of syllables for the three samples.
4. Plot on the graph the average number of sentences per hundred words and the average number of syllables per hundred words. Most plot points fall near the heavy curved line. Perpendicular lines mark off approximate grade level areas.

Example

	Sentences per 100 words	Syllables per 100 words
100-word sample page 5	9.1	122
100-word sample page 89	8.5	140
100-word sample page 160	7.0	129
	3)24.6	3)391
AVERAGE	8.2	130

Plotting these averages on the graph, we find they fall in the 5th grade area; hence the book is about 5th grade difficulty level. If great variability is encountered either in sentence length or in the syllable count for the three selections, then randomly select several more passages and average them in before plotting.

From Fry E: *J Reading* 11:514, 1968.

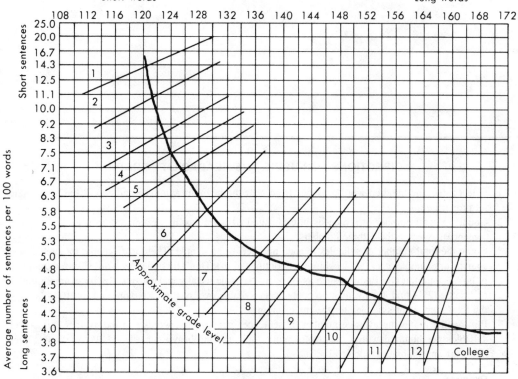

FIGURE 7-1. Graph for estimating readability. Directions: randomly select three 100-word passages from a book or an article. Plot average number of syllables and average number of words per sentence on graph to determine area of readability level. Choose more passages per book if great variability is observed. (From Fry E: *J Reading* 11:514, 577, 1968.)

THE GUNNING FOG INDEX

1. Select a sample of writing 100 to 125 words long. If the piece is long, take several samples and average the results.

2. Calculate the average number of words per sentence. Treat independent clauses as separate sentences. "In school we studied; we learned; we improved" counts as three sentences.

3. Count the number of words of three syllables or more. In your count, omit capitalized words; combinations of short words like *bookkeeper* or *manpower;* or verbs made into three syllables by adding "—*es*" or "—*ed*." Divide the count of long words by the passage length to get the percentage.

4. Add 2 (average sentence length) and 3 (percentage of long words). Multiply the sum by the factor 0.4, and ignore the digits following the decimal point.

    The result is the years of schooling needed to read the passage with ease. Few readers have over 17 years of schooling, so any passage over 17 gets a Fog Index of "17-plus."

From Gunning R: *The technique of clear writing,* rev ed, New York, 1968, McGraw-Hill.

FLESCH FORMULA

1. For short pieces, test the entire selection. For longer pieces, test at least three randomly selected samples of 100 words each. Do not use introductory paragraphs as part of the sample. Start each sample at the beginning of a paragraph.
2. Determine the average sentence length *(SL)* by counting the number of words in the sample and dividing by the number of sentences. Count as a sentence each independent unit of thought that is grammatically independent, that is, if its end is punctuated by a period, question mark, exclamation point, semicolon, or colon. In dialog, count speech tags (e.g., "he said") as part of the quoted sentence.
3. Determine the word length *(WL)* by counting all the syllables in the sample as if reading the words aloud. Divide the syllables by the number of words in the sample and multiply by 100.
4. These indices are then applied to the formula to compute the reading ease,

$$RE = 206.835 - 1.015\ SL - 0.846\ WL$$

where *RE* is the reading ease score, *SL* is the average sentence length in words, and *WL* is the average word length measured as syllables per 100 words.

INTERPRETATION OF THE FLESCH READING EASE SCORE

Reading ease	Grade	Description of style	No. syllables/ 100 words	Average sentence length
90-100	5	Very easy	123	8
80-90	6	Easy	131	11
70-80	7	Fairly easy	139	14
60-70	8-9	Standard	147	17
50-60	10-12	Fairly difficult	155	21
30-50	College	Difficult	167	25
0-30	College graduate	Very difficult	192	29

From Flesch R: *The art of readable writing*, New York, 1974, Harper & Row, pp 184-186, 247-251.

SMOG TESTING

The SMOG formula was originally developed by G. Harry McLaughlin in 1969. It will predict the grade-level difficulty of a passage within 1.5 grades in 68% of the passages tested. That may be close enough for your purposes. It is simple to use and faster than most other measures. The procedure is presented below.

Instructions

1. You will need 30 sentences. Count out 10 consecutive sentences near the beginning, 10 consecutive from the middle, and 10 from the end. For this purpose, a sentence is any string of words punctuated by a period (.), an exclamation point (!), or a question mark (?).
2. From the entire 30 sentences, count the words containing **three or more syllables,** including repetitions.
3. Obtain the grade level from the table below, or you may calculate the grade level as follows: Determine the nearest perfect square root of the total number of words of three or more syllables and then add a constant of 3 to the square root to obtain the grade level.

Example:

Total number of multisyllabic (3 or more syllables) words	67
Nearest perfect square	64
Square root	8
Add constant of 3	11 This is the grade level.

TABLE A. SMOG CONVERSION TABLE

Word count	Grade level
0–2	4
3–6	5
7–12	6
13–20	7
21–30	8
31–42	9
43–56	10
57–72	11
73–90	12
91–110	13
111–132	14
133–156	15
157–182	16
183–210	17
211–240	18

Developed by: Harold C. McGraw, Office of Educational Research, Baltimore County Public Schools, Towson, Maryland.

From McLaughlin GH: *J Reading* 12:639-646, 1969; Doak CC, Doak LG, Root JH: *Teaching patients with low literacy skills,* Philadelphia, 1985, JB Lippincott.

SPECIAL RULES FOR SMOG TESTING

Hyphenated words are **one** word.

For numerals, pronounce them aloud and count the syllables pronounced for each numeral (e.g., for the number 573, five = 1, hundred = 2, seventy = 3, and three = 1, or 7 syllables).

Proper nouns should be counted.

If a long sentence has a colon, consider each part of it as a separate sentence. However, if possible, avoid selecting that segment of the passage.

The words for which the abbreviations stand should be read aloud to determine their syllable count (e.g., Oct. = October = 3 syllables).

SMOG on shorter passages

Sometimes it may be necessary to assess the readability of a passage of less than 30 sentences. You can still use the SMOG formula to obtain an approximate grade level by using a conversion number from Table B and then using Table A to find the grade level.

First count the number of sentences in your material and the number of words with three or more syllables. In Table B, in the left-hand column, locate the number of sentences, and locate the conversion number in the column opposite. Multiply the word count found earlier by the conversion number. Use this number in Table B to obtain the corresponding grade level.

For example, suppose your material consisted of 15 sentences and you counted 12 words of three or more syllables in this material. Proceed as follows:

1. In Table B, left-hand column, locate the number of sentences in your material. For your material, the number is 15.
2. Opposite 15 in the adjacent column, find the conversion number. The conversion number for 15 is 2.0.
3. Multiply your word count, 12, by 2 to get 24.
4. Now look at Table A to find the grade level. For a word count of 24, the grade level is 8.

TABLE B. SMOG conversion for samples with fewer than 30 sentences

Number of sentences in sample material	Conversion number
29	1.03
28	1.07
27	1.1
26	1.15
25	1.2
24	1.25
23	1.3
22	1.36
21	1.43
20	1.5
19	1.58
18	1.67
17	1.76
16	1.87
15	2.0
14	2.14
13	2.3
12	2.5
11	2.7
10	3

From McLaughlin GH, *J Reading* 12:639-646, 1969; Doak CC, Doak LG, Root JH: *Teaching patients with low literacy skills,* Philadelphia, 1985, JB Lippincott.

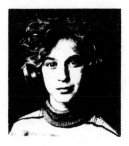

Ask your Lung Association for any of these leaflets

Air Pollution
Asthma
Bronchiectasis
Chronic Bronchitis
Chronic Cough
Cigarette Smoking
Cocci (Coccidioidomycosis)
Common Cold
Dust Disease
Emphysema
Farmer's Lung
Flu (Influenza)

Hay Fever
Histoplasmosis
Lung Cancer
Pipe & Cigar Smoking
Pleurisy
Pneumonia
Sarcoidosis
Second-Hand Smoke
Shortness of Breath
TB Outside the Lungs
Tuberculosis
Your Lungs

A community service paid for by Christmas Seals.®
Take care of your lungs.
They're only human.

A

AMERICAN ✝ LUNG ASSOCIATION
The Christmas Seal People ®

#0151   PUBLISHED BY AMERICAN LUNG ASSOCIATION   7/84

Chronic Cough

How many bottles of cough medicine did you buy last winter? Do you usually carry a package of cough drops?

A cough may seem like such a common thing—you just dose it and ignore it.

***Don't do that.* Your cough, if it is a chronic one, may be serious. It depends on**

The Facts About Your Lungs ✝

FIGURE 7-2. Sample pamphlet to be used with the public. **A,** Back and front. **B,** Inside. (Courtesy American Lung Association.)

WHEN A COUGH IS CHRONIC

Has your cough been hanging around for a month or more? Then you have a *chronic* cough. It doesn't matter that you cough only in the morning when you get up, or only at night when you lie down. If you've been coughing for more than a month, your cough is chronic.

Maybe you cough only during winter and feel fine the rest of the year. That cough is a chronic cough.

WHAT ABOUT SHORT-TERM COUGHS?

Just about everybody coughs from time to time. The common cold, for instance, is often followed by a cough that can last as long as two or three weeks. But if your cough following a cold hangs on longer than usual, it may be developing into a chronic cough.

If there is shortness of breath with a cough, or any pain, or blood in the stuff you cough up, you should see your doctor immediately, even though your cough may not have lasted more than a few days.

WHAT ABOUT SMOKING?

Do you smoke a pack or more of cigarettes a day? If you do, you're considered a heavy smoker. Heavy cigarette smoking can cause a chronic cough.

But don't dismiss a cough that hangs on as "just a cigarette cough." That cigarette cough of yours is serious in itself. It means that your excessive smoking has already damaged your breathing passages. In fact, the smoker who coughs is the person most likely to get lung cancer. And more likely to get emphysema.

You may be so used to your cigarette cough that you can't tell when something new has been added. Are you coughing more than you used to? For longer at a time? Or has your cough changed its character? Maybe you're coughing up streaks of blood or more phlegm (mucus). Any of these happenings may be a sign that something is wrong.

CHRONIC COUGH IS A SYMPTOM

A chronic cough is not a disease in itself. It is a sign of something wrong with the breathing system. That's why it isn't smart to take cough medicine for more than a week or two unless your doctor tells you to. Medicine may help with the cough, but meanwhile the underlying illness can be getting steadily worse.

The most likely causes of chronic cough are: lung cancer . . . bronchitis (inflammation in the lung tubes) . . . bronchiectasis (in which pus pockets form along the tubes) . . . tuberculosis . . . other lung diseases.

WHY GO TO THE DOCTOR?

The instant you realize you have a chronic cough, go to your doctor. The doctor can make a number of tests to find out if a lung disease is causing your cough. Then he can start treatment early in the game. That is when most lung diseases can be dealt with successfully.

If you're coughing too much, find out why. It may be something minor or it may be serious. Until you know for sure, it's nothing to fool around with or neglect.

Be sure—or you may be sorry!

B

FIGURE 7-2, cont'd. For legend see opposite page.

ference required to understand the text, whether it is explicit or whether it has inconsistencies in its logic. Normal text has short inferential chains with many close clues. Defective text includes many unclear inferences about meanings of words, motives, and actions, as well as the structure of the text itself. Content density involves the amount of information packed into the text and the amount of information the reader has read and must hold in mind to comprehend the text. A chemistry text is very dense.[3]

Although ways of measuring and further conceptualizing these elements of readability for comprehension need to be developed, the approach is most promising.

Analysis of sample instructional materials

A sample of a pamphlet for use by the lay public is shown in Figure 7-2.[2] Using the study questions at the end of this chapter, the reader is encouraged to make an assessment of the objectives that this pamphlet might meet. Its statements seem to be correct. No pictures are used to create interest or explain content; however, pictures would not seem particularly useful for this subject matter. Although the illustration does not show it, red is used on the covers and for the headings of the sections on content in the body of the pamphlet. Color catches attention and helps to make clear the sectioning of material into topics that follow a train of thought.

The organization of this pamphlet is excellent. Note that it centers on a single concept—cough. The sequence begins with definitions, differentiating the concept "chronic cough" from the overall concept "cough" and relating it to symptoms readers might have had. The sequence goes on logically to implications and action. Check the readability level.

Many health agencies prepare some teaching aids of their own, often incorporating schedules or procedures specific to that agency. These written materials must also be considered in light of the objectives they must meet, the validity of the material, and the likelihood of patient comprehension.

A number of journals regularly publish these teaching tools so that they may be used by others. The aid, "Difficult Decisions," was developed for families considering consenting to a no-code order.[4] It provides written material that the family can refer to during an emotional time when they cannot remember well, and it tries to clarify the clinical language involved. The aid is meant to reassure the family on three important points: that a no-code order can be reversed, that the patient is kept comfortable while the order is in effect, and that supportive medical and nursing care is not withheld.

The "Bone Marrow Procedure Guide" follows.[36] The guide is organized around questions likely to be asked by patients. It applies research that indicates that procedure preparation should include the feelings that patients will have and offers advice and ways for the patient to practice coping with feelings. Is the use of the analogy of bone marrow to a wet sponge useful? Will patients understand "at risk for bleeding"? Will they know that marrow is inside bone?

Materials and illiterate patients

One out of five adult Americans is functionally illiterate, reading at or below the fifth grade level. These individuals understand little if any of the written materials provided for them by health professionals. Five percent of the adult population is unable to read. The use of audiotaped instructions taxes the language and thinking skills of these individuals. Another 33% reads between the sixth and tenth grade levels.[14,23]

Many individuals who are illiterate have normal or above normal IQs. They will nearly always try to conceal their illiteracy and will use excuses such as not having time or having left their eyeglasses at home. They may be articulate and well dressed. Frequently, they "go along" and react positively even when they do not understand.[50] However, illiterate individuals cannot use reference documents or catalogs effectively, cannot follow instruction sheets, or cannot comprehend simple road maps.[23]

BONE MARROW PROCEDURE GUIDE

What is a bone marrow procedure?

Withdrawal of bone marrow through a needle for examination under a microscope. Think of your bone marrow as a wet sponge. *Aspiration* sucks out some fluid from the sponge. *Biopsy* cuts out a tiny piece of the sponge (marrow). You may have one or both procedures.

What is the purpose of a bone marrow procedure?

To examine how your blood cells are being formed, the number and type of blood cells, the amount of iron, *or* if there is any evidence of tumor or infection. You have three types of blood cells: red blood cells, white blood cells, and platelets. Their parent cells are in your bone marrow where they multiply, mature, and exit into the blood. A sample of blood cannot reveal all aspects of this process, and it becomes necessary to obtain cells from your bone marrow.

How long will it take?

About 20 minutes including the time needed to wash your skin.

Will I have to make any special preparations?

No, you do not have to prepare in any special way. However, if you are at risk for bleeding, you may receive a platelet transfusion prior to the procedure.

Where will it be done?

The bone marrow is taken from one of the shaded areas below. You will be asked to lie on your abdomen or back, close to the edge of the bed.

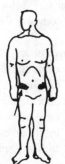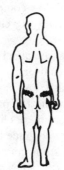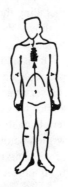

What will the procedure be like?

First, your doctor will press gently around the area. Next, he will wash it with a cleansing agent such as iodine, which will feel cold. Sterile towels will be placed around the area. So you will feel less pain, your doctor will inject a local anesthetic similar to the medication used by dentists. You will feel a "stick" from the needle, and a burning feeling as the medication penetrates the area. It takes a minute for the anesthetic to take effect.

Aspiration

Once the area is numb, a special needle will be put through your skin. The doctor will put slight force on the needle as it enters. You may feel some pressure. After the needle is in, a syringe will be attached to take some of the fluid. You may feel a sharp pain, deep inside, *but it lasts only a few seconds*. Taking a deep breath or using a relaxation technique often helps. Ask your nurse about this.

Biopsy

Through the same spot, a special needle will cut out a tiny piece of marrow, called a core. This usually does not cause any pain, but you may feel pressure as the needle is turned. The needle will then be removed and a Bandaid or dressing will be applied. The entire procedure usually takes no more than 8 to 10 minutes.

Is there any special care afterwards?

Bleeding occurs RARELY after this procedure. You may be asked to lie on the site for about 30 minutes, and the site will be checked for bleeding. If you have a low platelet count, you will need to put pressure on the site longer.

INPATIENTS: Call your nurse if you feel the dressing is wet.

OUTPATIENTS: If you see bleeding more than the size of a quarter in 1 hour, lie on the site on the floor for 30 minutes. If there is still bleeding, call: _____

_____.

The author gratefully acknowledges the assistance of Carolyn Bledsoe with the illustration. This booklet is reprinted with permission of the author. It may be reproduced and distributed.

BONE MARROW PROCEDURE GUIDE—
cont'd

Keep the dressing/Bandaid dry and in place for 24 hours. As the anesthetic wears off, you may need something for pain. Take ＿＿＿＿＿ for mild discomfort.

How long before the results are known?

Generally, your doctor will have the results in 48 to 72 hours. To learn the results of your bone marrow examination, call ＿＿＿＿＿＿＿＿.

TABLE 7-2. Readability of common OTC products as calculated using the FOG index and Fry readability graph

Product	FOG index	Fry graph
Advil	8.9	10.0
Afrin	7.8	10.0
Anusol	11.3	College
Ascriptin	9.5	11.0
Benylin DM	9.3	College
Cough Calmers	8.1	7.0
Debrox	4.3	4.0
Doxidan	9.8	College
Fleet	7.7	10.0
Liquiprin Infant Drops	12.6	College
Maalox Plus	15.4	College
Medipren	5.9	7.0
Metholatum	7.1	10.0
Metamucil	9.8	College
Primatene	8.2	10.0
Pronto	6.4	8.0
Rheaban	6.8	7.0
Tempra	5.4	7.0
Tinactin	7.5	10.0
Vicks Formula 44M	9.9	9.0
Zincfrin	7.6	9.0

From Holt GA and others: *Am Pharm* 30(11):51-54, 1990.
Numbers represent school grade level of reading skills required.

Because litigation initiated by a patient acting without knowledge that should have been provided is a possibility, the best-known techniques should be used to teach these individuals[15,50]:

1. Eliminate everything that is extraneous.
2. Build to complexity when it is necessary; break content into components; and build with review, feedback, and questions.
3. Require patients to demonstrate what they have learned.
4. Those who are insecure in their ability to learn need more rewards than do others to accomplish small tasks.
5. To reduce the reading level and literacy demand, use a conversational style, active voice, short words, and short sentences.
6. Use visuals, especially line drawings, with one idea portrayed by the picture; use captions not longer than ten words.
7. Show only correct behavior.
8. Organize material in the order the patients will use it, and use words that are familiar to them.
9. Pretest all materials.

Unfortunately, illiterate patients are greatly handicapped in many health care situations. Consider the labels for over the counter (OTC) drugs. Food and Drug Administration regulations require that drug companies label their products in terms that can be read and understood by the consumer, including those with low comprehension. Table 7-2 shows the readability levels of common OTC products.

Davis and others[12] obtained a convenience sample of patients from university and community clinics serving poor and low-income families. This author found that of the 150 patient education materials analyzed from these clinics, only 6% were written below the ninth grade level. Informed consent forms ranged from grades 13 to 31. Letters from physicians to patients required an average

EXAMPLE OF BRANCHING PROGRAMMING, BOOK FORMAT

(page 31)

See if you can tell the difference between performances (*doing* words) and abstractions (*being* words). *Circle the words below that describe performances:*

stating	listing
writing	appreciating
valuing	internalizing
drawing	smiling

When you have finished, turn to page 33.

(page 33)

Check your responses with mine. The performances are circled.

(stating)	(listing)
(writing)	appreciating
valuing	internalizing
(drawing)	(smiling)

The circled words describe things that people might do. The words not circled describe internal states or conditions. Valuing, for example, is not something that someone does; rather, it is something that is felt.

Now let's look at some statements and practice recognizing which ones include *performances*. Read the statements below, and turn to the page whose number appears beside the statement containing a *performance*.

Be able to understand mathematics.   *(page 35)*

Be able to sew a seam.   *(page 37)*

(page 35)

You said that "be able to understand mathematics" included a performance. Not for a minute . . .

From Mager RF: *Preparing instructional objectives*, ed 2, Belmont, Calif, 1984, David S Lake.

reading level of grades 16 to 17. Only 14% of the public clinic patients tested were reading at or above the eleventh grade level. Over sixty percent of participants were reading at least three grade levels below the grade they last attended. Average reading comprehension of public clinic patients was grade 6.5, yet most patient education materials required grades 11 to 14.

Clearly, it is essential to have teaching materials that are appropriate for patients with average reading levels as well as for those who are illiterate.

Programmed and computer instruction

Programmed instruction is a written sequential presentation of learning steps requiring learners to answer questions about the material presented and telling them whether they are right or wrong. It is primarily verbal, although pictures and diagrams are also used. An example of programmed materials in book format may be seen on p. 157. Answers appear on another page or in a covered column until the student wishes to compare his or her answers with the suggested ones.

Use of programmed instruction takes advantage of learning principles that are often difficult to apply with other teaching techniques, particularly with a large group of learners. It requires that the learner be active rather than passive, providing immediate feedback, correcting wrong answers, and reinforcing correct answers with knowledge of success. It allows students to work at their own pace.

Although programmers essentially agree on these facts, two major philosophies have grown up regarding the effect of errors: the resulting size of the learning step; and the importance of recognition versus recall. Proponents of the linear construction believe that learning should be as errorless as possible and that, to accomplish this, steps in the program should be small. Questions require recall (construction of the learner's own answers) rather than recognition of the correct answer in a multiple-choice type of question. Branching, or intrinsic, programming (p. 157) contains more explanation before questioning to refrain from fragmenting the material. Its proponents are not so concerned that

learning be errorless. Rather, the questions assume a diagnostic function to discover where learning has not occurred. A learner who chooses a wrong response is directed to a branch of the main program for supplemental instruction.[25] It is not unusual to find programs that combine features of both linear and branching techniques.

Programmed material is also presented by computers that have the added capability of storing response patterns for a particular learner and of selecting further lessons on the basis of these patterns.

Another example of a text lesson designed with correction for patients with rheumatoid arthritis appears on p. 159.[51]

Ways in which computers are used in education have been variously categorized and might include the following:

1. *Computer-assisted instruction.* The computer provides drill and practice or tutorial instruction.
2. *Computer-managed instruction.* The computer evaluates a test of performance, guides students to appropriate educational resources, and keeps records of their progress.
3. *Computer-enriched instruction.* The computer serves as simulator or calculating tool.[27]

The ability of the computer to simulate (imitate some aspect of reality) is valued.

A more complex use of computers for patient education is being implemented. For example, a computer game called "Asthma Command" focuses on how to recognize symptoms of asthma, as well as the allergens that might initiate an attack. The game also shows the appropriate use of medications and teaches information about the emergency room and the physician's office. The program allows entry of the names of the subjects' own specific medications and allergens into the memory of the game.[42] A behavioral treatment program for obesity uses an interactive microcomputer small enough to be carried by subjects during their normal daily routines. Learners make self-reports on consumption of food and exercise. If they forget to do so they are reminded by the computer. The

**AN EXCERPT FROM THE COMPUTER-BASED LESSON FOR PATIENTS WITH RHEUMATOID ARTHRITIS.
THE PATIENT'S RESPONSE IS FOUND TO THE RIGHT OF THE > SYMBOL.**

Aspirin has two important effects. First, it decreases and controls inflammation. Inflammation is the cause of pain, stiffness, swelling, heat, redness, and most importantly, joint damage. Therefore, by reducing inflammation, you relieve pain and help prevent damage to the joints. Secondly, aspirin is an effective drug for relieving other arthritis pain that is not caused by inflammation—pain like muscle tightening and muscle spasms.

What dosage of aspirin is usually needed to control inflammation?

1. 10 tablets a day
2. 12-25 tablets a day
3. 6 tablets a day

>3

No, to decrease inflammation larger amounts of aspirin are needed. Depending on the individual patient, doctors will prescribe 12-25 tablets a day. A dose under 12 tablets per day will not usually control inflammation. A dose over 25 tablets per day will not usually be necessary or tolerated. The most common dose is 12-18 tablets daily.

The goal of aspirin therapy is to keep the aspirin level in the blood at a level that will work against inflammation. This is a continuous process. It requires that aspirin medication be taken faithfully on schedule, every day.

Imagine that your doctor has prescribed 16 aspirin tablets per day on a continuous basis. You have been taking this dose for the past week and as a result, you are feeling much better. In fact, you have no more pain. What would you do next week?

1. Continue taking the aspirin as your doctor prescribed.
2. Cut down to 12 aspirin because you are feeling well, but you do not think that you need all 16 tablets.
3. Stop taking aspirin because you are already feeling better. Since your pain is gone, there is no need to continue taking medication.

>2

No, that would not be a good idea. Even when you feel no pain, you need to continue taking the aspirin exactly as your doctor prescribed to maintain the aspirin level in your blood. Only by maintaining this level will you keep inflammation under control.

> Remember, aspirin must be taken regularly as prescribed. It is not a pain medication to be taken only as needed. It is continuously preventing joint inflammation. If you stop taking aspirin when you feel well, you may have a flare of your disease!!!

Modified from Wetstone SL and others: *J Rheumatol* 12:909, 1985.

computer displays a count of the calories consumed, as well as a count of calories remaining for the day. If the data indicate that caloric intake exceeds daily limits for meal, snack, or total food consumption, the computer displays positively phrased instructions to stop eating and recommends alternative behaviors. If the number of calories is within the allotted amount, the computer message praises the learner. This approach produced greater weight loss at 8 months after treatment than did a paper-and-pencil approach used with the control group.[8]

Computers also can help care for persons with diabetes. A pocket computer has been used to calculate insulin dose[10] and to create a meal program based on the diet prescription, usual daily eating pattern, and subject food preferences.[52] Pernick reports development of a personal computer program that can provide an "electronic notebook" for storage and retrieval of information on blood glucose, insulin dosage, hypoglycemia reactions, urinary ketones, diet, activity, weight, and illness. The program produces: (1) apparent explanations for hypoglycemic reactions or glucose values outside target ranges; (2) graphic displays of glucose and insulin versus date; (3) a "glucose profile" versus time of day or day of week; (4) suggestions regarding compensatory supplements and adjustments of routine insulin dosage; (5) explanations of why various insulin dosages should or should not be altered; and (6) explanations of why various glucose values should be tested. The program can make comparisons of the insulin dosage administered by the patient and the dosage recommendations of the program with explanations for discrepancies offered by the patient, the ability to help evaluate compliance, and other features. Figure 7-3 displays a customized algorithm or computerized prescription from this program.[39]

Some systems can store data on self-monitored blood glucose, urine glucose, and insulin for as long as 28 days. Others analyze and interpret nutritional data, including computer-generated menus and grocery shopping lists. Another program breaks recipes into exchange list values.[44] An arcade-style game provides a safe opportunity for children with diabetes to practice and evaluate skills in food and insulin dose selection and to exercise. The child is led through a series of decisions typical of those in the life of a child, and remediation is available after each decision.[53]

Computer games can help adolescents understand the responsibilities parents face, as well as the costs of childbirth and childrearing. Throughout the game, the teen's readiness for parenting is visually displayed on a thermometer gauge. The program simulates, for example, a 1-year-old with a fever who cries persistently at night or a 2-year-old with temper tantrums. A similar game called "Romance" addresses sex and birth control. It provides simulated outcomes and realistic information. After these games were introduced in clinics, teenage pregnancy rates declined by 15%. Computer-assisted instruction uses role modeling and desensitization to raise teens' self-esteem. As teens gain new information, they are empowered with new ways to make decisions.[45]

Computers can generate individualized information leaflets. They incorporate new information easily. On-line, computer-based information systems can educate college students about topics such as AIDS—information that students might not seek at the health centers. Computer information systems can answer questions, offer recent research updates, and display guides to community services. They provide a useful and confidential source of information within a broader AIDS education program.[54] More sophisticated computer learning systems might assemble a variety of learning and assessment tools for those trying to solve problems, such as how to deal with stress.[21] These systems might offer a tutorial; a general health hazard appraisal; an assessment of an individual's beliefs (including the person's possible interest in changing); a computer program that branches to provide specific information based on a particular patient's health appraisal; an observation of what happens to body organs under stress; or support for a program of stress reduction based on priorities and life-style.

Despite these innovative uses of computers for

I.   Physician:
     Regimen: REGULAR and **NPH** at breakfast, **REGULAR** at dinner, **NPH** at bedtime. Insulin suggestions are available.

II. TARGET GLUCOSE LEVELS:

2-4 AM	95 to 150
before breakfast	80 to 175
after breakfast	80 to 200
before lunch	80 to 175
after lunch	80 to 200
before dinner	80 to 175
after dinner	80 to 225
bedtime	80 to 175

III. CALL THE DOCTOR IF:
glucose is below 30
glucose is above 400
glucose is above 350 with medium ketones
4 hypoglycemic reactions in 7 days
2 nighttime hypoglycemic reactions in last 7 days
Sick 2 days in a row

IV.   SUPPLEMENT TABLES

WELL-BEFORE MEALS		WELL-BEDTIME		SICK-BEFORE MEALS		SICK-BEDTIME	
Glucose	Supp.	Glucose	Supp.	Glucose	Supp.	Glucose	Supp.
below 69	−1	below 69	−1	below 109	0	SAME	
70 to 110	0	70 to 110	0	110 to 150	1		
111 to 150	1	111 to 150	1	151 to 200	2		
151 to 200	2	151 to 200	2	201 to 250	3		
201 to 300	3	201 to 300	3	251 to 300	4		
above 301	5	above 301	4	301 to 350	6		
				above 351	8		

V.   CHANGES in ROUTINE INSULIN if UNEXPLAINED HYPOGLYCEMIA:
     If unexplained hypoglycemia (low blood sugar) in the:

night-time	• REDUCE BEDTIME-NPH by 1 unit.
morning	• REDUCE BEFORE-BREAKFAST-REGULAR by 1 unit.
afternoon	• REDUCE BEFORE BREAKFAST-NPH by 1 unit.
evening	• REDUCE BEFORE DINNER-REGULAR by 1 unit.

VI. CHANGES in ROUTINE INSULIN if PERSISTENT UNEXPLAINED HYPERGLYCEMIA:
     If all 3 conditions (1-3) are met, then follow the instructions (below) for the appropriate time of day.
     1. Hyperglycemia is not due to obvious changes in meals, stress, illness, etc.
     2. Do not change more than one type of routine insulin every 4 days.
     3. NO Hypoglycemia reaction(s) in the past few days.

If hyperglycemic BEFORE BREAKFAST:
If 3 of the last 4 before breakfast glucose values, including the last one, were greater than 175 and unexplained, and if at least 1 of the last 4 2-4 am glucoses were checked and not less than 125, then increase the BEDTIME NPH insulin by 2 units.

If hyperglycemic BEFORE LUNCH:
If 2 of the last 3 before lunch glucose values, including the last one, were greater than 175 and unexplained, and if at least 1 of the last 3 after breakfast glucoses were checked and not less than 110, then increase the BEFORE BREAKFAST REGULAR insulin by 1 unit.

If hyperglycemic BEFORE DINNER:
If all of the last 3 before dinner glucose values, were greater than 175 and unexplained, then increase the BEFORE BREAKFAST NPH insulin by 2 units.

If hyperglycemic BED TIME:
If 3 of the last 5 bedtime glucose values, including the last one, were greater than 175 and unexplained, then increase the BEFORE DINNER REGULAR insulin by 1 unit.

FIGURE 7-3. Customized algorithm or computerized prescription. (From Pernick NL, Rodbard D: *Diabetes Care* 9:61-69, 1986.)

management and instruction, a survey of hospital promotion programs showed that only 4% were using computer education.[41]

NONPRINT MATERIALS

Audiovisual aids, sometimes combining sight and hearing with touch, smell, and taste, represent additional ways to communicate. The teacher must choose a form (from the many forms offered) that is likely to aid in meeting particular objectives. Usually the choice relates to the degree of reality needed to ensure transfer to the real situation. As with written materials, completeness and correctness affect learning.

Research on instructional materials has not recognized a distinction among three separate design elements: the medium, the presentation form, and the content. Presentation form is the structure that

carries the information by a medium. For example, a picture of an elephant in a book and verbal description of it by a teacher differ in both medium and presentation form. However, a picture of an elephant on a slide and the one in the book have the same presentation form but a different medium.

Consider the presentation form of programmed instruction: (1) its stimuli are presented in verbal or illustrated form, (2) it demands written or selected response, (3) the presentation lasts as long as the learner desires, and (4) the learner must make some response before proceeding to the next item. This form is really independent of both content and medium. A workbook is an obvious medium; however, others, such as slide-tapes, TV, problem books, and peer-tutor scripts, are possible. A classification system of presentation is shown in Figure 7-4. The primary disadvantage of transient presen-

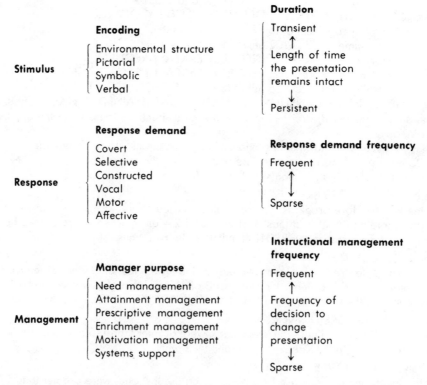

FIGURE 7-4. The dimensions of presentation. (From Tosti DT, Ball JR: *AudioVis Commun Rev* 17:5-25, 1969.)

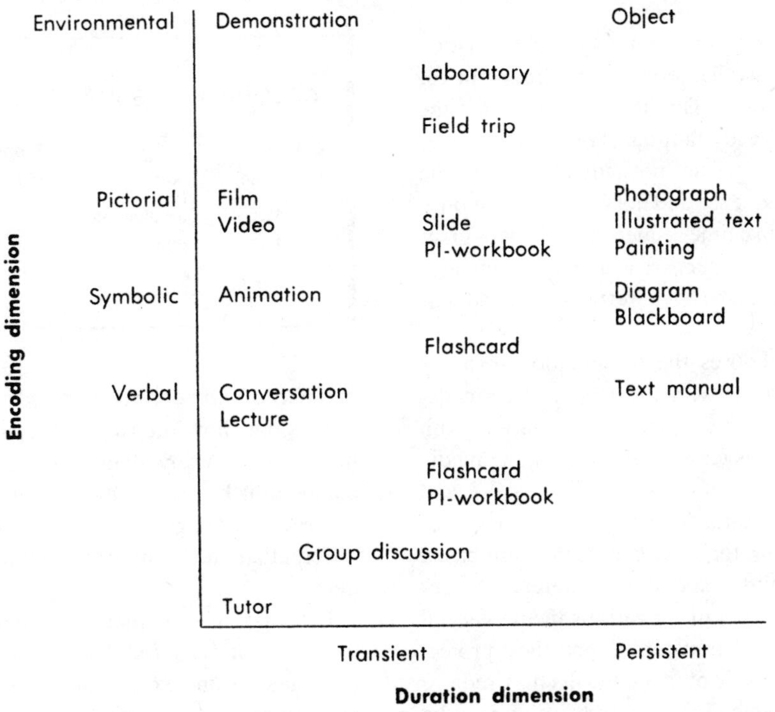

FIGURE 7-5.

Encoding dimension	Transient	(middle)	Persistent
Environmental	Demonstration		Object
		Laboratory	
		Field trip	
Pictorial	Film / Video	Slide / PI-workbook	Photograph / Illustrated text / Painting
Symbolic	Animation		Diagram / Blackboard
		Flashcard	
Verbal	Conversation / Lecture		Text manual
		Flashcard / PI-workbook	
		Group discussion	
	Tutor		

Duration dimension

FIGURE 7-5. Media classified by encoding versus duration. (From Tosti DT, Ball JR: *AudioVis Commun Rev* 17:5-25, 1969.)

FIGURE 7-6.

Encoding dimension	Covert	Selective	Vocal	Constructed	Motor
Environmental	Demonstration	Item sort			
	Field trip				
Pictorial	Film / Video / Slide / Painting / Photograph	Multiple-choice teaching machine		Illustrated PI-text	Laboratory
Symbolic	Blackboard / Diagram	Card-sort	Flashcard		Diagram
Verbal	Lecture / Audiotape	PI-workbook	Conversation / Role-playing / Audiotape		
	Text	Tutor	Tutor	Tutor	Tutor

Response demand dimension

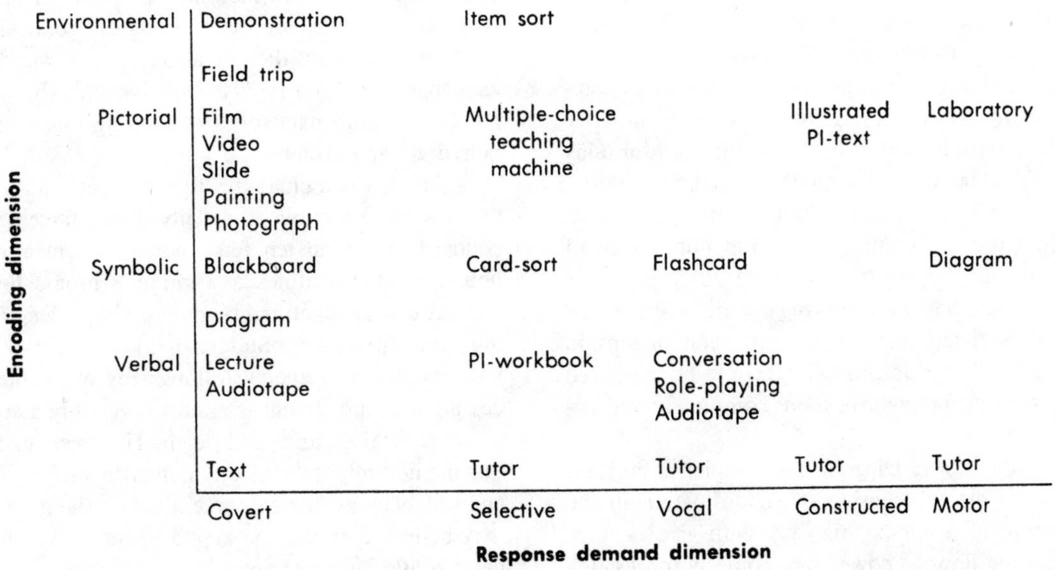

FIGURE 7-6. Media classified by encoding versus response demand. (From Tosti DT, Ball JR: *AudioVis Commun Rev* 17:5-25, 1969.)

tations is that the learner must store information because it is not available in the environment for a long period of time. This is not important if the presentation is already familiar. For persistent media, the disadvantages are not indicating real time in a behavioral sequence and not requiring response from the learner in a time sequence. It is, of course, possible to combine persistent and transient presentations to overcome their respective disadvantages.

The teacher chooses the presentation form by making it congruent with the response form described in the objective. A medium consistent with the response form is chosen; although some media can connect with several forms (Figures 7-5 and 7-6). Often the criteria for choosing the best medium or media mix for a given objective are based on cost, availability, and user preference.[49] Because the symbol systems in various media vary in the kinds of mental transformations they project and the different levels of mental skills they require to extract knowledge, difficulty in learning may be overcome by switching to a different medium that better matches the learner's mental skills.

Types of nonprint materials
Diagrams and charts

Although human relationships are not physical objects, well-designed diagrams using circles, lines, and arrows can portray the essence of a relationship vividly. A single diagram can summarize and clarify the concept of the health team for a lay individual better than a lengthy verbal description. In Figure 7-7, Diagram 1, placement of personnel around a circle communicates the importance of all roles of the health team. The circle indicates that the health team is working toward health goals, but it does not make clear their relationships in doing so. Therefore, its design could be improved to represent the concept more completely and accurately.

The concept in Diagram 2 is simpler to portray. It shows the relationship of subordination in the structure of a nursing service, with arrows indicating the flow of power. For some purposes this

CALORIE AND SUGAR VALUE OF FOOD		
Calories (per gram)	Food	Proportion converted to blood sugar
4	Carbohydrates	100%
4	Protein	58%
9	Fat	10%

diagram would not be considered complete because it does not show the two-way communication that must occur. Many diagrams can be made more compelling by using drawings instead of words; however, in Diagram 2 it would seem difficult to differentiate the various health workers with drawings.

Diagram 3 was first constructed without the words *fire* and *insulin*. These words were added in the course of the explanation. This tactic is meant to focus the learner on the essence of the relationship between insulin and the use of sugar for body energy.

A chart may be seen as an organized group of facts about something. The box on p. 164 is an arrangement of basic facts that explain, in part, why carbohydrates are the most rigidly controlled foods in a diabetic diet. It also explains why fat exchanges need not be distributed as equally over meals as would exchanges containing much carbohydrate and protein.

Figure 7-8 is a chart for high-risk antenatal patients with directions for daily fetal movement count. Fewer than ten fetal movements in a 12-hour period constitutes a warning. Chronic fetal distress can be identified by progressively decreasing fetal movement. Sudden marked increase in violent fetal movements followed by a complete cessation of movement is almost invariably a sign of acute fetal distress and death. However, using this method might cause the mother to suffer guilt and self-blame if the outcome is poor. The mother may believe that had she kept a better record, her baby would have survived.[28]

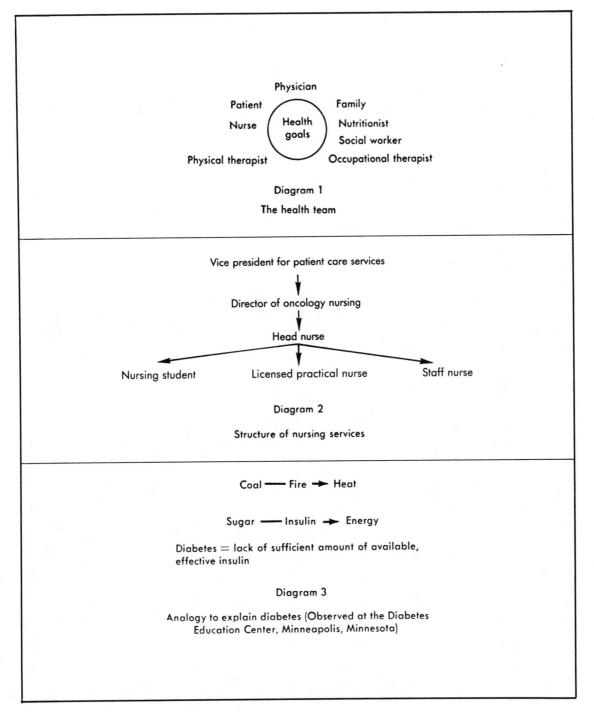

Diagram 1

The health team

Diagram 2

Structure of nursing services

Diagram 3

Analogy to explain diabetes (Observed at the Diabetes Education Center, Minneapolis, Minnesota)

FIGURE 7-7. Examples of teaching diagrams.

Daily Fetal Movement Count: Instructions for Pregnant Women
(Cardiff Method)

We would like you to help us check the health of your baby by keeping a record of the number of times your baby moves during the day.

Some babies are more active than others, and each baby tends to have its own pattern of activity, The total number of movements per day are significant only if they are less than 10 movements in 12 hours or if there is a change in the usual pattern of fetal movements.

Starting at 9:00 a.m., or whenever your day usually begins, count the number of movements until the total equals 10. After 10 movements are left, record on the graph the time elapsed since you started counting. For example, if you start on Wednesday, March 30, and count 10 movements by 10:20 a.m., block out the whole square between 10:00 a.m. and 10:30 a.m. Rather than recording the exact time, you record the half-hour period in which the tenth movement falls. It is not necessary to do any further counting until the next day, when you start again again at 9:00 a.m. (or at your usual time).

If you feel less than 10 movements within a 12-hour period, record the actual number of movements felt and **call your health care provider immediately.** Also call immediately if you 1) felt no movements in eight hours; 2) observe that the pattern of the fetal movements has changed from the usual pattern; and 3) if there is a sudden violent increase in fetal movements followed by complete cessation of movements.

The Cardiff "Count-To-Ten" Fetal Activity Chart

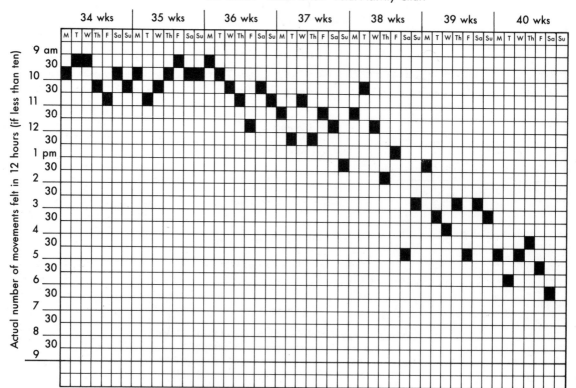

A typical normal completed chart showing the characteristic diminution of fetal activity as delivery becomes imminent.

FIGURE 7-8. Daily Fetal Movement Count Chart. (From Lehman AE, Estok PJ: *Nurse Pract* 12:40-44, 1987.)

Diagrams and charts such as these can serve as motivators for patients and can provide them with factual knowledge. Provision of all the necessary information in one easy-to-understand form can help the patients understand and focus their attention on what to do.

Physical objects

When one teaches about actual physical objects, it is often preferable to use the real thing. Nothing but a baby can act like a baby during a bath. However, models are useful when the third dimension must be retained but (1) the real thing is too small, large, complicated, or expensive; (2) the real thing is unavailable; (3) the desired view cannot be exposed; or (4) the object cannot be manipulated. For example, for demonstrating the birth of a fetus, a doll may be advanced through an actual-size model of the bony structure of the pelvis. Many times, anatomy and physiology cannot be adequately visualized with the use of a real person because other tissues are in the way or a body part, such as the eye, is too small and complex. A dummy can be useful for showing the position of a tracheostomy and how to remove and reinsert parts of the tube. It can also be used for practicing general movements with the suction tube. The dummy is clearly limited because it lacks functioning muscles and secretions. Some teachers would insist that it would be better to start the learner working with a real tracheostoma. However, if none is available, or if one that is available is difficult to care for, early practice on a model may be helpful. Models in the form of dummies are used to teach resuscitation techniques because someone whose heart or breathing has stopped is not usually available.

Thus models may be used because they can teach better than real objects can or because they are more practical to use. At times they are absolutely essential. However, models frequently are expensive and may not be easily available in many places where patients are being taught.

Pictures

The research literature on pictorial learning is sparse in comparison with that on verbal learning. Theory about how people learn from pictures is not completely developed. Pictorial learning is superior to verbal for recognition and recall. However, when the subject matter is abstract, it is difficult to communicate with pictures. Media used to convey pictures always distort the various visual dimensions—resolution, color fidelity, and size—to some degree. For example, paintings may eliminate or exaggerate various parts of an object. These distortions may or may not be important to a particular learning task.

Photographs and drawings lack the third dimension but are readily available or can be produced by the teacher. The third dimension is not imperative when the teacher is showing familiar objects or those in which shape and space are not the primary considerations. Examples that fall into these categories and are frequently not available include an infected finger or an abnormal stool in infants. However, the learner must be aware that odor can be important in recognizing abnormal stool. In both of these examples, photographs would be more desirable than diagrams because they more accurately portray the details of the real item.

Drawings are particularly pertinent for removing superfluous detail present in real objects. During an explanation to a patient about diverticulitis, visualization is obviously desirable. Whereas a photograph shows details of the tissue that the patient does not need to know, a simple line drawing can communicate the concept of a pouch in the intestinal wall. In other instances, drawings in the form of cartoons are used to create interest in a topic.

Pictures may be presented in many ways, depending on the size of the audience and equipment available. For a single individual, visuals on paper 8½ by 11 inches can be used. For small groups, posters can be prepared. Drawings can be made with crayons or felt-tipped pens on flip charts (pads of paper approximately 32 by 26 inches) supported on an easel or chair back. Cutouts can be attached by magnets or flannel to metal or flannel boards. Drawings can be done on the blackboard. Suitable for both large and small groups are 2 × 2 inch slides or filmstrips that can be projected on a screen or wall. Overhead projectors use transparencies

How to breathe easier, using your diaphragm

Dear patient:
The diaphragm is a dome-shaped muscle between your lungs and abdomen. When you breathe in, your diaphragm drops so your lungs can fill with air. When you breathe out, it rises and pushes the air out of your lungs. The illustration at right shows how your diaphragm changes position as you breathe.

You can breathe more deeply and with less effort by letting your diaphragm work for you. Learn to use it effectively by following these steps:

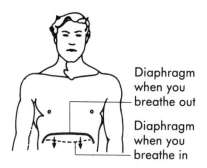

Diaphragm when you breathe out

Diaphragm when you breathe in

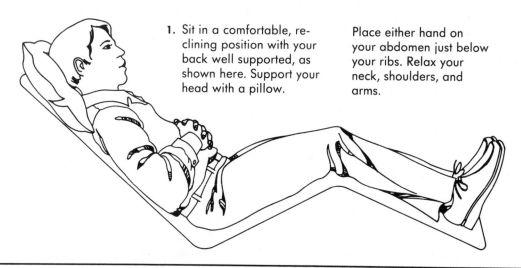

1. Sit in a comfortable, reclining position with your back well supported, as shown here. Support your head with a pillow.

Place either hand on your abdomen just below your ribs. Relax your neck, shoulders, and arms.

FIGURE 7-9. Teaching aid for patient with chronic obstructive pulmonary disease (COPD). (From *Nurs Life* 5[3]:332, 1985.)

(sheets of plastic) prepared with diagrams or drawn at the time of presentation and projected. When teaching is a regular part of the nursing activities, these materials and equipment may be readily available. More commonly, caregivers interact with an individual patient and use an easily obtained visual, such as the pictures in the *Birth Atlas*, sketch the objects needed for a given lesson, or use a prepared teaching aid.

Two examples of prepared teaching aids with print and visuals may be seen in Figures 7-9 and 7-10. In the aid on diaphragmatic breathing, note how movement is described with arrows and verbal descriptions.[47] "A Patient's Guide to the Implanted Port" is used with real ports and catheters available for patients to handle.[24] According to the FOG formula, the reading level of the guide is between grades 11 and 13.

Motion pictures and television

If motion is necessary, as it may be for teaching procedures, motion pictures and television are

2. Breathe in gently through your nose. Concentrate on feeling your abdomen rise, which allows your diaphragm to drop. Stay relaxed, and don't arch your back.

3. Purse your lips as if you're about to whistle. Breathe out gently without letting your cheeks puff out. Concentrate on feeling your abdomen sink, which allows your diaphragm to rise.

If you have trouble making your diaphragm drop, take a quick sniff through your nose—you'll feel your abdomen rise. Now, try to produce the same effect when you take a longer and slower breath.

After you can do this exercise in a sitting position, practice it in other positions: lying flat on your back with a pillow under your head, sitting upright, and standing.

Use this exercise whenever you feel short of breath. With practice, you can even use it to help you breathe more easily while walking.

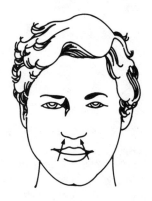
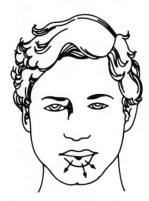

This patient-teaching aid may be reproduced by office copier for distribution to patients; © 1985 Springhouse Corporation.

FIGURE 7-9, cont'd. For legend see opposite page.

available. Videotapes are efficient tools for delivering instruction to a hospitalized population. In a 940-bed hospital, the pharmacy department developed a series of video tape recordings demonstrating 22 medications or drug classes on the basis of frequency of use and perceived difficulty with patient compliance for closed-circuit television. Without this mechanism, educating the patients about their medications would have been very difficult.[7]

Not only are films and videotapes available for rental or purchase, but patient education programming also has become part of national satellite networks originally developed for provider education.[38] In addition, some hospitals make their own videotapes, or they broadcast live programs.

Teaching by television requires many of the same skills as doing an in-person demonstration. It also involves obtaining camera shots that show the picture the teacher wants the viewer to see. TV demonstrations have the advantage over regular demonstrations because they can show a close-up or an over-the-shoulder view to many people at the same time. This enlarging feature can show labels on packaged foods, as well as various amounts and combinations of foods, to entire classes rather than only to a few individuals. Videotapes can be used as "triggers," providing an instructional stimulus that can be followed by discussion groups.

Most motion pictures and television presentations combine audio and visual communication. Although these media are valuable because of their ability to store visual images of motion, the audio portion teaches also. The way in which the audio explains and enhances the visual may be more or less well done. Strictly audio presentations are gen-

Your current treatment plan requires that you receive drugs into your veins. As part of your care, drawing blood samples on a regular basis is also necessary. The insertion of needles is painful and can be damaging to your veins. After weeks of treatment, you may find that you need to be stuck several times to get a blood sample or to give you your medicine. This booklet was designed to describe the implanted infusion port as a method for lessening the discomfort you may have when receiving I.V. treatments.

The implanted port consists of a silastic catheter (a special soft plastic tube) that is threaded into a large vein in your upper chest. The catheter is attached to a small, disc-like "port" (See Figure 1). The port has a metal base and a rubber-like top that seals itself off after needle sticks. You will then be able to receive your I.V. medications through this port, and in most cases blood samples can also be drawn. Patients usually feel little or no discomfort when needle sticks are made through the port.

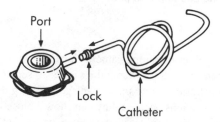

FIGURE 1. The implanted port.

How is the implanted infusion port inserted?

The catheter and port are inserted in the operating room. You will be awake during the procedure. The surgeon will numb the skin where the catheter will be inserted using a local anesthetic. Two small incisions are made. One will usually be made just above the collarbone, although there are several common locations as shown in Figure 2. This is where the catheter will be inserted and threaded into a large vein. A second small

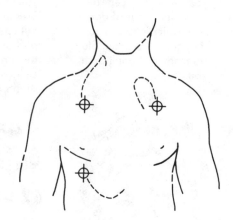

FIGURE 2. Common locations for catheter insertion.

incision will be made several inches below the first to make a "pocket" under the skin. This is where the port is placed and sutured to underlying tissues. The port is then attached to the soft plastic catheter and the pocket is sewn closed.

You may feel some pressure during the procedure, but it should not be painful. Placement of the implanted port takes about one hour. An X-ray is taken after the procedure to check for proper placement of the catheter. The incisions will be bandaged at first. Once the bandages are removed, you will be able to feel a small "bump" about an inch in size under the skin where the port is located. This area may be swollen and slightly tender for the first few days. Several days may be allowed for healing before the implanted infusion port is used for your blood tests and treatments. After 24 hours a dressing is no longer needed and the stitches will usually dissolve after 2 weeks or so.

How is the implanted infusion port used?

The implanted port is used much like a regular I.V. A special needle is inserted through the skin into the rubber-like top of the port. Insertion of the needle is usually

FIGURE 7-10. Patient's guide to the implanted port. (From Kilbride SS: *Oncol Nurs Forum* 13:83-85, 1986.)

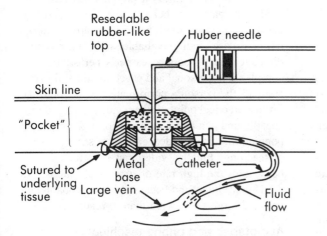

Resealable rubber-like top

Huber needle

Skin line

"Pocket"

Sutured to underlying tissue

Metal base

Large vein

Catheter

Fluid flow

FIGURE 3. Side view of the implanted port.

not painful, but if it is uncomfortable for you, the area may be numbed first. The needles are made straight or bent; the bent shape permits delivery of fluids or medications over a period of time. You may even receive your medicine at home using an ambulatory infusion pump. Blood samples can also be drawn from the port. When the treatment is completed, the needle can be removed. If you are on a treatment that goes for several days, the same needle can stay in for up to a week before it needs to be changed (see Figure 3).

How do I care for the implanted infusion port?

Since no part of the catheter or port is outside of your body, you can carry on with your normal activities, including showering and swimming, provided you are not receiving treatment. In caring for your implanted port, you will need to:

1. **Watch for infection**
   Notify your doctor or nurse if you develop any of the following symptoms:
   —Temperature/chills
   —Pain or redness around the port
   —Drainage at incision site
   —Shortness of breath
   —Chest pain

2. **Prevent blocking off the catheter**
   To keep the catheter from becoming blocked between uses, it must be "flushed" monthly. The nurse can do this for you during your regular clinic or doctor's office visits. Heparin is the drug used; it can keep the blood from clotting inside the catheter.

3. **Protect the needle during infusion and maintain the dressing**
   You may receive your treatment over a number of days using an ambulatory infusion pump. During the infusion it will be necessary for you to make certain the needle does not become dislodged. You may need to reinforce the dressing with tape or even change the dressing. If you notice any swelling about the port or experience unusual stinging or pain in the area of the port, call your doctor or nurse right away.

4. **Have the needle removed from the port**
   When your treatment is completed, your nurse will remove the needle after flushing the port with a heparin solution. Once the needle is removed, a dressing is no longer necessary.

5. **Protect the skin over the port**
   In order to protect the skin over the port from irritation, avoid bra straps and seat belts that may rub or place pressure on the port area.

How long will I have the implanted infusion port?

The implanted port can stay in place as long as your physician feels it is necessary. It can be surgically removed when you no longer need it. With good care and in the absence of infection, the port can remain in place for years, if desired.

The implanted infusion port is one way to help make your treatments easier. If you have any questions, be sure to ask your primary nurse _____ .

FIGURE 7-10, cont'd. For legend see opposite page.

erally less useful for the content that health care providers teach because so much that they do is visual. Audio presentations have special pertinence in teaching speech patterns.

Videotaped feedback was found in one study to have improved the degree of motor learning and ambulation performances of amputee patients. A group of similar patients were videotaped but did not see a playback of their performances until their last session. Their performances had not improved as much. Videotaping seems to have several advantages over using a mirror. When patients are asked to walk while observing themselves in mirrors, they must divide their attention between two tasks. Patients reported that when viewing was separated from doing, they were able to pay full attention to the activity presented. In addition, videotaping allows patients to observe their gait from different perspectives as often as they want.[1]

A fascinating approach to the use of movies in patient education has been developed in one setting, with production of instant color movies taken through the endoscope during procedures. Before surgery, patients can see films of similar procedures to help them understand how the procedure can be done without an incision. After surgery, viewing their own films can help them understand how the surgery was done and help them know why they should follow discharge instructions even though they do not feel sick.[37]

In addition the teacher can use the patient's own cardiac catheterization film to teach him and his family about the extent of or the absence of cardiac problems. This approach eliminates generic information in other educational tools that may not be immediately useful to a particular patient. The information can be particularly helpful when a decision has to be made. Often, patients need concrete evidence to accept their diagnoses or before they can consider treatment options.[6]

Two reviews have summarized studies of television's power to produce an effect in patient education.[19,35] Video is as effective as other presentations. The most suitable educational applications

of television are that (1) it presents powerful role models of particular behavior, attitudes, and values; (2) it presents vivid, active illustrative material not otherwise readily available; and (3) it provides direct feedback about a learner's performance of complex interpersonal and psychomotor skills (this assumes the person's performance is videotaped). From a practical point of view, videos are produced cheaply and can be tailor-made for a given patient population. Using video ensures a standard level of teaching. Finally, video can be effective now because of the high rate of functional illiteracy in the United States and because people probably are oriented more to viewing than to reading.

Audiotapes and phone teaching

In earlier sections of this book, the Cancer Information Service, a toll-free phone information program, was described. In addition, local hospitals, associations, and medical societies have sponsored dial-access systems that play audiotapes for callers. Such systems serve as links between symptomatic people and the health care system.

In some instructional situations audiotape is the best technique to use. For example, it provides an accurate portrayal of verbal behavior without the distraction of the accompanying nonverbal behavior that is a part of communication. The audiotape was used well by a nurse whose patient had to learn to do long-term (16 months) parenteral hyperalimentation at home. The nurse, in addition to supervision, dictated the entire procedure onto a cassette audiotape to assist the patient in managing the numerous complicated steps. The tape allowed time for the patient to perform each step. When the patient became more adept, the tape was redictated at a faster pace. After several weeks, the patient was able to proceed confidently without the tape.[5]

Screening and preparing teaching materials

All materials must be viewed and evaluated before they are used for teaching. If a teacher rents the video, a preview is necessary because video catalogs usually do not comment on the quality of the presentation. Also, catalogs do not provide sufficient description of the content of the video so that a teacher can know before viewing whether a particular video supports the objectives of a lesson. If the teacher wants children to know the kinds of agents to use to clean their teeth, he or she needs to know ahead of the class if the video on toothbrushing presents this information adequately. If it does not, the teacher needs time to find other ways of presenting the material. This kind of detail is necessary for planning the class.

Previewing is also necessary to identify material that the teacher believes is incorrect or is contradictory to other sources being used. If the children have been taught that both nylon and natural bristles on toothbrushes are acceptable, yet the movie strongly recommends only natural bristles, the learner is confused. If the teacher must explain too many contradictions, it may be better to omit the video and substitute another video or substitute a teacher presentation. It also is possible, of course, that the error may have been in the teacher's presentation—a circumstance that underscores the need for careful preparation. It may be necessary to reject an audiovisual aid because it is beyond the level of the learners' understanding or because the aid may be peripheral to the objectives. A video that explains the chemical and microbiologic formation of calculus may only detract if the main objective is to learn the motions for brushing the teeth.

Figure 7-11 shows a visual aid poster made by a student. It was originally done with white lettering and pink lungs on a black background—a good combination for catching the learner's attention. The size was 28 by 22 inches—large enough to be seen by several viewers at once. The objective of this poster was to increase understanding of the role of coughing, turning, and deep breathing to ensure health in the lungs.

Presenting the lungs drawn inside the chest in a series of posters or presenting the lungs in motion on video can demonstrate the process of coughing, turning, and deep breathing and the subsequent effect this movement has on secretions in the lung. Such a demonstration would explain the differences and similarities in the lungs' functions. In this poster all three drawings look alike. The error in drawing three lobes for the left lung is not serious in the attainment of the objective. Extension of the alveoli and bronchioles to the entire lung surface could clutter the drawing; however, it should have been made clear that other areas of the lung could become involved.

These errors could have been anticipated by a knowledgeable teacher, particularly if he or she had asked a colleague to check the materials. Other errors resulting in learner misconceptions do not become evident until the materials are used. It is difficult for even an experienced teacher to view the materials from numerous perspectives. Thus constant evaluation of audiovisual aids, as well as other teaching techniques, determines which methods best contribute to learning.

Care providers design and approve visual and written materials for both class and home use. Once these materials have been used by a number of patients, the providers can then review and revise them. Good design, particularly for home use, is important. Those who are most confident in taking their medications often have a schedule posted on the wall at home that describes each medication, the dosage needed, and the time of day that the medicine must be taken. Directions for taking medications that are written on prescription blanks turned in to pharmacies rather than on the containers of medicines that patients receive are not useful. This unhappy occurrence demonstrates the need for carefully planned visual aids, especially those that patients can take with them.

Materials must also be culturally relevant. Hall[22] describes designing materials for Mexican-American clients in the California Diabetes Control Program. Nutrition and diabetes educational materials written in Spanish were frequently literal translations of the English language version. For example, a booklet on diet showed one bread exchange equal to one slice of bread, one half of a bagel, or one half of a cup of cooked cereal. Many Mexican-

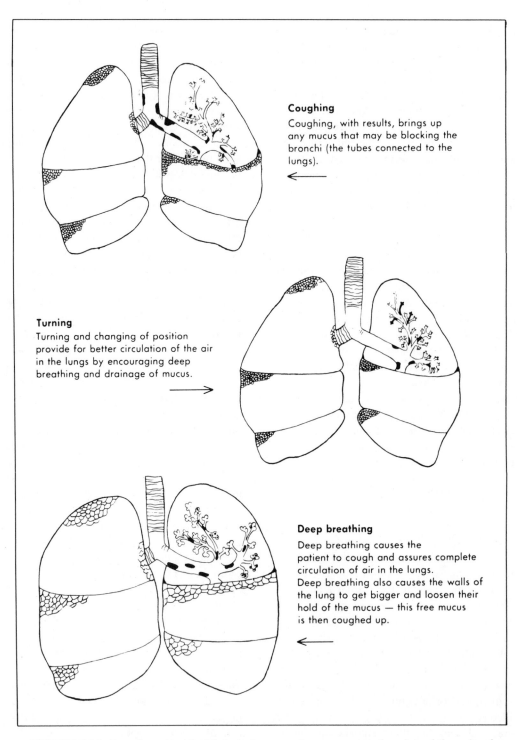

FIGURE 7-11. Sample poster that fails to increase learner comprehension of the role of coughing, turning, and deep breathing in health of the lungs.

Americans have never heard of bagels. Tortillas, the starchy food they use daily, were not mentioned. In the new educational package, pictorial exchange lists were modified to reflect Mexican food habits. If possible, the portion sizes on the exchange list were reworked so that one piece of food (banana) represented one exchange. A simplified measuring system was adopted, using only common household measures. For example, three ounces of meat could be estimated by modeling the palm of the hand. Field testing this new material with a target population should determine its effectiveness.

Developing, testing, and improving teaching materials

Presumably trial and improvement procedures would not be necessary if we had a comprehensive theory of learning that would enable us to design teaching strategies. Using the bits and pieces of partial theories that are available, a teacher constructs the best possible teaching event, tries it out, and, insofar as it fails, improves both the procedure and the materials on the basis of the experience. The following stages are used.[34]

1. *Product formulation.* Focus on the target audience and their perceptions or performance;

IMPORTANT! PLEASE READ THIS NOW AND READ IT AGAIN WHEN YOU GET HOME

Dear patient:

One of your prescriptions is for a medicine called **ampicillin.** There are certain things you should know about this medicine which will help you get well and stay feeling well.

Your doctor wants you to take ampicillin because you may have an infection. There are many kinds of infections, and everybody gets an infection at one time or another.

Infections are caused by germs growing in your body. These germs grow very fast and make more germs just like themselves. Naturally, the way to get rid of the infection is to kill the germs which cause the infection.

When you take your ampicillin medicine it will kill these germs, but it will kill the weakest ones first. After a few days you may begin to feel better, even though the ampicillin has not killed all the strong germs yet. If you stop taking your ampicillin before it kills all of these germs, they will grow fast again and make more strong germs again. **And you may get sick again.**

That is why it is important for you to take **every** capsule of this medicine at the time of day when you are supposed to take it, and why you must keep taking the ampicillin until it is all gone.

Remember, **take every capsule of the ampicillin at the time you are supposed to take it.** If you are going to be away from home for part of the day, take the medicine with you so you won't miss taking the ampicillin during the day.

Remember also, take the ampicillin **until all the capsules are gone.**

Take your ampicillin like this:

Take one capsule **when you get up** in the morning.

Take one capsule **a half hour before lunchtime,** even if you don't eat.

Take one capsule **a half hour before suppertime,** even if you don't eat.

Take one capsule **before you go to bed** at night.

Keep taking the medicine until all of it is gone.

Please save this and refer to it again when you get home.

From Sharpe TR, Mikeal RL: *Am J Hosp Pharm* 31:481, 1974.

prepare a list of tentative objectives and a general strategy for content, media, and presentation.

2. *Product preparation.* List the various teaching tools to be prepared, with objectives for each; develop prototype materials and procedures; field test and revise them.

3. *Product verification.* Arrange a tryout of the materials under conditions approximating those in which the finally developed product will be used, using a pretest measure on each instructional objective; record time spent on program components, teacher-learner behavior, and other relevant measures of student use of the material; use a postassessment measure and release the materials for general use if performance is high on all objectives.

4. *Product revision.* Identify the objectives not well met; from data gathered in the verification step, propose revisions; test the revised version.

In the first two stages it is important to use experts in determining whether the content is important and theoretically sound and whether the objectives are likely to be attainable.

Student data are most important in judging learnability. A more complete testing program should be used when there is no precedent for either the content or teaching method; when learning materials are more complex and expensive; when the materials seek to change attitudes rather than increase knowledge; when materials are designed for long-term rather than short-term use; and when the target audience is large. This involves repetitive tryouts with individuals to identify major errors, repetitive tryouts with small groups, and a field test when the materials are well developed. In preparation of a series of after care instructions developed for emergency room use, developers first investigated the patient population profile (discharge diagnosis, education level). They developed a draft and had the staff review it. Then they pilot tested it with patients and revised it.[11] These forms were also reviewed by the legal department. These clinicians used a form of product development appropriate for the kinds of materials they were developing, especially if revision cycles were pursued as long as necessary to obtain a good product.

SUMMARY

Providers doing patient education will find a plethora of certain kinds of educative materials for patients but almost none for other patient needs. No comprehensive mechanisms exist for cataloging or evaluating the effectiveness of patient education materials. Therefore it is important for individual providers to analyze and possibly alter those that exist or to construct new materials, using a process that optimizes their teaching effectiveness.

STUDY QUESTIONS

1. Consider the pamphlet in Figure 7-2 (pp. 152 and 153). What objectives could be met or partially met by use of this pamphlet?

2. The following terms were used in the index of a catalog of community nurse services. Each of these words or phrases was found by some patients to be difficult to understand. Indicate an alternative for each item, and then turn to the suggested answers in the Appendix for a list of the alternatives suggested by the users of this index.[48]

Maternity care
a. Menstruation
b. Father's role
c. Adjustment to parenthood
d. Uterus
e. Episiotomy care
f. Signs of illness in pregnancy
g. Fetal growth
h. Conception
i. Antepartum
j. Postpartum
k. Mood swing
l. Anesthesia
Infant care
a. Layette
b. Genitals
c. Weaning
d. Immunizations
e. Growth and development
Child care
a. Sibling rivalry
b. Enuresis
c. Communicable disease
d. Peer relationships
e. Socialization

Family planning
   a. Birth control
   b. How to control pregnancy
   c. IUD
   d. Condom
   e. Anatomy and physiology
3. Provide a critique of the information sheet on p. 175 used with adults who received a prescription of ampicillin.
4. Patients with gout were tested for knowledge based on having read a particular booklet on gout, half having used an unillustrated booklet and half a booklet with the same text but illustrated with 89 cartoons. No significant difference was observed either in the overall test scores between the two groups or between individual question scores. The author suggests that possible reasons for these findings include a strong interest factor of patients reading about their own disease and technical factors such as page layout and picture-text imbalance.[33] What other possible reasons for these findings can you think of?

REFERENCES

1. Alexander J, Goodrich R: Videotape immediate playback: a tool in rehabilitation of persons with amputations, *Arch Phys Med Rehabil* 59:141-144, 1978.
2. American Lung Association: *Chronic cough: the facts about your lungs,* New York, 1986, The Association.
3. Amiran MR, Jones BF: Toward a new definition of readability, *Educ Psychol* 17:13-50, 1982.
4. Anthony ML: Difficult decision—a family teaching aid, *Nursing* 16(8):55, 1986.
5. Baker DI: Hyperalimentation at home, *Am J Nurs* 74:1826-1829, 1974.
6. Billiard SJ, Beattie S: A nontraditional approach to cardiac education: the use of cardiac catheterization films, *Prog Cardiovasc Nurs* 5:21-25, 1990.
7. Burkle WS, Lucarotti RL: Videotaped patient medication instruction program using closed-circuit television, *Am J Hosp Pharm* 41:105-107, 1984.
8. Burnett KF, Taylor CB, Agras WS: Ambulatory computer-assisted therapy for obesity: a new frontier for behavior therapy, *J Consult Clin Psychol* 53:698-703, 1985.
9. Carroll JB: *The potentials and limitations of print as a medium of instruction,* National Society for the Study of Education Yearbook, Part I, Chicago, 1974, The Society.
10. Chanoch LH, Jovanovic L, Peterson CM: The evaluation of a pocket computer as an aid to insulin dose determination by patients, *Diabetes Care* 8:172-175, 1985.
11. Danis DM: Aftercare instruction: an overview, *J Emerg Nurs* 7(1):31-32, 1981.
12. Davis TC and others: The gap between patient reading comprehension and the readability of patient education materials, *J Fam Pract* 31:533-538, 1990.
13. Dixon E, Park R: Do patients understand written health information? *Nurs Outlook* 38:278-281, 1990.
14. Doak CC, Doak LG, Root JH: *Teaching patients with low literacy skills,* Philadelphia, 1985, JB Lippincott.
15. Doak LG, Doak CC: Lowering the silent barriers to compliance for patients with low literacy skills, *Promoting Health* 8(4):6-8, 1987.
16. Evanoski CAM: Health education for patients with ventricular tachycardia: assessment of readability, *J Cardiovasc Nurs* 4(2):1-6, 1990.
17. Fry E: A readability formula that saves time, *J Reading* 11:513-516, 575-577, 1968.
18. Fry E: A readability formula for short passages, *J Reading* 33:594-597, 1990.
19. Gagliano ME: A literature review on the efficacy of video in patient education, *J Med Educ* 63:785-792, 1988.
20. Glanz K, Rudd J: Readability and content analysis of print cholesterol education materials, *Pat Educ Counsel* 16:109-118, 1990.
21. Gustafson DH and others: Computer-based health promotion: combining technological advances with problem-solving techniques to effect successful health behavior changes, *Annu Rev Public Health* 8:387-415, 1987.
22. Hall TA: Designing culturally relevant educational materials for Mexican American clients, *Diabetes Educator* 13:281-285, 1987.
23. Holt GA and others: OTC labels: can consumers read and understand them? *Am Pharm* NS30(11):51-54, 1990.
24. Kilbride SS: A patient's guide to the implanted port, *Oncol Nurs Forum* 13:83, 85, 1986.
25. Klausmeier HJ: *Educational psychology,* ed 5, Philadelphia, 1985, Harper & Row.
26. Kozma RB: Learning with media, *Rev Educ Res* 61:179-211, 1991.
27. Kulik CC, Kulik JA, Shwalb BJ: The effectiveness of computer-based adult education: a meta-analysis, *J Educ Computing Res* 2:235-251, 1986.
28. Lehman AE, Estok PJ: Screening tool for daily fetal movement, *Nurs Pract* 12:40-44, 1987.
29. Mager RF: *Preparing instructional objectives,* ed 2, Belmont, Calif, 1984, David S Lake.
30. Mathews PJ, Thornton L, McLean L: Reading-level scores of patient education materials and the effect of teaching special vocabulary, *Respir Care* 33:245-249, 1988.
31. Meade CD, Smith CF: Readability formulas: cautions and criteria, *Pat Educ Couns* 17:153-158, 1991.
32. Meade CD, Wittbrot R: Computerized readability analysis of written materials, *Comput Nurs* 6:30-36, 1988.
33. Moll JMH and others: The cartoon in doctor-patient communication: further study of the Arthritis and Rheumatism Council handbook on gout, *Ann Rheum Dis* 36:225-231, 1977.
34. Nathanson MB, Henderson ES: *Using student feedback to improve learning materials,* London, 1980, Croom Helm.
35. Nielsen E, Sheppard MA: Television as a patient education tool: a review of its effectiveness, *Pat Educ Couns* 11:3-16, 1988.

36. O'Rourke A: Bone marrow procedure guide, *Oncol Nurs Forum* 13:66-67, 1986.

37. Parker CF: Endoscopic movies for patient teaching, *AORN J* 34:(2):254-257, 1981.

38. Patient America news release, Los Angeles, 1986, Hospital Satellite Network.

39. Pernick NL, Rodbard D: Personal computer programs to assist with self-monitoring of blood glucose and self-adjustment in insulin dosage, *Diabetes Care* 9:61-69, 1986.

40. Richwald GA and others: Are condom instructions readable? Results of a readability study, *Pub Health Rep* 103:355-359, 1988.

41. Ross CK and others: Health promotion programs flourishing: survey, *Hospitals* 59:128-135, 1985.

42. Rubin DH and others: Educational interventions by computer in childhood asthma: a randomized clinical trial testing the use of a new teaching intervention in childhood asthma, *Pediatrics* 77:1-10, 1986.

43. Sharpe TR, Mikeal RL: Patient compliance with antibiotic regimens, *Am J Hosp Pharm* 31:479-484, 1987.

44. Smith JM and others: Survey of computer programs for diabetes management and education, *Diabetes Educator* 15:412-415, 1988.

45. Starn J, Paperny DM: Computer games to enhance adolescent sex education, *MCN Am J Matern Child Nurs* 15:250-253, 1990.

46. Steiff LD: Can clients understand our instructions? *Image* 18:48-52, 1986.

47. Teaching your patient to live with c.o.p.d., *Nurs Life* 5(3):332, 1986.

48. Tiede J and others: *Report of the evaluation of a community nurse's catalogue*, Minneapolis, 1970, Combined Nursing Service.

49. Tosti DT, Ball JR: A behavioral approach to instructional design and media selection, *Audio Vis Commun Rev* 17:5-25, 1969.

50. Walker A: Teaching the illiterate patient, *J Enterostomal Ther* 14:83-86, 1987.

51. Wetstone SL and others: Evaluation of a computer based education lesson for patients with rheumatoid arthritis, *J Rheumatol* 12:907-912, 1985.

52. Wheeler LA and others: Evaluation of computer-based diet education in persons with diabetes mellitus and limited educational background, *Diabetes Care* 8:537-544, 1985.

53. Wheeler LA and others: Betakid—lessons learned while developing a microcomputer pediatric case simulation, *Diabetes Educator* 13:403-405, 1987.

54. Wolitski RJ, Rhodes F: AIDS info on-line: a computer-based information system for college campuses, *J Am Coll Health* 39:90-93, 1990.

55. Zion AB, Aiman J: Level of reading difficulty in The American Colleges of Obstetricians and Gynecologists patient education pamphlets, *Obstet Gynecol* 74:955-959, 1989.

CHAPTER 8

Teaching: planning and implementing

PLANNING

All items necessary for constructing a teaching plan have been introduced. Evaluation, which is also part of the plan, is discussed thoroughly in Chapter 9. Since the purpose of a teaching plan is to force the teacher to examine the relationships among learner receptivity, objectives, content, teaching methods, tools, and evaluation, a plan should be written for all but incidental teaching.

Instructional design

Many instructional design models have been published that were developed mostly from general systems theory and used in job analysis and military training. However, few models have been validated in terms of their ability to improve instruction and reduce the cost of education. The successful models assist greatly in structuring development of educational procedures and materials. An outline for such a model is included in Chapter 7 in the section on materials preparation. An instructional design model described by Merrill, Kowallis, and Wilson includes these elements[3]:

1.1 Analyze job; 1.2 Select task functions; 1.3 Construct job performance measures; 1.4 Analyze existing courses; 1.5 Select instructional setting.
2.1 Develop objectives; 2.2 Develop tests; 2.3 Describe entry behavior; 2.4 Determine sequence and structure.
3.1 Specify learning events/activities; 3.2 Specify instruction management plan and delivery system; 3.3 Review/select materials; 3.4 Develop instruction; 3.5 Validate instruction.
4.1 Implement instructional management plan; 4.2 Conduct instruction.

5.1 Conduct internal evaluation; 5.2 Conduct external evaluation; 5.3 Revise system.

Other approaches, such as hierarchy analysis, are used to break an objective into simpler skills and identify the tasks that can be developed through instruction. Recent trends reflect a switch of focus in learning theory from behavioral to cognitive theory. In an attempt to develop a technology to improve learning and to test theories of cognitive learning, attention is being paid to strategies for analyzing the logical structure of the subject matter to be learned, including ways of mapping an individual learner's schemata or ways of organizing a thought.

Reports indicate that using the systems approach for designing instruction has not had a major impact on education except for organizations doing major materials development. Although use of a design can be expensive for individual teachers and small teams working on educational development projects,[12] functioning without a design model does not provide structured analysis of an educational problem or feedback on its solution. An analysis and feedback system should be initiated for teaching plans that will be used extensively, just as resources are used to validate instructional materials that are widely used.

Designing instruction plans that will motivate learners is important. Keller[2] has developed a model describing four conditions that enable people to become and to remain motivated: attention, relevance, confidence, and satisfaction (ARCS). Strategies to incorporate these motivating elements in the design of instruction are detailed in Table 8-

1. Using appropriate stimuli is central to getting and sustaining attention. Relevance is established by the content of the lesson or by the way the subject is taught. Such a device helps the learner form an impression that some degree of success is possible if effort is exerted. Satisfaction involves providing appropriate contingencies for the learner.

To begin, the caregiver must identify motivational gaps in the audience and use the model to prepare instruction that will address those gaps. If people are already motivated, motivational strategies need not be included in the instruction.

Text continued on p. 185.

TABLE 8-1. The ARCS model by Keller

Attention strategies

A1: *Incongruity, Conflict*
    A1.1   Introduce a fact that seems to contradict the learner's past experience.
    A1.2   Present an example that does not seem to exemplify a given concept.
    A1.3   Introduce two equally plausible facts or principles, only one of which can be true.
    A1.4   Play devil's advocate.

A2: *Concreteness*
    A2.1   Show visual representations of any important object or set of ideas or relationships.
    A2.2   Give examples of every instructionally important concept or principle.
    A2.3   Use content-related anecdotes, case studies, biographies, etc.

A3: *Variability*
    A3.1   In stand up delivery, vary the tone of your voice, and use body movement, pauses, and props.
    A3.2   Vary the format of instruction (information presentation, practice, testing, etc.) according to the attention span of the audience.
    A3.3   Vary the medium of instruction (platform delivery, film, video, print, etc.)
    A3.4   Break up print materials by use of white space, visuals, tables, different typefaces, etc.
    A3.5   Change the style of presentation (humorous-serious, fast-slow, loud-soft, active-passive, etc.).
    A3.6   Shift between student-instructor interaction and student-student interaction.

A4: *Humor*
    A4.1   Where appropriate, use plays on words during redundant information presentation.
    A4.2   Use humorous introductions.
    A4.3   Use humorous analogies to explain and summarize.

A5: *Inquiry*
    A5.1   Use creativity techniques to have learners create unusual analogies and associations to the content.
    A5.2   Build in problem solving activities at regular intervals.
    A5.3   Give learners the opportunity to select topics, projects, and assignments that appeal to their curiosity and need to explore.

A6: *Participation*
    A6.1   Use games, role plays, or simulations that require learner participation.

From Keller JM: *J Instruc Dev* 10(3):2-10, 1987.

TABLE 8-1. The ARCS model by Keller—cont'd

<hr>

Relevance strategies

R1: *Experience*
  R1.1 State explicitly how the instruction builds on the learner's existing skills.
  R1.2 Use analogies familiar to the learner from past experience.
  R1.3 Find out what the learners' interests are and relate them to the instruction.

R2: *Present Worth*
  R2.1 State explicitly the present intrinsic value of learning the content, as distinct from its value as a link to future goals.

R3: *Future Usefulness*
  R3.1 State explicitly how the instruction relates to future activities of the learner.
  R3.2 Ask learners to relate the instruction to their own future goals (future wheel).

R4: *Need Matching*
  R4.1 To enhance achievement striving behavior, provide opportunities to achieve standards of excellence under conditions of moderate risk.
  R4.2 To make instruction responsive to the power motive, provide opportunities for responsibility, authority, and interpersonal influence.
  R4.3 To satisfy the need for affiliation, establish trust and provide opportunities for no-risk, cooperative interaction.

R5: *Modeling*
  R5.1 Bring in alumni of the course as enthusiastic guest lecturers.
  R5.2 In a self-paced course, use those who finish first as deputy tutors.
  R5.3 Model enthusiasm for the subject taught.

R6: *Choice*
  R6.1 Provide meaningful alternative methods for accomplishing a goal.
  R6.2 Provide personal choices for organizing one's work.

Confidence strategies

C1: *Learning Requirements*
  C1.1 Incorporate clearly stated, appealing learning goals into instructional materials.
  C1.2 Provide self-evaluation tools that are based on clearly stated goals.
  C1.3 Explain the criteria for evaluation of performance.

C2: *Difficulty*
  C2.1 Organize materials on an increasing level of difficulty; that is, structure the learning material to provide a "conquerable" challenge.

C3: *Expectations*
  C3.1 Include statements about the likelihood of success with given amounts of effort and ability.
  C3.2 Teach students how to develop a plan of work that will result in goal accomplishment.
  C3.3 Help students set realistic goals.

<hr>

Continued.

TABLE 8-1. The ARCS model by Keller—cont'd

Confidence strategies—cont'd

C4: Attributions

C4.1 Attribute student success to effort rather than luck or ease of task when appropriate (i.e., when you know it's true!).

C4.2 Encourage student efforts to verbalize appropriate attributions for both successes and failures.

C5: *Self-Confidence*

C5.1 Allow students opportunity to become increasingly independent in learning and practicing a skill.

C5.2 Have students learn new skills under low risk conditions, but practice performance of well-learned tasks under realistic conditions.

C5.3 Help students understand that the pursuit of excellence does not mean that anything short of perfection is failure; learn to feel good about genuine accomplishment.

Satisfaction strategies

S1: *Natural Consequences*

S1.1 Allow a student to use a newly acquired skill in a realistic setting as soon as possible.

S1.2 Verbally reinforce a student's intrinsic pride in accomplishing a difficult task.

S1.3 Allow a student who masters a task to help others who have not yet done so.

S2: *Unexpected Rewards*

S2.1 Reward intrinsically interesting task performance with unexpected, non-contingent rewards.

S2.2 Reward boring tasks with extrinsic, anticipated rewards.

S3: *Positive Outcomes*

S3.1 Give verbal praise for successful progress or accomplishment.

S3.2 Give personal attention to students.

S3.3 Provide informative, helpful feedback when it is immediately useful.

S3.4 Provide motivating feedback (praise) immediately following task performance.

S4: *Negative Influences*

S4.1 Avoid the use of threats as a means of obtaining task performance.

S4.2 Avoid surveillance (as opposed to positive attention)

S4.3 Avoid external performance evaluations whenever it is possible to help the student evaluate his or her own work.

S5: *Scheduling*

S5.1 Provide frequent reinforcements when a student is learning a new task.

S5.2 Provide intermittent reinforcement as a student becomes more competent at a task.

S5.3 Vary the schedule of reinforcements in terms of both interval and quantity.

CATEGORIES OF THE EXPERIENTIAL TAXONOMY

1.00 Exposure

Consciousness of an experience. This involves two levels of exposure and a readiness for further experience.

1.10 *Sensory*

Through various sensory stimuli one is exposed to the possibility of an experience.

1.20 *Response*

Peripheral mental reaction to sensory stimuli. At this point, one rejects or accepts further interaction with the experience.

1.30 *Readiness*

At this level one has accepted the experience and anticipates participation in it.

2.00 Participation

The decision to become physically a part of an experience. There are two levels of interaction within this category.

2.10 *Representation*

Reproducing, mentally and/or physically, an existing mental image of the experience, that is, through visualizing, role playing, or dramatic play. This can be done covertly or overtly.

2.20 *Modification*

With the input of past personal activities, the experience develops and grows. As there is a personal input in the participation, one moves from role player to active participant.

3.00 Identification

The coming together of the learner and the idea (objective) in an emotional and intellectual context for the achievement of the objective.

3.10 *Reinforcement*

As the experience is modified and repeated, it is reinforced through a decision to identify with the experience.

3.20 *Emotional*

The participant becomes emotionally identified with the experience. It becomes "my experience."

3.30 *Personal*

The participant moves from an emotional identification to an intellectual commitment that involves a rational decision to identify.

3.40 *Sharing*

Once the process of identification is accomplished, the participant begins to share the experience with others, as an important factor in his life. This kind of positive sharing continues into and through Category 4.00 (internalization).

4.00 Internalization

The participant moves from identification to internalization when the experience begins to affect the life-style of the participant. There are two levels in this category.

From Steinaker NW, Bell MR: *The experiential taxonomy: a new approach to teaching and learning,* New York, 1979, Academic Press. *Continued.*

CATEGORIES OF THE EXPERIENTIAL TAXONOMY—cont'd

4.00 Internalization—cont'd

4.10 *Expansion*

The experience enlarges into many aspects of the participant's life, changing attitudes and activities. When these changes become more than temporary, the participant moves to the next category.

4.20 *Intrinsic*

The experience characterizes the participant's life-style more consistently than during the expansion level.

5.00 Dissemination

The experience moves beyond internalization to the dissemination of experience. It goes beyond the positive sharing that began at Level 3.00 and involves two levels of activity.

5.10 *Informational*

The participant informs others about the experience and seeks to stimulate others to have an equivalent experience through descriptive and personalized sharing.

5.20 *Homilectic*

The participant sees the experience as imperative for others.

Taxonomic level	Teaching role model	Learning principles
1.00 Exposure	Motivator	1. Extrinsic motivation
		2. Focusing
		3. Anxiety level
2.00 Participation	Catalyst	1. Initial guidance
		2. Meaning exploration
		3. Chance for success
3.00 Identification	Moderator	1. Personal interaction
		2. Knowledge of results
		3. Reinforcement
4.00 Internalization	Sustainer	1. Overlearning
		2. Intrinsic transfer
		3. Differentiated input
5.00 Dissemination	Critique	1. Extrinsic transfer
		2. Reward
		3. Intrinsic motivation

Experiential taxonomy

Patients who need to make major changes in their lives will discover that experiential taxonomy[9] (box on pp. 183 and 184) is useful in guiding long-term development. It describes the sequential stages of a person's experiences with an issue or problem. These descriptions are particularly important in health teaching. Major changes may take a long time, and patients are seen by the caregiver intermittently, making it difficult to keep track of their progress (or lack of it) as they experience health problems or health strengths. The table below the taxonomy summarizes major teaching tasks and learning principles applicable to each stage.

The experience referred to in this taxonomy is a positive educational experience that also may be a health experience with a planned educational component. A program for rehabilitation of a group of patients might produce instruction for the full experiential development, follow patients longitudinally, and assist with appropriate instruction to help move each patient to the next stage when possible. This is preferable to giving each patient instruction at the time of an acute physical problem and considering future interactions to be primarily supportive instead of developmental.

TEACHING PLANS

Teaching plans can be written in many formats. The major criterion for judging a format is whether it clearly states the various elements of the teaching process. Are the relationships among assessment-readiness, objectives, teaching actions, and content and evaluation clear? Is the format easy to follow in the urgent state created by teaching in a busy clinical situation? When teaching and learning are a major intervention, it is possible to construct a separate teaching plan. Usually, teaching-learning will be incorporated into the general nursing care plan. Two examples appear in the boxes on pp. 186 through 191.

Both examples use nursing diagnoses, desired or expected outcomes, and nursing actions or interventions.[8,11] The examples by Shotkin, Boer, and Norton use a columnar format that allows eas-

ier visualization of the relationships among the elements. Although not explicit, both care plans assume an assessment of need and a readiness to learn—a desirable element when coupled with assessment questions or tools. Both examples include clearly stated outcomes that serve as objectives, as well as criteria for evaluation; however, they do not include helpful evaluation tools. If the patient does not meet crucial outcomes, reteaching with altered strategies is necessary. Clearly, the level of organized detail in these plans is preferable to sketchy notes or to no plan whatsoever.

The curriculum for the sibling-to-be program (Table 8-2) provides a plan for a teaching program and includes objectives, content, teacher activity, and learner activity.[1] The objectives include the outcomes desired from the lesson, as well as the process the child must follow to learn. Note how learning principles are used. Reinforcement and attention build motivation. Puppetry, storytelling, imitative role playing, and play are necessary to enable the child to express feelings about newborns and to feel as important as the new baby. This lesson plan format does not direct evaluation. Neither plan focuses on assessment of learner motivation and readiness. Clearer evaluation activities would be helpful.

Keeping a log book of lesson plans is useful. After each class the provider can write comments describing which approaches and teaching tools worked and which ones did not work, noting ideas for improvement.

Forms that are specific to education are often developed to aid communication among health team members about teaching. An example of such forms used by St. Francis Hospital may be seen in Figure 8-1.[4] The form demonstrates a more detailed teaching plan. Some institutions have attempted to use generic teaching chart forms. A provider fills in the content.

Because hospital stays have been made as brief as possible, both preadmission teaching and good preparation for discharge have become tremendously important. Rice and Johnson found that patients provided with preoperative, preadmission

Text continued on p. 197.

TEACHING PROGRAM FOR PATIENTS WITH LOW-BACK PAIN

Nursing care plan

Nursing diagnosis	Expected outcomes	Nursing interventions
1) Knowledge deficit related to:		
a) Diagnostic procedures	Patient will authorize diagnostic procedures based on informed consent	Provide written teaching modules and discuss information regarding all diagnostic procedures
b) Anatomy of the back	By discharge, patient will verbalize knowledge of anatomy of the back By discharge, patient will verbalize relationship of nerves and muscles to back pain	Assess readiness of learner Offer written teaching modules "Anatomy of the Back" and "Anatomy of the Intervertebral Disc" when appropriate Reinforce teaching as required
c) Self-care related to home care	By discharge, the patient will: Demonstrate proper body mechanics related to sitting, lifting, and work activities Demonstrate proper posture Demonstrate proper exercise program Verbalize importance of lifetime back and abdominal exercise program Verbalize importance of proper weight in controlling back pain Verbalize action and side effects of any prescribed medications	Provide and review teaching module "Back Facts" with patient Observe posture during activities and make appropriate recommendations Observe patient performance of exercises Provide written teaching module "Home Care Advice" Weigh patient weekly; consult the dietician if needed Provide written teaching modules regarding medication patient is receiving
2) Potential for anxiety/ineffective coping related to stressor of chronic illness	By discharge patient will: Demonstrate adaptive coping strategies and behavior responses Verbalize role stress plays in pain intensity	Refer patient as appropriate to the Wellness Center Reinforce relaxation techniques Psychiatric referral as necessary
3) Alteration in comfort: Chronic low-back pain related to unknown origin	By discharge the patient will: Experience comfort by using a variety of pain relief measures Verbalize five keys to preventing back pain: rest, exercise, proper body mechanics, proper lifting, and proper posture	Provide written teaching module "The Pain Cycle" Have patient verbalize activities and situations that increase and decrease pain Have patient verbalize proper use of prescribed medications

From Shotkin JD, Bolt B, Norton DA: *J Neurosci Nurs* 19:240-243, 1987.

TEACHING PROGRAM FOR PATIENTS WITH LOW-BACK PAIN—cont'd

4) Potential for maladjustment due to changes in lifestyle secondary to chronic back pain

Patient will adjust to lifestyle on an ongoing basis

At discharge patient will state resources if not coping effectively

Provide written teaching module "Sexual Information" as appropriate

Have patient verbalize resources available if pain increases

Assist patient in prioritizing activities, setting aside time for rest periods

Emphasize importance of using most rested times to accomplish tasks of highest priority

---

STANDARD NURSING CARE PLAN

1. Nursing diagnosis   **Difficulty adapting to life-style changes related to peripheral arterial occlusive disease**

Desired outcomes
1. Accepts the necessary life-style changes
2. Maintains a positive self-concept
3. Uses support available within the family and community

Nursing actions
1. Assesses patient's strengths and abilities
2. Assesses family's strengths and nature of support available
3. Explains reasons for the life-style changes
4. Discusses with patient and family members their fears, hopes, and frustrations
5. Explains importance of using existing family and community resources
6. Involves patient in decision-making to help maintain a feeling of control
7. Arranges a family conference
8. Refers to community health nurse

Evaluation
1. Initiates necessary life-style changes
2. Uses positive coping behavior in adapting to life-style changes and family role relations
3. Exhibits feelings of self-sufficiency and control
4. Explains plans for using existing resources

2. Nursing diagnosis   **Progressive peripheral arterial occlusive disease related to cigarette smoking**

Desired outcomes
1. Understands the effect of smoking on the peripheral arterial system
2. Stops smoking
3. Knows available community support groups

From Warbineck E, Wyness MA: *Cardiovasc Nurs* 22:6-11, 1986.   *Continued.*

STANDARD NURSING CARE PLAN—cont'd

Nursing actions	1. Encourages discussion of feelings related to smoking. If appropriate, involves family
	2. —Explains the effects of smoking on the heart and arteries: —tobacco constricts blood vessels —inhibits ability of blood to carry oxygen
	3. Explains that more exercise will be tolerated if smoking stops
	4. Provides literature on the hazards of smoking
	5. Discusses ways to decrease the number of cigarettes smoked or to stop smoking entirely
	6. Provides information on community support groups
	7. Explains that individual may experience increased warmth in legs and feet
Evaluation	1. States accurately the effects of smoking on the heart and arteries
	2. States names of community support groups
	3. Describes plans to stop smoking
	4. Stops smoking and displays a positive attitude towards it
3. Nursing diagnosis	Increased blood lipids related to dietary fat intake
Desired outcomes	1. Knows relationship between lipids and atherosclerosis
	2. Participates in developing a low-fat diet plan
	3. Before discharge, describes how he will adhere to his diet
	4. Maintains a desirable body weight
	5. Knows names of community support groups
Nursing actions	1. Teaches patient and family the importance of reducing total fat intake to less than 30% of total caloric intake by restricting eggs, meat, and whole-milk products
	2. Encourages the patient and family to eat poultry, fish, and skim-milk products
	3. Discusses substituting margarine and other vegetable fat for animal fat, thus reducing saturated fat intake
	4. Teaches importance of reducing sugar consumption to 10% of total calories
	5. Teaches importance of no added salt in the diet
	6. Arranges consultation with a dietician
	7. Provides written information on accepted diet plan
	8. Reinforces dietary pattern which maintains desirable body weight
	9. If patient is overweight, discusses weight reduction, including the following: —reducing portion sizes rather than eliminating favorite food in order to enjoy the taste and eat the same foods as the family —curtailing the use of margarine and butter —reducing consumption of alcohol —increasing fiber content, vegetables and fruit providing bulk but few calories —joining a support group such as a weight control group

STANDARD NURSING CARE PLAN—cont'd

Evaluation	1. Knows why dietary fat should be decreased

Evaluation
1. Knows why dietary fat should be decreased
2. Suggests ways to decrease fat intake
3. States plans for keeping track of caloric intake, including amounts of fat, sugar and salt
4. Weighs self weekly and continues to lose weight to reach and maintain desirable weight
5. States names of at least two community resources

4. Nursing diagnosis   **Lack of exercise related to peripheral arterial occlusive disease**

Desired outcomes
1. Explains the importance of a regular exercise program in maintaining patency of arteries
2. Participates in the development of a realistic exercise program

Nursing actions
1. Gives patient a diagram of the arteries in the legs and marks sites of blockage
2. Explains how collateral circulation develops
3. Plans with physician an appropriate exercise program
4. Discusses the importance of physical activity in improving mental outlook
5. Explains the importance of walking as a stimulus for collateral circulation if performed twice a day for 20 minutes or more, including the following points:
   —Flat surface walking is best
   —Walking at an easy pace to warm up
   —If pain occurs, stopping and resting, then continuing
   —Slowing down (cool down phase) rather than stopping suddenly to avoid cramps
   —Gradually increasing distance walked
6. Gives information on planned activity programs in the community

Evaluation
1. States the importance of daily exercise
2. Plans activities to include regular flat surface walking
3. Experiences less claudication pain
4. Reports improved mental outlook; feels and looks better

5. Nursing diagnosis   **Impotence caused by ischemia or surgery**

Desired outcomes
1. Understands the reason for the impotence
2. Knows alternative ways of providing sexual fulfillment for his partner
3. Maintains a positive self-concept

Nursing actions
1. Encourages patient and partner to discuss their feelings about this loss of sexual functioning
2. Discusses with the physician the possibility of a penile prosthesis
3. Discusses with patient and partner alternative ways of expressing affection, other than through sexual intercourse
4. Arranges consultation with sex therapist

Continued.

STANDARD NURSING CARE PLAN—cont'd

Evaluation	1. Discusses feelings about his sexual role
	2. Is willing to express feelings and to try alternative ways of demonstrating affection

6. Nursing diagnosis   **Calf pain caused by muscle ischemia during exercise**

Desired outcomes
1. Understands the reason pain occurs
2. Takes appropriate action to cope with pain

Nursing actions
1. Explains that during exercise the calf muscles receive an inadequate amount of blood because of narrowing or blockage of the arteries
2. Explains that rest reduces the need of muscles for blood and relieves pain
3. Explains that exercise promotes adequate circulation and formation of collateral (secondary) blood vessels
4. Reinforces patient's current exercise pattern if it is appropriate
5. Identifies with the patient ways to cope with pain including the following:
   —Rest when pain occurs and until it is relieved
   —Alter pace of walking
   —Walk on flat surfaces
   —Combine activities to reduce distance walked
6. Designs with the patient a regular exercise routine within limits of claudication pain

Evaluation
1. Makes accurate statements of cause of pain and ways to cope with pain
2. Uses behaviors to reduce pain and promote circulation

7. Nursing diagnosis   **Persistent throbbing leg pain caused by ischemia**

Desired outcomes
1. Understands chronic nature of pain
2. Develops ways to prevent social isolation and depression

Nursing actions
1. Explains that pain is caused by inadequate blood supply to tissues because of narrowing or blockage of arteries
2. Asks patient to try distraction and relaxation techniques to reduce pain
3. Designs with the patient an appropriate plan for analgesic use
4. Reinforces patient's current coping behaviors for pain if effective
5. Identifies with the patient ways to promote circulation and reduce pain
   —Elevate head of bed on 4 to 6 inch blocks
   —Sit with feet dependent
   —Use padded bed cradle or footboard if weight of bedcovers increases pain
   —Maintain warm environment without extremes of heat and cold
6. Expects patient to participate in decision-making regarding measures to reduce pain
7. Positively reinforces independence in activities of daily living
8. Designs activities to provide variety and stimulation throughout the day
9. Communicates caring concern regarding patient's pain

```
┌─────────────────────────────────────────────────────────────────────────────┐
│                      STANDARD NURSING CARE PLAN—cont'd                        │
│                                                                               │
│   Evaluation        1. Gives accurate statements of cause of pain and degree  │
│                        of pain relief that is achievable                      │
│                     2. Utilizes techniques that are effective in reducing pain│
│                     3. Demonstrates interest in various activities and        │
│                        appropriate level of independence                      │
└─────────────────────────────────────────────────────────────────────────────┘
```

TABLE 8-2. Curriculum for the sibling-to-be program

Objectives	Content	Methodology—teacher activity	Learner activity
Session one			
The child will be involved in class activities and discussions; watch a film about a sibling-to-be; identify an image of family and the interrelationships within a family; identify feelings and concepts of newborn, family, and siblinghood; express feelings verbally and through play; and complete an at-home play activity	Introduction of teacher, Ernie, and siblings-to-be Prebirth and postbirth experiences Characteristics and concepts of newborn Concept of family Common feelings about siblinghood	Demonstration/show Audiovisual presentation: *Nicholas and the Baby* Puppetry Informal discussions Play activity: draw family Experience story about family drawing Read experience story to class Application and reinforcement through at-home play activity and lending library Handouts: annotated bibliography of children's literature and class narrative for parents Encourage group involvement	Sits on floor with group of children Verbalizes name Writes name tag or dictates to teacher Watches film in the group Verbalizes about film Expresses concept of drawing and verbalizes feelings through experience story Completes play project at home (cutouts of pictures of family, mothers, fathers, and babies)

From Honig JC: *MCN* 11:37-43, 1986.   *Continued.*

TABLE 8-2. Curriculum for the sibling-to-be program—cont'd

Objectives	Content	Methodology—teacher activity	Learner activity
Session two			
The child will become familiar with the birth process, some child care techniques, and characteristics and concepts of newborns; role-play and imitate child care techniques; express feelings about newborns, verbally and nonverbally; and be involved in class activities.	Reintroduction of teacher, Ernie, and siblings-to-be Discussion of the cutouts Children and teacher's concept of pregnancy, birth, and newborn Techniques of child care, including diapering, holding, breast-feeding, and bottle-feeding Newborn characteristics, including crying, feeding, sleeping, limited communication, not a playmate at first	Reinforcement of at-home project; application of continued project Reading of picture book on prebirth, birth, and newborn Use of vicarious sensory experiences with visual and symbolic representations (three-dimensional, life-sized pelvis; stuffed fetus with umbilical cord and placenta that detach; knitted uterus with doll that emerges as in birth; vivid photographs covered with clear plastic to encourage touching and feeling) Informal discussion and questions Imitative role playing and symbolic play with "infant" (doll or stuffed animal for each child) Puppetry and storytelling about concepts of newborn	Participates in show-and-tell about cutouts Listens to and looks at a picture book about pre-birth, birth, and newborn while in the group Assimilates concepts through looking at, touching, and interacting with visual and symbolic aids Participates individually in role playing and imitation Listens to Ernie's story Answers and asks questions and verbalizes feelings and concepts about newborns, birth, and sibling-hood Completes play project at home by pasting cutouts on large white paper

TABLE 8-2. Curriculum for the sibling-to-be program—cont'd

Objectives	Content	Methodology—teacher activity	Learner activity
Session three			
The child will identify consistent and transient aspects of his or her life; verbalize consistent objects, "special" people, and transitory objects and express feelings about them; be aware of future separation from mother at the time of birth; identify with Ernie and feel as important as the new baby; participate actively in the expectant family; and make a present to give the new sibling	Reintroduction of teacher, Ernie, and siblings-to-be Discussion of the collage, including the notion of it as a gift for the new baby Aspects of child's life that are consistent (grandparents, aunts and uncles, school, teachers, classmates, and special toys) Aspects of child's life that are transient ("baby things," bottles, pacifiers, crib, carriage, and high chair) Separation from mother (necessity, not a punishment, fatigue of mother and baby after "work" of birth, body is made for this "work," loneliness, sadness and anger, availability of telephone calls, and sibling visitation) Aspects of being a "big" brother or sister, advantages of an older sibling, and capabilities of an older sibling Birthday party to celebrate becoming a "big" sibling	Reinforcement of at-home project Informal discussion and questions Puppetry and storytelling on consistency and transition, separation, and being a "big" sibling Birthday party Formal acknowledgement of class participation with a certificate and a T-shirt imprinted with "I am a big brother or big sister"	Participates in show-and-tell about collages Listens to and identifies with Ernie's story Thinks about and verbalizes consistent and transient aspects of own life Assimilates concepts of separation and its individual impact on child Begins conceptualization of being a sibling through verbalizing, participating, and asking questions Participates in party for family Receives certificate and T-shirt to take home

TEACHING PLAN: Radiation Therapy, Management of Side Effects Implemented: Revised: GENERAL GOALS: Pt./family will understand side effects which may occur with radiation therapy and will have information to manage them.							INIT	SIGNATURE
	IMPLEMENTATION				EVALUATION			
PLANNED LEARNING OBJECTIVES	QUESTIONS ANSWERED	INFORMA-TION PROVIDED	TASK DEMON-STRATED	NOT APPLI-CABLE	NEEDS INSTRUC-TIONS	OBJECTIVE MET		REMARKS
After instruction and review of ACS booklet, "Radiation Therapy and You"								
1. Patient/family will describe expected side effects of radiation therapy.								
2. Patient/family will recognize signs and symptons of dose limiting toxicities for which they should notify physician.								
3. Patient/family will discuss methods to prevent or manage side effects using appropriate instruction sheets as reference:								
—skin reaction —nausea/vomiting —loss of appetite/taste changes —leukopenia —thrombocytopenia —stomatitis —constipation —diarrhea —fatigue —hair loss								

FIGURE 8-1. Sample teaching plan for patient receiving radiation therapy. (From Myers JS and others: *Oncol Nurs Forum* 14:95-99, 1987.)

Teaching content	Time frame	
	Initiated	Completed
1. Community health nursing referral	_____	_____
2. Social service referral	_____	_____
3. Assessment	_____	_____
a. Family assessment	_____	_____
b. Family and babysitter roles	_____	_____
c. Family member's physical conditions	_____	_____
d. Parental feelings regarding home monitoring	_____	_____
e. Motivation for home monitoring	_____	_____
f. Identified supports/coping strategies	_____	_____
g. Financial status; insurance coverage	_____	_____
h. Access to medical care	_____	_____
i. Educational level (reading skills, ability to learn)	_____	_____
Planning	_____	_____
1. Interdisciplinary conference with family	_____	_____
Implementation	_____	_____
1. Meeting with another apnea monitoring family in home	_____	_____

	Initial instruction completed	Parents verbalize and demonstrate
2. Preparing the home environment		
a. Adequate electrical outlets or adaptors	_____	_____
b. Solid/flat surface for monitor placement	_____	_____
c. Plan for phone access 24 hr/day	_____	_____
d. Supplies available near the monitor: record sheets, pen, batteries, flashlight	_____	_____
e. Parents have contacted appropriate departments: telephone company, electric company, fire department (emergency medical services), police department	_____	_____
3. Care of the monitored infant:	_____	_____
a. Attaching the child to the monitor: lead or belt placement	_____	_____
b. Responding to alarms: 10 seconds	_____	_____
c. Infant resuscitation techniques:		
1. Observe color, chest movement, precipitating events, alleviating factors, response to treatment, length of episode.	_____	_____
2. First stimulate gently, then more vigorously.	_____	_____
3. CPR	_____	_____
d. Using log at home to record above data	_____	_____
e. Troubleshooting techniques with the monitor	_____	_____
1. Loose lead	_____	_____
2. Improper lead or belt placement	_____	_____
3. Infant movement/pulling off lead	_____	_____
4. False alarms	_____	_____

FIGURE 8-2. Nursing discharge planning tool for families planning home apnea monitoring. (From Norris-Berkemeyer S, Hutchins HK: *Pediatr Nurs* 12:259-304, 1986.)

Continued.

Teaching content	Time frame	
	Initiated	Completed
5. Dry electrodes	_____	
6. Sensitivity adjustment	_____	
4. Safety measures	_____	
a. Electrical safety (such as, no bathing)	_____	
b. Supervision of infant, siblings	_____	
c. Ensuring that monitor alarms are audible (such as not placing next to drapes or walls)	_____	
d. Use of intercoms	_____	
5. Medications	_____	
a. Discharge dose (_____ mg/hr); draw up to _____ cc on syringe	_____	
b. Home time schedule: _____	_____	
c. Rationale for use	_____	
d. Demonstrate administration with syringe.	_____	
e. Side effects (increased heart rate, increased respiratory rate, increased urine output, feeding intolerance, irritability)	_____	
f. Rationale for drawing monthly blood levels	_____	
6. Economic issues	_____	
a. Costs/reimbursements	_____	
b. Plans for employment/child care	_____	
7. Family lifestyle changes	_____	
a. Plan for observing infant	_____	
b. Plan for hearing monitor alarms (no vacuuming or hair drying if infant is not seen)	_____	
c. Plan for training support people/babysitters	_____	
d. Plan for traveling	_____	
e. Developmental stimulation plans	_____	
f. Family plans for their own social needs	_____	
8. Support systems	_____	
a. Support group numbers given to parents	_____	
b. Heart Association phone numbers (for community CPR course) given to parents	_____	
c. Parents describe their emergency support plan with names and phone numbers for:		
1. Hospital emergency room _____	_____	
2. Primary physician _____	_____	
3. Emergency squad ambulance _____	_____	
4. Monitor company _____	_____	
5. Transportation to hospital _____	_____	
d. Medical follow-up plans	_____	
e. Nursing follow-up plans	_____	

FIGURE 8-2, cont'd. For legend see p. 195.

self-instruction booklets required significantly less teaching time in the hospital than did patients who did not receive the booklets. The authors conclude that many patients can learn postoperative exercise behaviors before hospital admission.[7] Figure 8-2 presents a discharge planning tool for families planning home apnea monitoring. The tool sets forth home environment preparation, family life-style changes, and a support system, as well as direct infant care and use of the monitor.[5]

Availability of good protocols, teaching tools, and forms for recording teaching are essential to ensure that teaching is actually delivering to patients the underlying support that produces these structures. The reinforcement for teaching will help to ensure that patient education does not slip to the bottom of the priority list.

IMPLEMENTATION

In purposeful, planned teaching, the caregiver carries out the plan. It cannot work perfectly, but it can be used as a guide unless feedback from the patient indicates clearly that it is inappropriate or ineffective. If this happens the planning process must be repeated and new data must be added. Experienced teachers can do that on the spot and move ahead. Others will need to break the teaching session and, if possible, to replan and to reimplement again. Questions that come up during implementation include substitution of learning experiences. The patient may request the substitution. The planned material may become unavailable, or something much better may appear. The caregiver can decide if the substitution is a good one.

Lessons cannot be memorized; however, the teacher should exercise enough control to carry out his or her intent.

Increasingly, in the health promotion area an agency may contract with an organization that provides programs that are already developed. The agency uses its own staff to deliver the program, or it employs training agency personnel to present the program. Before purchasing the program, it is important to determine if the materials are correct, if the program is successful, and if the cost is reasonable. Examining any accompanying marketing materials or marketing plans that might save the agency additional time and money is also wise. Are promotional materials such as fliers, advertising copy, posters, sales brochures, videotaped sales presentations, and press releases available? Will the vendor provide marketing expertise to help the agency determine how best to promote the program, attract media attention, encourage professional referrals, and increase attendance? Who provides the training if agency staff deliver the instruction? Are mechanisms built into the program to ensure that staff will conduct the program in the prescribed manner?[6]

Staff training is also important to implement programs. Traditional methods of teaching health professionals how to teach often focus only on the theoretic aspects of the teaching-learning process. Frequently, little is offered to help transfer this information into the practice setting. The guided decision-making model described by Strodtman is one attempt to provide actual practice with a problem-solving approach to patient education. The model uses typical practice situations with frequent feedback about the decisions caregivers are making. Detailed examples may be found in Strodtman's article.[10] Another approach involves apprenticing novice teachers to master teachers, allowing them to observe and participate and gradually do the teaching on their own with feedback from the master teacher. Videotaping teaching interactions provides an opportunity for self-evaluation as well as critique from a master teacher.

SUMMARY

Teaching involves creating conditions where learning can occur. This is accomplished first by a teacher-learner relationship that motivates. The teacher is also skilled in deciding which particular experiences will benefit certain individuals. The experiences should help learners reach and carry out objectives.

STUDY QUESTIONS

1. Following are descriptions of general teaching situations. Indicate ways in which you might alter teaching activities for patients with various levels of motivation to learn.

    a. The patient has had a hysterectomy and has been told that some blood flow will occur until the tissue heals; that if the odor becomes noticeable or if the flow increases or turns bright red, she should report this at once to her physician; and that unless specifically ordered, she should not douche.

    b. Assimilation of a disability includes shift to an asset value system as opposed to comparison by the patient with what he or she used to be able to do.

    c. A goal of patient education for labor and delivery is for patients to feel satisfaction with their behavior.

2. A mother comments to you, "My baby has clumsy fingers." You determine that the child's growth and development are normal for his or her age but that he or she could profit from environmental stimulation to develop his or her eye-hand coordination and prehension. What kinds of general teaching approaches might be used?

REFERENCES

1. Honig JC: Preparing preschool-aged children to be siblings, *MCN* 11:37-43, 1986.
2. Keller JM: Development and use of the ARCS model of instructional design, *J Instruc Dev* 10(3):2-10, 1987.
3. Merrill MD, Kowallis T, Wilson BG: *Instructional design in transition*. In Farley FH, Gordon NJ, editors: *Psychology and education: the state of the union,* Berkeley, Calif, 1981, McCutchan.
4. Myers JS and others: Standardized teaching plans for management of chemotherapy and radiation therapy side effects, *Oncol Nurs Forum* 14:95-99, 1987.
5. Norris-Berkemeyer S, Hutchins KH: Home apnea monitoring, *Pediatr Nurs* 12:259-304, 1986.
6. Powell DK: Sizing up the packaged program, *Promot Health* 6(4):4-5, 11, 1985.
7. Rice VH, Johnson JE: Preadmission self-instruction booklets, postadmission exercise performance, and teaching time, *Nurs Res* 33:147-151, 1984.
8. Shotkin JD, Bolt B, Norton DA: Teaching program for patients with low back pain, *J Neurosci Nurs* 19:240-243, 1987.
9. Steinaker NW, Bell MR: *The experiential taxonomy: a new approach to teaching and learning,* New York, 1979, Academic Press.
10. Strodtman LK: A decision-making process for planning patient education, *Patient Educ Couns* 5:189-200, 1984.
11. Warbinek E, Wyness MA: Peripheral arterial occlusive disease. II. Nursing assessment and standard care plans, *Cardiovasc Nurs* 22:6-11, 1986.
12. Wildman TM, Burton JK: Integrating learning theory with instructional design, *J Instruc Dev* 4(3):5-13, 1981.

CHAPTER 9

Evaluation of health teaching

Evaluation determines the worth of something by judging it against a standard. It is a process that can be explicit or implicit. In patient education patients are evaluated on how well they have learned the desired behavior—on how much their performance has improved since teaching began.

Evaluation can serve several purposes. It can direct and motivate learning because it provides evidence about patients' accomplishments or their lack of accomplishments. It can also judge whether someone ought to be selected or certified for having met a particular level of expertise. Patient education generally has not been used to provide a formal certification; however, evaluative judgments about learning commonly provide the basis for allowing a patient to progress to another setting, such as home. Evaluation also reinforces correct behavior on the part of the learner and helps teachers determine the adequacy of their teaching. In each situation it is important to think through the purpose of the evaluation first.

The next step is to assign learners evaluative tasks. Ambiguous tasks produce faulty evidence and lead to faulty conclusions concerning how much the patient has learned. As a result the learner is confused. Evidence is compared with criteria or standards of adequate performance, and a judgment of adequacy or inadequacy is made.[29] The teaching that follows a judgment of inadequate learning can correct errors in the patient's performance, present correct behavior, and explain the errors and correct behavior.

Evaluation of programs of patient education is also necessary for teaching large groups of patients over a period of time. Program evaluation provides direction for improvement of learning in individual patients and leads to judgments about whether the program should continue.

The goals of this chapter are (1) to explain situations in which various techniques for measuring patient behavior are appropriate, (2) to explain how to detect and correct major sources of measurement error, and (3) to develop additional skills in making evaluative judgments about individual learning and the performance of patient education programs.

OBTAINING MEASURES OF BEHAVIOR

All measurement involves observation of behavior. These observations are more or less direct. They are more direct if the method of measurement involves viewing actual behavior as it occurs and having access to its intended meaning. They are less direct if the method of measurement involves the subject's response to substitute situations that may be largely verbal and requires much inference of intended meaning. Each method contains certain weaknesses that can produce error in measurement.

Because one of the major purposes of measurement and evaluation activities is to predict how the individual will behave in the future, it is best to base this prediction on observation of actual behavior (direct measurement). The basis for this position is well known. Response to a situation is very complex. It involves conscious and subconscious levels of mental activity. Responses may vary according to the situation. For example, the individual's feelings, previous experiences with similar situations, and current circumstances must be considered.

Thus what people say they will do and what they

actually do may be different. People often respond in ways that are socially acceptable. Such response may or may not involve a conscious alteration. Behavior in the affective domain is, perhaps, the most difficult to measure because the individual can easily control the expression of feelings. Direct observation of behavior when the individual is unaware of being observed is the best opportunity for accurate assessment.

Although indirect measurements are risky, they also possess advantages that can contribute greatly to accurate assessment. Natural behavior is often inaccessible because it occurs in private: in family interactions. Natural behavior might occur infrequently and in various places. For example, it might surface in response to emergencies that require resuscitation measures, such as insulin shock, diabetic coma, or ingestion of poisons by a child.

Natural behavior might also occur infrequently, such as when a parent provides sex education for a child. Therefore the observer might not be present, or it might be inconvenient for him or her to be present, when natural behavior occurs. The strategy behind most tests used in indirect measurement is to control the situation in such a way that the provider can rouse the desired behavior in a written, an oral, or a performance response to a mock situation. Test results for complex behaviors are more accurate if the learner responds to situations on videotape rather than responds to written test situations.

Thus far in this chapter several major sources of error in measurement have been identified. One source of error is the constant possibility that indirect measures may present a false picture of the individual's behavior. A second source of error rests in the complexity of behavior. An observer may be unable to identify the causes of a particular behavior or be unable to measure thought patterns and attitudes even by direct observation. A third source is the bias of human observers. Observers cannot attend to or record all stimuli. They tend to assign meanings according to their own views. A fourth source of error is sampling. It is often not feasible in terms of time and effort expended to observe an individual's or a group's behavior repeatedly to account for the variation in performance from day to day and from situation to situation. It is not possible to inventory all aspects of an individual's knowledge about a particular subject. Getting samples over a period of time and in general areas of subject matter decrease error to an acceptable level.

The degree of error allowable depends on the predictions and decisions made and on the precision of the best measuring tool available. The provider should be more concerned with the person who needs to know what to do about a blood pressure drop or a blood leak during home hemodialysis than with the person who needs to know how to fold diapers with extra thickness for a boy baby. In both cases observing the learner doing the behavior would be appropriate for evaluation. However, for hemodialysis the teacher should observe many times, measuring the learner's behavior against objective criteria agreed on by experts. To evaluate the learner's understanding the caregiver can supplement the observation with oral or written questions asking what constitutes a blood pressure drop, what can cause it, and how it can be corrected. The caregiver might surreptitiously add some blood to the dialysate to see if the learner detects it and responds appropriately. All methods of measurement are prone to particular errors. To arrive at a decision the best information often can be gained by using a combination of methods.

Measurement involves obtaining a record of pertinent behavior. Not only is it quite difficult to record all that occurs, but this mass of information is not useful. The guideline for the pertinence of recording behavior is the objective. If this statement has met all the specifications for preciseness and clarity that were outlined in Chapter 4, it is much easier to decide which information is useful to record. Envision the difference in trying to evaluate these two objectives: (1) to know injection sites; and (2) to draw on his or her own skin five areas suitable for injection of insulin. It is difficult to identify and measure the content and behavior of objective number one. Also the teaching may have been haphazard because of the lack of specificity. Note that no time is stipulated in this objective. Tests limiting time are appropriate only if the learned behavior requires speed.

The taxonomy of educational objectives in Chapter 4 provides a general classification of behaviors and may be used as a guide or a method of measurement.

USING MEASUREMENT TECHNIQUES

Behavior can be measured in a number of units: speed, accuracy, probability of occurrence, originality, persistence, amount, and correctness. Of these, measurement of persistence is often neglected, leaving little knowledge about retention of health teaching. These measures are made through a variety of techniques.

Direct observation of behavior

As in much of health care practice, observation skills are often used in teaching. However, observation is more effective in evaluating learning in some areas than in others. In the absence of many well-developed, readily available tests for the measurement of attitudes, the best course is to become skilled in examining behavior that expresses feelings and values. Cognitive skills are more difficult to observe because thinking is an internal act that may or may not be expressed in actions. Cognitive skills underlie motor acts. For example, cognitive skill is evident when the learner decides that the irrigated catheter is patent. An example of behavior more completely cognitive is a mother's reasoning for bringing her child to the health care provider. Thought processes are most often measured by verbal means through oral questioning or by written tests.

The recording of observations (necessary when observation is being used in the evaluation of learned behavior) varies with the type of learning being evaluated. Because attitudes often change slowly and are expressed in many different ways, the form for recording observations can be relatively unstructured and adaptable to long-term use. Motor skills, in contrast, are much more uniform in their expression, so that the recording observation form can describe specific steps that every learner will do. The products and processes of learned behavior also can be described. For example, how the diaper looks after it has been secured and the process of putting it on can be described. Indeed, some products are difficult to evaluate without seeing the process, as in the case of a paraplegic patient learning to irrigate his catheter.

Rating scales and checklists

The most complete recording of behavior is obtained from videotape. Replaying the performance is an advantage that aids in obtaining an accurate description of what happened and in pointing out relevant behavior to learners. However, this tool is expensive and rarely available. By itself it does not summarize the kind of behavior seen or identify its meaning in relation to objectives. To fill this need, a rating scale that describes pertinent behavior in words (anchored) can be constructed.

To reduce error in measurement, the words must be precise so that misinterpretation is avoided. For example, the rating scale on p. 202 can be refined so that several teachers who are observing a learner's behavior can independently classify it at one of the three points with little variation. If the raters cannot agree, the wording probably needs to be clarified. After the scale is refined, individual caregivers can use it by itself. As a prerequisite the caregivers should know the subject matter well enough to be able to make the observations of behavior required by the rating scale quickly.

Of course, it is possible for an individual to be displaying behavior from two different levels of functioning (see descriptions of behavior in sample rating scale). For example, the patient may contaminate the syringe and needle fairly often (lowest level) but be quite skilled at removing bubbles from the syringe and measuring accurately (highest level). Usually, the behaviors are at adjacent levels on the rating scale because certain skills involve comparable levels of coordination. The difference may be that the learner is careless about contaminating. Checks can be made beside individual

---

SAMPLE RATING SCALE

Subobjective: To obtain 1 ml of aqueous fluid for injection from a 2 ml vial with a 2 ml syringe, 22-gauge needle, using sterile technique.

•   •   •

Consistently uses contaminated syringe, needle, or top of vial. Cannot push needle through diaphragm. Is rarely aware of erring and if so usually does not know how to correct the error.	Occasionally contaminates. Can push needle through diaphragm. Has difficulty withdrawing all the fluid and obtaining accurate measurement (within 0.1 ml). Can usually diagnose errors while doing the procedure and correct them.	Rarely contaminates. Can obtain last few drops out of vial without damaging needle. Can measure within 0.1 ml even if bubbles present. Can change needle or syringe if defective or contaminated. Corrects errors by self.

(Other scales can be developed for other subobjectives of the skill of giving an injection.)

---

statements at various levels of the description. This will ensure that the teacher does not lose information about the learner's performance by checking just one of the categories on the line.

Another alternative is construction of several scales for this particular subobjective, each dealing with one set of behaviors—maintenance of sterility, obtaining and measuring fluid, or handling errors. Space is usually left below each rating scale for comments. A well-developed scale will include all pertinent points and will rarely require extra written comments. The form is developed to preclude recording behavior by writing it out at great length.

Other factors in the construction of a rating scale besides preciseness of the descriptions contribute to its quality as a measuring instrument. One factor is the number of levels of achievement represented in the behavior descriptions. The sample rating scale given here uses three steps because it is difficult for an observer to discriminate among more than five levels of achievement. Four or five steps could have been used. Note that the kinds of behaviors described in the scale are those that are crucial to the success of the skill as described in the objective: asepsis, accuracy of measurement, and ability to perceive and correct errors. Concerns such as inserting the needle precisely through the center of the rubber stopper or the particular manner in which the syringe is grasped are not considered crucial.

The rating scale is designed to summarize a series of trials; for example, the learner may have practice sessions in learning how to obtain fluid for injection. The scale also has the advantage of describing levels of attainment. This information calls the teacher's and learner's attention to faulty skills. If the skill is complex, it is advisable to subdivide the task into a series of skills and to test for each one sequentially (wipes bottle, injects air, draws correct dosage).

An instrument closely related to the rating scale is the checklist. In the example given crucial steps are chosen. Remember that subobjectives deal with other behaviors crucial to giving an injection. Directions for using a checklist should indicate that a check or a letter means that the step was either done or not done and, if done, was satisfactory or

Directions: Give one point if step is done correctly, no point if done incorrectly

1. Puts inhaler together correctly.   _____

2. Shakes inhaler.   _____

3. Holds inhaler correctly.   _____

4. Gives full expiration with pursed lips through mouth.   _____

5. Places mouthpiece in mouth correctly.   _____

6. Breathes in deeply through mouth.   _____

7. Activates aerosol while breathing deeply.   _____

8. Holds breath after activating aerosol.   _____

9. Waits between puffs.   _____

10. Shakes inhaler again.   _____

11. Replaces cap when finished with entire procedure.   _____

FIGURE 9-1. Vanceril Inhaler Performance Evaluation. (From Heringa P, Lawson L, Reda D: *Health Educ Q* 14:309-317, 1987.)

unsatisfactory. The following is an example of a checklist that could be used in lieu of the sample rating scale given on p. 202:

☐ Scrubbed top of vial with disinfectant sponge
☐ Punctured rubber vial with needle without contaminating
☐ Withdrew all of fluid from vial
☐ Expelled excess air from syringe without losing fluid
☐ Measured fluid to within 0.1 ml of the correct dose

To determine progress in learning the skill, a check may be done periodically. Checking as the skill is performed reduces the likelihood of error in trying to summarize several trials. Learner and teacher can see the steps in which errors occur, particularly if successive ratings show the errors that are consistent.

Using either a rating scale or a checklist, an acceptable level of performance must be determined. The learner should reach the top performance level to give an injection alone. However,

the second level is sufficient if supervision is provided. To satisfy the checklist, the individual should consistently be performing all steps satisfactorily to function independently; however, he or she might perform fewer of the steps satisfactorily if competent supervision is given.

Figure 9-1 provides an example of a performance evaluation tool.[22] Can it elicit critical data? Are the most important steps in this procedure included? Are some steps more crucial than others? If so, should these steps be marked so that patients who cannot do critical steps are identified? Would two health care providers watching a patient perform this procedure give him or her the same number of points? Might it help to include further descriptors of a correct performance for each step?

Anecdotal notes and critical incidents

Other behaviors do not lend themselves as easily to the kind of preset description found in the rating scale, particularly behaviors expressing attitudes in which the context is often significant to interpre-

---

SAMPLE ANECDOTAL NOTES

Subobjective: To accept the restriction on activity and smoking.

January 19,1992, 1:30 P.M. Patient: James Jones

    Diagnosis: Myocardial infarction

    Recorded by: S. Smith, L.P.N.

    Found Mr. Jones in his room leaning over the bed to get urinal out of bedside stand. I asked him why he was doing that, since he was supposed to be on bedrest. He states, "Dr. won't let me have cigarettes, so I didn't see why I should lie still for him." I said, "But you're making such good progress, and rest is essential for that." Pt. turned head and looked at wall. He did not answer when I called his name three times. I left the room.

January 21, A.M. Patient: James Jones

    Recorded by: M. Jones, R.N.

    When I was giving bath, patient said he hoped Dr. would come in soon so he could discuss with him why he could not smoke.

January 21, 4 P.M. Patient: James Jones

    Recorded by: M. Jones, R.N.

    Pt.'s wife came to visit. He seemed very cocky with her—like a banty rooster. Bragged that he was going to tell the Dr. off because he wasn't going to be confined to bed and be told he couldn't smoke.

tation. A more useful form for recording such behaviors is perhaps the anecdotal note.

This technique consists of recording pertinent behavior described in objective terms. After a period of time, the anecdotes are compared, noting change or lack of it. Especially important are critical incidents that starkly portray the behavior of major interest. Again, too much time and effort are needed to record all kinds of behavior. Pertinent behavior is related to the objective. The objective in the sample anecdotal notes above need not discuss the patient's knowledge of toothbrushing or the patient's conversation with a roommate about the time that breakfast is served. Such information is not pertinent. The patient's explanation to the roommate about why he or she is in the hospital may have relevance if it expresses feelings regarding the illness, the treatment, or the physician. The third anecdote contains material that is not objective. The expressions "cocky," "like a banty rooster," and "bragged" are definitely colored with the provider's feelings toward this patient. Such biased

reporting prevents those who read the reports from drawing their own conclusions. In addition, the wife's response during this situation is important to an assessment because it might explain the patient's behavior; yet, it is omitted.

The only interpretation that can be made on the basis of the three notes in the sample is that Mr. Jones is not accepting activity and smoking restrictions and, in particular circumstances, his feelings seem to have been stronger than in others. These notes and others may serve as a baseline to compare behaviors during teaching. Anecdotes similar to those in the sample anecdotal notes appear on patients' charts; however, the notes do not appear consistently, particularly if the learning objective is not clearly defined. The notes also tend to be scattered among the daily notes and thus are difficult to find. It is wise to collect notes specific to teaching-learning on a special form that would outline the entire teaching-learning plan. To obtain more valid measurements of learning, notes should be written within an hour or so after events occur and should be collected regularly. The records may be reviewed periodically to determine progress and plan teaching tactics. Measurements are continued until the goal is reached or until it appears that the behavior is static over a period of several observations. Then a reassessment of the goal should take place.

It is fortunate that caregivers usually deal with individuals or with small groups of learners because observation procedures using the rating scale, checklist, or anecdotal notes are expensive in time. Observing one learner at a time requires the caregiver's full attention. Opportunities for observing cannot always occur at the staff's convenience. For example, a patient can be asked to demonstrate a motor skill almost any time; however, interaction with the patient's family can happen only when the family is present.

After these methods of observation are used to collect data, interpretation of the data begins.

Evidence of behavior change

It is easy for staff to err as they decide whether evidence indicates that a behavior change (learning) has occurred. For example, in teaching coughing, turning, and deep breathing to a patient who is going to have surgery, the caregiver may have absence of complications as a criterion for successful learning. Such a criterion encompasses too much. Many factors contribute to development of atelectasis besides the patient's failure to do the prescribed exercises. If a decreased absentee rate, for instance, is used as a criterion of successful health teaching in an industrial nursing situation, evidence must be present that the decreased rate resulted from the teaching and not other factors, such as change in administrative policy about absences.

Too many other elements affect these criteria to make them the sole measures of the effectiveness of teaching and learning unless elaborate measures are taken to control or account for other possible causes of the behavior change. Evaluations of learning with such controls could become experimental studies. However, practicing health care professionals are usually not equipped to do such

studies; therefore they gather as many clues as possible and proceed. In the previous example the practicing nurse would note that the atelectasis had occurred, review the available medical evidence about the cause, and perhaps review with the nursing staff and the patient how the coughing, turning, deep breathing, and patient teaching has been carried out. The evidence is most supportive of teaching effect when the behavior occurs soon after the teaching action or when the intervention seems to be the major change in the situation.

The provider who is less effective than the one who errs in determining the criteria of learning is the provider who uses a pamphlet as the major means of teaching and evaluates the learning only by asking patients if they have read the pamphlet. Similar comments can be made about considering the number of patients attending teaching sessions as a criterion of successful teaching. This kind of criterion is often cited as evaluative of teaching programs. Such statistics may indicate valuable interest in the program; however, they are not likely to be an accurate indicator of learning. Providers must also be wary of statements implying that considerable behavior change has taken place without presenting supporting evidence.

Oral questioning

Oral questioning is a flexible form of measurement often used in combination with techniques such as observation. It attempts to reach those behaviors that cannot be easily observed. For example, the caregiver may ask patients questions to determine if they understand the basis for their actions in performing a psychomotor skill. Oral questioning also allows construction of hypothetic situations that are not present in the actual teaching environment. Examples of these practices include asking a man learning to irrigate his colostomy why he is preparing the equipment as he is or asking a mother what she would do if her baby turned blue, which may include a demonstration of resuscitation techniques.

The method of oral questioning can be expensive in time, particularly if done in a one-to-one teacher-student relationship. The strength of oral questioning over written testing is that the teacher knows immediately whether the learner understands the question, and the teacher can let the learner know immediately whether the answer is right. In a group teaching situation this kind of direct interchange is limited—although the reaction of one learner responding to another learner's answer can be very educational. In large groups the advantages of oral questioning are somewhat lost because every individual cannot respond to an oral question unless that response is in writing.

The verbal nature of both oral and written questioning may handicap individuals who have difficulty expressing themselves. People probably find it easier to express themselves orally than in writing. In addition, those who are verbally fluent may *seem* to know more. For these reasons combinations of methods, such as observation of behavior and oral questioning, can often provide a truer picture than a single method can.

It is a common misconception that oral questioning does not require much preparation on the part of the teacher. Questions must be very care-

---

SAMPLE OBJECTIVES AND ORAL QUESTIONS FOR EVALUATION

Objectives	Questions
To state what effect worry in the mother may have on her breast milk (level of knowledge)	"What effect can worry have on a mother's breast milk?" (This question presumes that the learner has read or been told of this relationship.)
To translate instructions for time and route on a medicine bottle into appropriate action (level of comprehension)	Present to learners several medicine bottles with directions for time and route different from those on their own bottles. "How and when should these be taken?"
Given general knowledge of safety, to plan how to rid a house of safety hazards (level of application)	"How would you make your kitchen safer?" Repeat the question for bathroom and other rooms, being certain that areas covered include fire safety, electrical hazards, safety from poisons, safety from falling.
To distinguish how a quack's argument differs from scientific reasoning (level of analysis)	This can be analysis only if the individual has not been told or has not discussed the difference. Otherwise, he or she will repeat thoughts that are not original thoughts and will be at the level of knowledge or comprehension. Several examples of quack and scientific reasoning may be presented and the learner asked to state differences based on those samples.
To design an ileostomy bag that suits one's needs better than do available commercial ones (level of synthesis)	"For what reasons did you design the bag this way?" This would be combined with observation of the bag.
To assess the health care one is receiving in terms of its completeness, one's satisfaction with it, and the results obtained (level of evaluation)	"What quality of care would you say you have received? Consider its completeness, your satisfaction with it, and the results that have occurred."

fully phrased so that the learner can understand them and so that they test the objective. With knowledge of the individual's previous exposure to an idea, questions can be phrased to stimulate thinking at any level of the cognitive domain. The box on p. 206 shows sample objectives taken from Chapter 4 and questions that should test various levels of thinking.

A series of questions is often needed to encourage the learner to do the entire evaluation task. An example is the question on safety (testing application) shown in the boxed material. At other times the learner may not remember the entire question or may need the continued interest of the teacher to complete the answer. If the patient who designed an ileostomy bag talked only about how he or she had designed the appliance so that it had a better seal, the nurse might prompt him or her to suggest its characteristics with regard to cost, odor control, and strength—all of which are important to an adequate ileostomy appliance. Additional questioning may also serve the purpose of determining the extent of an individual's knowledge. After the mother has correctly answered the question about the effect of worry on breast milk, she might then be asked, "Does this mean that this mother should not allow herself to become angry?" Such a question requires a higher level of thinking than the previous question.

Any question, whether written or oral, can be stated in such a vague manner that the learner does not know what the teacher wants and becomes frustrated trying to guess. An example of a vague question is: "How do you take care of Jimmy?" It is not clear whether this question refers to who takes care of Jimmy, how his mother manages to care for him, or what theories of child rearing the mother believes are useful.

A clearly stated, broad question, such as "What do you think is the most important thing to do in caring for a child?", serves the purpose of obtaining general attitudes and values. Some less educated or less motivated people would find it difficult to answer such a broad and abstract question. They respond best to specific questions about concrete items: "What do you do when Jimmy uses improper words?" Only the more mentally adept individuals can assess their thoughts about the many areas of child care, summarize them, and state them.

Tact must be used in presenting questions. People do not like to be grilled. They will not be as accepting of the traditional teacher-in-authority role in health care situations as they are of formal school classroom situations. This does not mean that evaluation should not be done with patients who seem resistant and somewhat forbidding. It can be done subtly by noticing questions or comments that arise naturally during a discussion or by observing a motor skill when it is practiced. For example, a woman discussing a booklet she has read on breast self-examination may say to other learners or to the nurse, "I don't see why it's necessary to look at the breasts besides feeling them"—a comment that may indicate an emotional rejection of observing the breasts. It may mean that this point was not explained in the booklet, or it may mean that it was explained and the woman forgot it or didn't understand it. The provider should know the book's text and observe and question the learner further.

In addition, questions need to be carefully phrased to avoid leading the patient to the socially desirable answer or to "the answer" the provider wants that may be an inappropriate reiteration of the information just presented by the provider. Such a circumstance may indicate that the patient has not comprehended the material well enough to express the idea in alternative ways.

Written measurement

Written measurement is indirect and demands at least some reading skill and knowledge of test taking on the part of the learner. Written measurement offers an excellent opportunity to measure learning at all levels of the cognitive domain with considerable efficiency of teacher time, after the items are constructed. Written tests seem most appropriate in teaching situations involving learners who are well because learners must be able to concentrate for a certain length of time.

General considerations

Tests are prepared by individuals or groups of teachers in a particular institution and are used within that institution. They may be adapted to and published by other institutions, or they may be developed by test experts and sold. Tests sold commercially should provide a manual with information that explains the purposes of the test. Also, the manual should give evidence that it accurately measures the goals it claims to measure. Evidence should include information that describes how well the test covers the subject matter. If, for example, the test is meant to evaluate knowledge of nutrition, it should include items on all the major concepts in nutrition today. This quality of a test is called *content validity*. Additional information should describe how closely the test score is related to actual patient behavior in the present *(concurrent validity)* or the future *(predictive validity)*. For example, if a diabetic patient scores high on the test, is he or she giving good self-care now, and will he or she

be giving good self-care in the future? A similar kind of statement about future self-care would be needed for those doing less well on the test. If a test contains a high degree of validity, its value for decision making is greater than that of a test with a low degree of validity.

It is very rare that tests developed locally by teachers are this carefully studied. The teachers who use their own tests and have continuing contact with the same patients gain a feeling for how closely the test relates to their patients' actual behavior. However, these teachers rarely perform studies that provide them with accurate test-validity information. Measurement characteristics of certain knowledge tests in the patient-education field have been carefully studied. Garrard and others[14] report on psychometric study of the Diabetes Information Test, and Devins and others[9] report on the initial development of a psychometrically sound instrument for measuring understanding of end-stage renal disease (ESRD). The ESRD test accurately dis-

---

THE KIDNEY DISEASE QUESTIONNAIRE:

A TEST FOR MEASURING PATIENT KNOWLEDGE ABOUT END-STAGE RENAL DISEASE

Form A*

1. (1) People normally have two kidneys in the body.
   (a) True
   (b) False
   (c) Don't know
2. (5) When a person has kidney disease, his kidneys must be removed from his body before he can get treatment with a dialysis machine.
   (a) True
   (b) False
   (c) Don't know
3. (3) Kidneys do many important things in the body, but they function only at night while the person is sleeping.
   (a) True
   (b) False
   (c) Don't know
4. (25) What is the term used to describe the vibration or buzzing sensation that can be felt over the vein of a shunt or fistula?
   (a) Hypoplasia
   (b) Lobulation
   (c) Enervation
   (d) Thrill or bruit
   (c) Don't know

From Devins GM and others: *J Clin Epidemiol* 43:297-307, 1990.

*Correct responses for Form A of the KDQ are as follows: item 1 (alternative A), 2 (B), 3 (B), 4 (D), 5 (A), 6 (A), 7 (C), 8 (C), 9 (B), 10 (C), 11 (D), 12 (A), 13 (D). Individual item scores (i.e. 0 vs 1) are summed to generate a total score which can, thus, range between 0 and 13.

criminates between groups that differ in relevant knowledge of kidney disease. The test's reading level is grade 9. Consultation with nephrology nurses and physicians determined the content validity. One question arises: "Why was content validity not determined in consultation with patients who have ESRD?" This test comes in parallel forms (see boxes on pp. 208, 209, 210, and 211): that is, patients can be retested for the same content without using the exact same items. Such tests would need regular updating because knowledge about kidney disease and its treatment changes.

Commercially produced, standardized tests with norms indicating the scores of large numbers of students are widely used in school settings. No such market exists in patient education. Measures of patient education outcomes have been seriously flawed, even in research literature. In reviewing

---

THE KIDNEY DISEASE QUESTIONNAIRE—cont'd

5. (11) In CAPD, waste substances pass from the blood, across the peritoneal membrane and into the dialysate fluid by a process called:
   (a) Diffusion
   (b) Transport
   (c) Excretion
   (d) Chemical breakdown
   (e) Don't know

6. (17) In addition to removing wastes from the blood, the artificial kidney also functions to remove excess water from the blood. This water-removal process is called:
   (a) Ultra-filtration
   (b) Ultra-refraction
   (c) Osmosis
   (d) Catharsis
   (e) Don't know

7. (9) A patient with kidney disease can experience high blood pressure, swelling, and rapid weight gain when his body becomes overloaded with:
   (a) Protein
   (b) Urea
   (c) Water
   (d) Don't know

8. (7) Which one of these foods has a lot of potassium?
   (a) Rice
   (b) Ice cream
   (c) Bananas
   (d) Don't know

9. (15) Approximately how many times a week do hemodialysis patients usually have their sessions on the kidney dialysis machine?
   (a) 1
   (b) 3
   (c) 6
   (d) Don't know

10. (14) A patient with chronic kidney diseases may have a living relative who wants to donate a kidney to the patient for transplantation. Which one of the following items about the donor is *FALSE?*
   (a) The donor will have to undergo a series of medical tests before the transplant operation.
   (b) The donor runs very little risk to his own health when he donates one kidney.
   (c) The donor will need to take immunosuppressive drugs for life.
   (d) After the transplant operation the donor's remaining kidney will enlarge in size.
   (e) Don't know

11. (18) Which one of the following items about kidney transplantation is *FALSE?*
   (a) Sometimes a transplanted kidney will begin to function as soon as the blood vessels are connected on the operating table.

Continued.

THE KIDNEY DISEASE QUESTIONNAIRE—cont'd

(b) Kidney transplants are placed in the patient's pelvis rather than in the usual kidney location.

(c) A person who has recovered from transplant surgery and has a new well-functioning kidney will no longer need dialysis treatment.

(d) A patient can receive a kidney from a living relative but the donor's kidney must be removed one week before the transplant for close observation.

(e) Don't know.

12. (20) CAPD is a form of dialysis treatment which is used as an alternative to hemodialysis. One *advantage* of CAPD is that:

(a) It allows the patient to walk about freely during the course of treatment.

(b) It only needs to be performed once a week.

(c) It does not involve any preparatory surgical procedure.

(d) It makes it easier for the patient to bathe and swim.

(e) Don't know

13. (23) Patients with chronic kidney disease are advised to eat limited quantities of potassium-rich foods. Elevated potassium levels in the blood is dangerous because:

(a) It can cause fluid overload.

(b) It can raise the patient's hematocrit.

(c) It can decrease the production of white blood cells.

(d) It can cause the heart to beat irregularly and even stop.

(e) Don't know.

Form B†

1. (2) Kidney disease is a problem that comes with old age—young people do not get this disease.

(a) True

(b) False

(c) Don't know

2. (4) Most types of kidney disease last about 5 years. After this the kidneys start to work normally again.

(a) True

(b) False

(c) Don't know

3. (6) Peritonitis, an infection of the abdominal cavity, is one of the major problems for patients on CAPD.

(a) True

(b) False

(c) Don't know

4. Kidney transplantation is the best form of treatment for patients with kidney disease because after the transplant the patients are less likely to get infections from bacteria or virus.

(a) True

(b) False

(c) Don't know

5. (24) There are about one million tiny filters in the human kidney. They are called:

(a) Ribosomes

(b) Ureters

(c) Glomeruli

(d) Organelles

(e) Don't know

6. (13) In kidney failure, waste products in the blood build up to abnormal levels and this causes a condition called:

(a) Absorption

(b) Uremia

(c) Libido

(d) Adaptation

(e) Don't know

†Correct responses for Form B of the KDQ are as follows: item 1 (alternative B), 2 (B), 3 (A), 4 (B), 5 (C), 6 (B), 7 (D), 8 (A), 9 (B), 10 (A), 11 (B), 12 (B), 13 (A). Individual item scores (i.e. 0 vs 1) are summed to generate a total score which can, thus, range between 0 and 13.

THE KIDNEY DISEASE QUESTIONNAIRE—cont'd

7. (16) The artificial kidney is also called:
   (a) Henle's loop
   (b) Transferrin
   (c) Bun
   (d) Dialyzer
   (e) Don't know

8. (21) A new type of dialysis for treating kidney disease is called CAPD. Which part of the body makes this type of dialysis possible?
   (a) Peritoneum
   (b) Bladder
   (c) Renal pelvis
   (d) Don't know

9. (8) Patients with kidney disease are told not to eat salty foods because salt has a lot of:
   (a) Potassium
   (b) Sodium
   (c) Calcium
   (d) Don't know

10. (10) Immunosuppressive drugs are given to transplant patients in order to:
   (a) Prevent and treat rejection of the kidney graft.
   (b) Treat blood clotting in the new kidney.
   (c) Prevent infection of the kidney by virus or bacteria.
   (d) Raise the patient's hematocrit.
   (e) Don't know.

11. (19) Bone disease is a medical problem that could result from chronic kidney disease. It can occur because:
   (a) The diseased kidney can no longer rid the body of excess water in a normal fashion.
   (b) The diseased kidney loses its ability to keep calcium and phosphate levels in the proper range in the body.
   (c) The diseased kidney loses its ability to excrete excess potassium from the bloodstream.
   (d) The body is no longer able to use protein foods.
   (e) Don't know.

12. (12) Which medication is sometimes prescribed to control the level of potassium in the patient's body?
   (a) Riopan
   (b) Kayexalate
   (c) Amphojel
   (d) Aldomet
   (e) Don't know

13. (22) In the regular procedure for CAPD, dialysate fluid is introduced into the patient's abdominal cavity through an implanted tube just below the navel. The dialysate fluid is then:
   (a) Left inside the abdominal cavity for several hours and then drained out.
   (b) Left inside the abdominal cavity until it is completely absorbed into the body.
   (c) Transferred into an artificial kidney through another tube.
   (d) Transferred into an artificial kidney through the same tube.
   (e) Don't know.

Note: Items that comprise the 25-item version of the KDQ, described in Study 1, are indicated in parentheses.

studies on diabetes patient education between 1954 and 1986, Brown concludes that authors often developed new instruments of their own but usually did not address reliability and validity issues.[5]

Nationally distributed tests can have a beneficial effect in widening the staff's view. It is easier to teach patients how something is done in the institution where they receive care than it is to teach them by broad principles that might help them to transfer knowledge to other institutions and situations. Examining the content of a national test can help staff recognize limitations in their own objectives by reviewing the objectives that others set for their learners.

Evaluation of patient's learning should be tailored to address the material that has been taught. Published tests may not reflect this material. Teachers may want to use a test item bank as an alternative. Banks contain large numbers of questions that have been keyed to lists of instructional objectives. The items are field tested, reviewed for content validity by experts, and judged technically sound. The developer of a new test on the subject matter covered by the item bank need only specify the objectives of a particular instructional program, suggest a desired number of items per objective, and allow a computer to select the items appropriate for the objectives. A test item bank for diabetes education has been described.[30]

Both so-called objective questions—multiple-choice, true-false, and matching items—and essay questions have their place in measuring health learning. Essay writing requires considerable skill in organizing and expressing ideas. It is more ap-

---

TEST ITEMS ON VARIOUS LEVELS OF THE COGNITIVE DOMAIN

Knowledge T F The hospital is required by law to use isolation with certain diagnoses.

Comprehension T F A patient will not be retained in isolation after a diagnosis is made.

Application Isolation is a means of containing the spread of micro-organisms. How can these methods be used with a person at home who has a cold?

Analysis The basic principle(s) of our society that relate(s) to the reason isolation is used is (are):

a. Certain institutions have the right to carry out certain functions for the society.
b. An individual has certain rights.
c. The majority rules.
d. *a* and *b*.
e. *a, b, c*.

Synthesis Suggest a set of rules for isolation that will maximize the well-being of staff, visitors, and patients.

Evaluation It seems necessary to isolate persons with communicable disease to varying extents in order to protect others from the disease. Which one of the following policies would best achieve protection of the public and the welfare of the ill individual?

a. After diagnosis allow the individual and family a choice of sites for care.
b. Have a team of health personnel to enforce the proper degree of isolation in a hospital and the reporting of communicable disease.
c. Allow individual physicians and health agencies considerable latitude in establishing such policies.

(NOTE: The answer must not be in terms of opinion but must show evidence of judgment in terms of particular criteria, such as safety and psychologic and sociologic well-being.)

propriately used in an academic setting than with patients. Thus essay questions for patients are usually shortened and made more specific. They are presented in oral or written form. An example is: "What should be done if your child eats poison, and why should it be done?" Note that this question, whether oral or written, requires recall of information. However, the response will elicit a different behavior than does discriminating among answers that are already present in multiple-choice, true-false, and matching items.

The ability to recall is desirable for information used frequently. It is essential for emergency situations, such as child poisoning, diabetic coma, or seizures. The objective is to be able to act on the information. A person must be able to produce the information from memory, not just recognize it among several alternatives. Periodic self-testing of memory for specific information will strengthen retention of infrequently used material. The strength of the recognition item is that it can enable learners to discriminate between ideas—ideas they might not otherwise consider—thus helping them test their depth of understanding.

As in the box on p. 212, items can be written to test all levels of cognitive behavior. The level measured by a particular question depends on the information the learner has received; therefore the questions are based on written material that is given first. The questions should ask for more information as the patient progresses upward through the levels of understanding. These questions are presented in the illustration as examples of questions that might be given to test learning on higher levels of thinking. The patient need not reach these higher levels of thinking for subjects or circumstances in which he or she does not function independently. Some patients may function at this level because their general level of knowledge and thinking is elevated. However, these objectives are not common. For home hemodialysis the patient and family function more independently, and objectives requiring complex levels of thinking are common.

The true-false item form is used to test knowledge or comprehension. The multiple-choice form is more flexible and can be used at all levels. Synthesis requires independent thought; therefore it is tested by methods that suggest no answers. At all levels, visual materials can be incorporated into written questions. For example, the provider can show a mother four photos of umbilical cords and ask her to indicate the one(s) that need(s) to be called to the attention of the nurse midwife and which one(s) will probably drop off soon.

Item construction

Numerous possible errors in the construction of single test items and groups of items can prevent an accurate assessment of an individual's knowledge. The skills required to construct written tests are complex. Without having additional training, many teachers cannot become accomplished in construction. However, they should learn to avoid obvious errors. The points considered in making oral questions specific and understandable for learners hold true for written questions. A good way to test whether these criteria have been attained with written (essay) and oral questions is to outline a suggested answer. Frequently, ambiguities that are not otherwise evident in many questions will be uncovered. The final test is presenting all items to learners to discover how the learners interpret them.

For open-ended questions the provider can develop criteria for correct responses. The following questions were asked of parents: (1) What would you do if you just saw your child drinking a poison? (2) What would you do if your child just drank some toilet bowl cleaner? (3) What would you do if your child just drank some Drano or Liquid Plumr? Criteria for evaluating answers to these questions are described as follows:

Incorrect response Immediately make child vomit
Use ipecac without medical
   clearance
Give home remedy without
   seeking medical advice
Call ambulance
Miscellaneous response without
   therapeutic merit
No answer

Partially correct	Rush child to ER or MD (for question 1)
	Follow directions on label of product ingested
	Check a home reference for instructions
	Neutralize, then call MD or poison control center
Correct	Call MD immediately
	Call poison control center immediately
	Rush to ER (for questions 2 and 3 only)[8]

In the box on this page is a list of guidelines for writing multiple-choice test items.[12]

Testing for trivia or for irrelevant material is an error to avoid. Consider the nurse who shows a film in conjunction with baby care classes. The following questions are irrelevant to the objectives of most baby care classes:

1. The name of the movie you saw about your baby's bath was
   a. "Your Baby's Bath"
   b. "Bathing Baby"
   c. "Morning Adventure"
   d. "Mother Loves Baby"
2. The company that sponsored the movie you saw was
   a. Pet Milk Company
   b. Carnation Milk Company
   c. Pampers
   d. Foremost Milk Company

Two examples of testing for trivia are to ask the size of the room in which the baby's bath is given or to ask whether the nurse held the washcloth in the right hand or the left hand during the demonstration. Notice that triviality and irrelevance are defined in terms of the learning objectives.

Clues in the language of the item give away the correct answer to someone who is test wise. The following example, based on the pamphlet explaining isolation care, suffers from one clue—exactly the same terminology as that used in the teaching presentation:

T F   Your illness may be transmitted to others.

GUIDELINES FOR WRITING MULTIPLE-CHOICE TEST ITEMS

1. Make all distractors plausible.
2. Avoid "None of the above" as an option.
3. Make all the options approximately the same length.
4. Avoid negatively stated items, especially double negatives.
5. Randomly vary the position of the correct answer.
6. Avoid grammatical mistakes. Each option should fit grammatically with the stem.
7. Avoid using "All of the above" as an option.
8. Put as much of the item as possible into the stem. Do not repeat words in the options.
9. The stem should present a definition problem and not lead into a series of unrelated true-false statements.
10. There should be only one correct or best answer.
11. Avoid superfluous wording and irrelevant material.
12. Attempt to measure higher order learning by using novelty.
13. Use three to five options, depending on how many can be logically created for each item.
14. Do not give irrelevant clues to the correct answer.
15. Avoid specific determiners, such as always, never, all, none.

From Ellsworth RA, Dunnell P, Duell OK: *J Educ Res* 83:289-293, 1990.

In such a case the individual learns to recognize the words without necessarily knowing what they mean. A similar clue occurs in the previously stated question 1. The correct answer occurs in the lead-in phrase (the "stem") before the choices. Grammatical clues, such as a plural subject used in the stem, can make some choices in a multiple-choice question grammatically incorrect. An example, using a plural subject and a plural verb, follows:

3. Areas under the scalp where bone has not yet filled are known as:
   a. Meconium
   b. An umbilicus
   c. Fontanels
   d. All of the above

The following matching item illustrates several problems with clues, ambiguity, and vocabulary level:

Directions: Match the body part with the action that best describes how to wash it.

Body part	Washing action
____ 4. Vulva	a. With a pointed object
____ 5. Neck	b. With a soft washcloth
____ 6. Soft spot	c. Vigorously but gently
____ 7. Ear	d. With a twisted piece of cotton

Mothers may not know the term *vulva* unless it has been specifically introduced to them. Some learners would eliminate choice *a,* because they would know that no one washes the body with pointed objects. The fact that choice *a* is so much easier an item than the others makes it less plausible— a clue. This does not mean that the idea is not important to test; however, it probably should be made into a separate item. The directions indicate that one single choice is better than any other: however, more than one of the washing actions given are equally good for several of the body parts. If the correct answer is not clear-cut to the teacher, the question will probably be ambiguous and frustrating to the learners. Therefore the teacher should try to form questions and answers that are free of confusion. This holds true with any item form. Such ambiguity is particularly difficult to avoid if the basis for a difference of opinion about what is correct lies in cultural belief.

T F   Meat should be eaten once a day.

True-false items are notorious for having clues and can also be ambiguous. Statements containing absolute terms such as *all, always, certainly,* and *entirely* are more often false than true. Statements with words that qualify, such as *generally, sometimes, as a rule,* or *may,* are more often true than false. Uncertainty about the correct answer ensues when part of a question is true and part of it is false, as in the following example:

8. T F   The umbilical cord may be swabbed with alcohol in order to dry it and sterilize it.

Directions should state that if any part of the item is false, the item should be marked false.

For all kinds of items, the best distractors (incorrect choices) are misconceptions that are common among learners. It is easy to learn about these misconceptions by listening to patients talk among themselves, talk with visitors, or talk with nurses or by watching them perform certain skills. The following is an example:

9. T F   The soft spot should not be touched when the baby is being bathed.

Learners' incorrect ideas may not be the same as providers' incorrect ideas because of frequent differences in training and cultural background.

Many times true-false items that are long in text are true. Figure 9-2 shows a test for cardiac patient learning. Does it suffer from this error in measurement?[6] All of these items test the cognitive domain at the lowest levels—a characteristic of true-false items. Sometimes an item format does not provide as much information about the learner's knowledge as the objective must require. An example follows:

Is there a treatment for diabetic retinopathy?
( ) no
( ) yes[23]

Although the following multiple-choice format can assess the patient's knowledge, it suffers from the problem of a high readability level:

Select the best description of diabetic retinopathy from the choices listed below (select only one)
( ) clouded lens
( ) corneal disease
( ) iris malfunction
( ) vitreous detachment
( ) blood vessel abnormality[23]

When constructing a test the goal is to produce items that will assess the learner accurately. Clues

This questionnaire will help evaluate teaching and learning about heart disease. The following statements pertain to various aspects of heart disease. Please read each statement. Next to each statement check T for *true*, F for *false*, and N for *not sure*. Do not guess at the answers.

1. T__F__N__ A heart attack means that part of your heart muscle has been permanently damaged.

2. T__F__N__ Heart attacks occur because the oxygen supply to the heart muscle is blocked.

3. T__F__N__ The buildup of cholesterol and other material in the arteries leading to the heart can cause a heart attack.

4. T__F__N__ The heart acts as a pump to circulate blood. It normally pumps from 30 to 40 times per minute.

5. T__F__N__ If you have chest pain that does not go away after taking 3 nitroglycerin tablets 5 minutes apart, you should go immediately to the hospital or call your doctor.

6. T__F__N__ Heart attack can be signaled by pain in the jaw or numbness in the left arm.

7. T__F__N__ Heart attack can be signaled by pressure in the center of the chest and shortness of breath.

8. T__F__N__ Heart attack can be signaled by a severe headache and sudden blind spot.

9. T__F__N__ The heart takes 6 months to heal after a heart attack.

10. T__F__N__ Regular walking is an excellent exercise in the prevention of heart disease. However, after having a heart attack, your walking will have to be limited for the rest of your life.

11. T__F__N__ Lifting weights is one good way to get your heart back in shape.

12. T__F__N__ Your sex life has to be greatly altered after a heart attack.

13. T__F__N__ After a heart attack, it is possible for you to surpass your previous level of physical fitness by gradually increasing your physical activity.

14. T__F__N__ Cooking with butter is better than cooking with corn oil if you are trying to control cholesterol.

15. T__F__N__ As long as you exercise, it doesn't matter how much animal fat you have in your diet.

16. T__F__N__ An occasional cocktail is bad for your heart.

17. T__F__N__ After a heart attack, weight control becomes especially important in managing your health.

18. T__F__N__ Cutting down on salt is important for you even if you don't have high blood pressure.

19. T__F__N__ Coffee drinking is usually discouraged for heart patients. However, one to two cups of coffee a day may be allowed.

FIGURE 9-2. Teaching effectiveness evaluation form. (From Budan LJ: *Focus Crit Care* 10[5]:16-22, 1983.)

20. T__F__N__ The heart attack rate is twice as high in men who are heavy smokers as it is in nonsmokers.

21. T__F__N__ If you have smoked regularly for 10 to 20 years, quitting now won't help much.

22. T__F__N__ Shortly after returning home from the hospital, you can expect to feel rested and ready to go.

23. T__F__N__ Your spouse should always be in the house with you during your first 2 to 3 months at home.

24. T__F__N__ After discharge from the hospital, your doctor will ask you not to drive for a couple of weeks.

25. T__F__N__ Many heart attack patients feel more depressed shortly after they go home than while they are in the hospital.

26. T__F__N__ After you return home, the best thing to do is to stay in bed most of the time.

27. T__F__N__ During your first month at home, you will be permitted to move furniture, cut the grass, or carry in the groceries.

28. T__F__N__ In general, people who develop heart attacks are hard driving, competitive persons who don't take time to relax.

and implausible distractors help the learner get the correct answer by guessing. People appear to know more than they do. By contrast, ambiguity makes it difficult for learners to demonstrate the knowledge that they actually have. Testing for trivia may be reliable in providing information, but it is information about unimportant learning. Such errors should be avoided.

All item-writing methods can be placed along a continuum that ranges from writing informal-subjective items to writing from instructional objectives, writing from detailed instructional objectives, writing from algorithms, writing from item forms, or writing by computerized methods. Current test theorists suggest generating a number of items representing a domain (an objective) and randomly drawing a sample of items from each domain. Of course each objective should contain the kind of measurements that could measure that behavior. For example, a major objective for instruction about bathing babies might be to cleanse the baby safely. First of all much of the evaluation of learning in this situation should be done by observing the mother's motor skills. For evaluation of cognitive skill a group of written items may be collected. Consider the previously stated items 1 through 9 as a test of the basic cognitive aspects necessary for meeting this major objective. Large areas of content are left untested, such as correct temperature of the water and reasons for care of the eyes and the genitals. All the questions test at the level of knowledge or comprehension. Subobjectives would be defined in the learning plan and would indicate more specific behaviors. However, it is possible that testing at the levels of knowledge and comprehension would be sufficient to evaluate learning. Again, careful definition of goals is essential to teaching; however, teaching must be supplemented with other skills.

A strong logical link between instructional intent as expressed by the objectives and test items has been stressed in this discussion. It is also important to examine the response patterns of patients. Instructional sensitivity is especially important. When subjects have not been taught, they will do

TABLE 9-1. Types of measurement

Technique	Advantages	Disadvantages
DIRECT OBSERVATION	Performance under real or simulated conditions can be assessed	Awareness of the observer may affect performance
	Task is credible to patient	Training, supervising, using observers are costly
	Measure has good content validity	Number of patients who may be studied and their locale may be restricted because of the high per-patient cost of observing
Observational checklist	Simple, objective task to record observations	Checklist may be long if a multifaceted behavior is measured
	Observer error low	
Anchored rating scale	Simple, objective task to record observations	Difficult to write behavioral descriptions that differ by equal amounts over an ordered scale
	Observer error low	
	More gradations of judgment allowed than typical of an observational checklist	Descriptions may introduce several dimensions into a single rating
Observational record	Permits routine recording of simple, repetitive behaviors	Inferences depend on sample of time and fineness of recording unit
Anecdotal notes	May provide unique insights, illustrations	May be irrelevant to outcomes of interest
Critical incidents	Characterize adaptive and maladaptive behavior	Time consuming to collect and analyze
	May serve as the basis for more structured measurement	Focus on behavioral extremes; ignore typical behavior that is not outstandingly adaptive or maladaptive
PHYSIOLOGICAL MEASURES	Measure is accurate	Measure may be multiply determined; not affected by teaching outcomes alone
	Measure is a good indicator of health status	Measure may depend on patient's willingness and ability to perform routine self-testing and recording
	Measure is responsive to compliance with health care regimen	Measurement may be costly to obtain and analyze
		Measurement may be invasive
SELF-REPORT	Provides data and insights not available from other sources	Subject to faking, socially desirable response set
	Measures cognitive, affective, and performance outcomes directly	Requires skill in construction of instrument
Oral self-report	Little reading and no writing required of patient	Recording burden for interviewer
	Contingent questions, probing, and question clarification possible	Responses may be biased by interviewer
		Data collection individualized and costly

From McSweeney M: *Diabetes Educator* 7(3):9-15, 1981.

TABLE 9-1. Types of measurement—cont'd

Technique	Advantages	Disadvantages
Written self-report	Cheap, group administration of instruments is possible	Reading and recording burdens are placed on patient Questions are fixed; probes and clarifications cannot be introduced Possible reduction in response rate or quality resulting from respondent burden
Open-ended questions	Respondent free to shape reply	Extent of reply depends on verbal fluency of respondent Heavy recording burden for respondent or interviewer Inconsistent dimensions of response across patients Responses difficult to code and analyze
Closed, fixed-alternative questions	Easy recording, coding, processing of data Limited dimensions for replies Relative insensitivity to verbal fluency	Construction of instrument is time consuming Dimensions on which choices will vary must be anticipated Choices may be forced among nonsalient options
Single questions per topic	Speed, ease of response	Instability of response
Scales of questions per topic	Stability of response	Increased length of instrument
SELF-MONITORING	Recording occurs concurrently with behavior Access to all behaviors, covert and overt, is possible	Recording process may be reactive Quality of record is dependent on patient's cooperation Self-monitored data may differ from externally observed data
RECORDS	*Noninvasive*—supply data without added demands on patients *Nonreactive*—relatively insensitive to external manipulation to claim desired outcomes Relatively low cost of collection	May not be organized to permit easy access retrieval Incomplete and/or inconsistent records Indirect measures; may not be directly relevant to teaching outcomes
Patient charts, physician records		May require health care professional to record and interpret relevant data Privacy considerations may restrict access to records or require hierarchy of obtained consents
Agency service records, public records and reports	Data may be collected by relatively unskilled workers	Data come from a variety of sources with varying degrees of accessibility, reporting standards, and variable conceptualization

poorly on the items; when they have been taught, they will do well on the items. Items that fail to reflect this pattern may be faulty, or, possibly, a particular area of content was not taught.[23]

Other measures

Patients, perhaps guided by a monitoring form or a checklist, provide information on their own via self-reports (oral and written) and via self-monitoring (written). Physiologic measures are relevant to patient education and are often determined by several causes. In themselves they may not be valid indicators of the effects of patient education. Table 9-1 presents advantages and disadvantages of various measures in evaluating patient education.[28]

Earlier chapters placed emphasis on the emerging importance of self-efficacy as an outcome measure of patient education. Three examples of measures of self-efficacy in particular areas and for particular tasks are shown in the boxes on pp. 220 through 223.[21,27,39]

Measurement of affective learning

Much of this discussion has been related to cognitive and psychomotor learning because measures in those areas are best developed. Affective learn-

---

THE COPD SELF-EFFICACY SCALE

Read each numbered item below, and determine how confident you are that you could manage breathing difficulty or avoid breathing difficulty in that situation. Use the following scale as a basis for your answers:

(a) = Very confident
(b) = Pretty confident
(c) = Somewhat confident
(d) = Not very confident
(e) = Not at all confident

1. When I become too tired.
2. When there is humidity in the air.
3. When I go into cold weather from a warm place.
4. When I experience emotional stress or become upset.
5. When I go up stairs too fast.
6. When I try to deny that I have respiratory difficulties.
7. When I am around cigarette smoke.
8. When I become angry.
9. When I exercise or physically exert myself.
10. When I feel distressed about my life.
11. When I feel sexually inadequate or impotent.
12. When I am frustrated.
13. When I lift heavy objects.
14. When I begin to feel that someone is out to get me.
15. When I yell or scream.
16. When I am lying in bed.
17. During very hot or very cold weather.
18. When I laugh a lot.
19. When I do not follow a proper diet.
20. When I feel helpless.
21. When I drink alcoholic beverages.
22. When I get an infection (throat, sinus, colds, the flu, etc).
23. When I feel detached from everyone and everything.
24. When I experience anxiety.
25. When I am around pollution.
26. When I overeat.
27. When I feel down or depressed.
28. When I breathe improperly.
29. When I exercise in a room that is poorly ventilated.
30. When I am afraid.
31. When I experience the loss of a valued object or a loved one.
32. When there are problems in the home.
33. When I feel incompetent.
34. When I hurry or rush around.

From Wigal JK, Creer TL, Kotses H: *Chest* 99:1193-1196, 1991.

SELF-EFFICACY IN ADOLESCENT GIRLS AND BOYS WITH INSULIN-DEPENDENT DIABETES MELLITUS

Self-efficacy for diabetes scale (SED)

Instruction: Read the following questions and decide how much you believe you can or cannot do.

1. Be the one in charge of giving my insulin injection to myself
2. Figure out my own meals and snacks at home
3. Figure out what foods to eat when I am away from home
4. Keep track of my own blood sugar levels
5. Watch my own sugar levels in my urine
6. Change the amount of time I get insulin when I get a lot of extra exercise
7. Judge the amount of food I should eat before activities
8. Figure out how much insulin to give myself when I am sick in bed
9. Prevent having reactions
10. Avoid or get rid of dents, swelling, or redness of my skin where I get my shot
11. Talk to my doctor myself and ask for the things I need
12. Suggest to my parents changes in my insulin dose
13. Sleep away from home on a class trip or at a friend's house where no one knows about my diabetes
14. Keep myself free of high blood sugar levels
15. Know how to make my urine tests look better or worse than they are
16. Avoid having acetones
17. Change my doctor if I don't like him/her
18. Feel able to stop a reaction when I am having one
19. Ask for help I need from other people when I feel sick
20. Tell a friend I have diabetes
21. Play baseball or other sports that take a lot of energy
22. Argue with my doctor if I felt he/she were not being fair
23. Prevent blindness and other complications from my diabetes
24. Tell my boyfriend or girlfriend I am diabetic
25. Do things I have been told not to when I really want to do them
26. Get as much attention from others when my diabetes is under control as when it isn't
27. Easily talk to a group of people at a party when I don't know them
28. Make a teacher see my point of view
29. Show my anger to a friend when he/she has done something to upset me
30. Take responsibility for getting my homework and chores done
31. Regularly wear a medical alert tag or bracelet which says I have diabetes
32. Sneak food not on my diet without getting caught
33. Believe that I have the ability to have control over my diabetes
34. Follow my doctor's orders for taking care of my diabetes
35. Run my life the same as I would if I didn't have diabetes

From Grossman HY, Brink S, Hauser ST: *Diabetes Care* 10:324-329, 1987.

ARTHRITIS SELF-EFFICACY SCALE*

Self-efficacy pain subscale

In the following questions, we'd like to know how your arthritis pain affects you. For each of the following questions, please circle the number which corresponds to your certainty that you can *now* perform the following tasks.

1. How certain are you that you can decrease your pain *quite a bit?*
2. How certain are you that you can continue most of your daily activities?
3. How certain are you that you can keep arthritis pain from interfering with your sleep?
4. How certain are you that you can make a *small-to-moderate* reduction in your arthritis pain by using methods other than taking extra medication?
5. How certain are you that you can make a *large* reduction in your arthritis pain by using methods other than taking extra medication?

Self-efficacy function subscale

We would like to know how confident you are in performing certain daily activities. For each of the following questions, please circle the number which corresponds to your certainty that you can perform the tasks as of *now, without* assistive devices or help from another person. Please consider what you *routinely* can do, not what would require a single extraordinary effort.

AS OF NOW, HOW CERTAIN ARE YOU THAT YOU CAN:

1. Walk 100 feet on flat ground in 20 seconds?
2. Walk 10 steps downstairs in 7 seconds?
3. Get out of an armless chair quickly, without using your hands for support?
4. Button and unbutton 3 medium-size buttons in a row in 12 seconds?
5. Cut 2 bite-size pieces of meat with a knife and fork in 8 seconds?
6. Turn an outdoor faucet all the way on and all the way off?
7. Scratch your upper back with both your right and left hands?
8. Get in and out of the passenger side of a car without assistance from another person and without physical aids?
9. Put on a long-sleeve front-opening shirt or blouse (without buttoning) in 8 seconds?

From Lorig K and others: *Arthritis Rheum* 32:37-44, 1989.

---

ing has been thought to develop automatically, although not directly, from knowledge and is private behavior. Although some providers worry about indoctrination, affective learning (attitudes, values, interests, preferences, anxiety, self-esteem) is critical to purposeful behavior and can be developed through instructional programs.

The measurement of affective learning[1] flows from critical features of affective characteristics: (1) they are typical ways of feeling, (2) they possess intensity, (3) they imply direction, and (4) they are directed toward some target. Table 9-2 provides comparison of specific affective characteristics in terms of these critical features. The higher the intensity, the more motivating the characteristic. Cognitive tests aim to measure maximum performance and correctness of response. Affective instruments test for typical performance and consistency across situations.

To start measuring affective characteristics, define the set of behaviors that can be used to make deductions about the characteristic. Define also the

ARTHRITIS SELF-EFFICACY SCALE—cont'd

Self-efficacy other symptoms subscale

In the following questions, we'd like to know how you feel about your ability to control your arthritis. For each of the following questions, please circle the number which corresponds to the certainty that you can *now* perform the following activities or tasks.

1. *How certain* are you that you can control your fatigue?
2. *How certain* are you that you can regulate your activity so as to be active without aggravating your arthritis?
3. *How certain* are you that you can do something to help yourself feel better if you are feeling blue?
4. As compared with other people with arthritis like yours, *how certain* are you that you can manage arthritis pain during your daily activities?
5. *How certain* are you that you can manage your arthritis symptoms so that you can do the things you enjoy doing?
6. *How certain* are you that you can deal with the frustration of arthritis?

---

*Each question if followed by the scale:

10	20	30	40	50	60	70	80	90	100
very uncertain				moderately uncertain					very certain

Each subscale is scored separately, by taking the mean of the subscale items. If one-fourth or less of the data are missing, the score is a mean of the completed data. If more than one-fourth of the data are missing, no score is calculated. (The authors invite others to use the scale and would appreciate being informed of study results.)

situations in which the behaviors occur. For example, a patient following a low-sodium diet might be in the situations of cooking for self, eating at a restaurant, or eating in social situations. The patient values the idea of adherence to the diet. However, the patient is still enjoying a social life by inquiring about the sodium content of food in question, abstaining from food that is questionable, and attending social functions of interest, even if appropriate food is not available. Data on affective learning are gathered through observational and self-report methods. Observations can be misinterpreted. Observations with clear operational definitions and with several trained observers—an expensive undertaking—can reduce the risk of faulty inference.

In a clinical setting a consistent perceptive caregiver (a primary nurse) could perform many observations. Self-report methods containing statements, questions, or adjectives that query the patient, asking him or her to agree or disagree, are useful. A scale can list responses of "strongly agree" to "strongly disagree" or list a scale of how many people are characterized by particular behaviors or thoughts. Following is an example of an item that might be answered on the former scale:

Illness isolates a person.

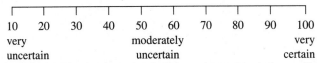

| Strongly disagree | Disagree | Uncertain | Agree | Strongly agree |

TABLE 9-2. A comparison of specific affective characteristics in terms of the critical features of affective characteristics

Specific affective characteristics*	Average intensity	Direction	Target
Attitudes	Moderate	Unfavorable or favorable	Any object, activity, or idea; most frequently an object
Interests	High	Disinterested or interested	Any object, activity, or idea; most frequently an activity
Values	High	Unimportant or important	Any object, activity, or idea; most frequently an idea
Preferences	Low	Target A or target B	Pairs (target A, target B) of objects, activities, or ideas
Locus of control	Moderately low	External or internal	A behavior or an activity that follows a behavior
Anxiety	High	Relaxed or tense	Any object, activity, or idea perceived as a threat
Health learning self-esteem	Moderately high	Negative or positive	The self in a health learning setting

From Anderson LW: *Assessing affective characteristics in the schools,* Boston, 1981, Allyn & Bacon, p 41.
*Characteristics defined as follows:
Attitude: A learned predisposition to respond in a consistently favorable or unfavorable manner with respect to a given object.
Interest: A disposition organized through experience that impels an individual to seek out particular objects, activities, understandings, skills, or goals for attention or acquisition.
Values: A conception of the desirable—that which ought to be desired, not that which *is* desired—influences the selection of behavior.
Preferences: A disposition to receive one object as opposed to another.
Locus of control: Extent to which individuals tend to accept responsibility for their own behavior, the consequences of their behavior, or both.
Anxiety: The experience of tension that results from real or imaginary threats to the individual's security.
Health learning self-esteem: The individual's evaluative perception of how good a learner he or she is in a health setting.

A number of such items could be used in an attempt to elicit expression of feeling about dependence, for example, or about a group of attitudes common to illness. The person who develops such a tool and interprets results must know a considerable amount about attitudes and how they are exhibited. This is particularly important because attitude scales are easily faked or answered in a socially desirable manner, and persons with the same attitudes can manifest different behaviors. Because of the skill needed and the limitations of this method, usually only standardized tests are used. These are combined with other behavior observations. Specialized texts are available to assist the caregiver in developing the various kinds of scales used to measure the affective characteristics by self-report. Because of the recent concern about the level of relationship between attitudes and behavior, perhaps direct measurement of behavior is a more useful approach when behavior change is the goal.

Goal attainment scaling

Goal attainment scaling[25] is a form of goal-oriented evaluation developed in the field of mental health that can be used with individual clients, staff, or programs. It can be adapted to patient education. A form bearing a grid with a succession of discrete five-point scales is used to assess attainment level. Each scale represents an individual

Check whether or not the scale has been mutually negotiated between patient and CIC interviewer.	SCALE HEADINGS AND SCALE WEIGHTS				
SCALE ATTAINMENT LEVELS	SCALE 1: Education Yes __ No X__ ($w_1 = 20$)	SCALE 2: Suicide Yes __ No X__ ($w_2 = 30$)	SCALE 3: Manipulation Yes __ No X__ ($w_3 = 25$)	SCALE 4: Drug Abuse Yes X__ No __ ($w_4 = 30$)	SCALE 5: Dependency on CIC Yes X__ No __ ($w_5 = 10$)
a. most unfavorable treatment outcome thought likely (−2)	Patient has made no attempt to enroll in high school. ✓	Patient has committed suicide.	Patient makes rounds of community service agencies demanding medication, and refuses other forms of treatment.	Patient reports addiction to "hard narcotics" (heroin, morphine).	Patient has contacted CIC by telephone or in person at least seven times since his first visit.
b. less than expected success with treatment (−1)	Patient has enrolled in high school, but at ime of follow-up has dropped out.	Patient has acted on at least one suicidal impulse since her first contact with the CIC, but has not succeeded. ✓	Patient no longer visits CIC with demands for medication but continues with other community agencies and still refuses other forms of treatment. ✓	Patient has used "hard narcotics," but is not addicted, and/or uses hallucinogens (LSD, Pot) more than four times a month. ✓	Patient has contacted CIC 5-6 times since intake. ✓
c. expected level of treatment success (0)	Patient has enrolled, and is in school at follow-up, but is attending class sporadically (misses an average of more than a third of her classes during a week).	Patient reports she has had at least four suicidal impulses since her first contact with the CIC but has not acted on any of them.	Patient no longer attempts to manipulate for drugs at community service agencies, but will not accept another form of treatment.	Patient has not used "hard narcotics" during follow-up period, and uses hallucinogens between 1-4 times a month. *	Patient contacted CIC 3-4 times since intake.
d. more than expected success with treatment (+1)	Patient has enrolled, is in school at follow-up, and is attending classes consistently, but has no vocational goals.	*	Patient accepts non-medication treatment at some community agency. *	Patient uses hallucinogens less than once a month.	
e. best anticipated success with treatment (+2)	Patient has enrolled, is in school at follow-up, is attending classes consistently, and has some vocational goal.	Patient reports she has had no suicidal impulses since her first contact with the CIC.	Patient accepts non-medication treatment, and by own report shows signs of improvement.	At time of follow-up, patient is not using any illegal drugs.	Patient has not contacted CIC since intake. *

FIGURE 9-3. Form for assessing goal attainment. (From Evaluation, Special Monograph No. 1, 1973, p 15.)

goal arranged along a qualitatively ordered series of possible outcomes. The nature of these outcomes ranges from the most unfavorable outcome possible to the best anticipated success with the treatment.

Each scale represents an area of need—perhaps an objective for education with an individual patient. The problem areas or goals are weighted to indicate their relative importance. A time is specified for goal follow-up, and scales are developed to assess the level of achievement reached. After specifying the outcomes relevant to each level of expectation, and after appropriate and effective action has been taken, the form (Figure 9-3) is used. The form describes whether the stated goals have been attained at the specified time of follow-up and allows calculation of a summary score. Indicators of goal attainment can range from client self-report to report of family and friends, clinical observations by health care professionals, results on lab tests, and scores on tests. Scaling can be done by clinicians, by clinicians with patients, or by patients, depending on the content of the scale. This system allows individualized problem definition and uses each client as his or her own control in the definition of success.

EVALUATING THE TEACHING-LEARNING PROCESS

Measurement is carried out so that the teaching-learning process can be evaluated more accurately than it could be by general impressions. Evaluation must go beyond measurement. It requires a value judgment about learning and teaching. Evaluation must summarize the evidence and determine how well the objectives are being met.

The goal-attainment scaling system described earlier puts measurements in an evaluative framework. Most measurements are not placed into such a clear framework but rather are compared with the stated outcome goals or with a set of standards.

Measurement and evaluation occur continuously during teaching, serving to redirect the activities of the teacher and the learner. Information about learners' progress is gathered by having learners respond to questions, perform periodically, or both.

The expressions of boredom, interest, confusion, or enlightenment on learners' faces give clues about their understanding of the material being taught.

Some individuals are able to tell the teacher that they do not understand. Others cannot identify or express their uncertainty. To identify material that is not clear to the learner, the provider can retrace the explanation or the skill demonstration, can ask questions at intervals, or can observe and critique the performance of a skill by the learner. Such technique will point up terms used by the teacher that the learners may not understand, or it may reveal that the learners are overloaded with complex instructions. Trying to reteach without determining the nature of the learning problem may cause the caregiver to make the same error again. It is unwise to teach for a very long period of time (or even one lesson period) without requiring the learner to respond so that teaching and learning errors can be corrected.

Adequacy of learning must eventually be evaluated in terms of meeting the final objectives. Of course, if satisfactory evaluation is done as the teaching is going on, the degree of attainment of final objectives or the time needed to meet the final objectives can be quite accurately predicted. Too often when staff are teaching hospital patients, flexibility in time is not available for teaching, and the entire teaching-learning process, particularly evaluation, gets short shrift. Having only a brief time for teaching imposes restrictions. Staff may assume that the patient who has been taught has learned. Do not take this for granted!

Crucial decisions regarding patients, such as whether they can live alone, rest on the outcome of learning. The minimum performance necessary for the individual to function must be identified. Certain basic information and skills must be learned because they are essential to the performance of a particular task. Other information and skills may also be crucial, depending on how independently the individual will be functioning. Therefore an adequate level of performance for one individual may not be sufficient for another.

When measuring, teachers focus on the element they have identified as crucial. In a test the learner should probably be able to answer or perform nearly 94% of all crucial behaviors. This figure allows for some error in the measurement tool. Patient education must be followed by questioning and the reteaching of crucial items when patients give incorrect responses. In giving a written test, the teacher may easily lose sight of the difference between essential learning and other items. The score may be added up, and the observer may decide that the learner, who has passed half the items, has learned adequately. The question may never be asked: Exactly what does he or she know? Observers of motor skills are more likely to realize intuitively that the individual who is not placing the crutches in the proper position will have difficulty learning to walk with them.

The person constructing the series of items must be sure that the plan measures an individual's ability to transfer knowledge and skills gained in the instructional situation to other situations described or suggested by the objectives. Thorough testing of transfer is necessary because knowledge about ways to produce and verify transfer without careful measurement is insufficient. Initial learning must be established well enough to allow for transfer. Stimulus variation (a variety of situations and tasks) in the initial learning produces transfer and determines how much time instruction and learning difficult tasks should take at various stages in the process of learning.

Suppose that related objectives are as follows:
- To take diuretic in the prescribed dosage and at the prescribed time
- To recognize desired and undesired effects of the medication
- To contact the nurse practitioner when undesired effects occur

Instruction for such objectives would no doubt include information about the purpose of the medication, the skills needed to take it, the monitoring of desired and undesired effects, the behavioral reinforcements for adherence, and the practice in problem situations related to taking the medication

correctly. It is not feasible to give instruction that represents all possible situations an individual will encounter. If representative situations are used for teaching, most individuals can transfer information to similar situations. To check the amount of transfer the patient actually can make, questions should be constructed that deal with variations or combinations of themes already presented that represent situations the patient might encounter. With a series of questions, it is possible to map the areas that the patient does and does not know. The following questions should require transfer (if they have not been used in original instruction):

1. Suppose you have intestinal flu with vomiting and diarrhea for several days. How would this affect the taking of your diuretic?
2. If the belts on your clothes feel tighter over a period of 3 days, what should you do?
3. You are visiting friends for a few days and find that they do not have any citrus fruit. What should you do?

The interpretation of evaluation by teacher and learner is of utmost importance. Learners will have varying degrees of insight into their progress. Allowing for teacher bias, teachers and learners will agree more or less on the amount of progress that has been made. Learners should assess their progress and should discuss differences and similarities with regard to the teacher's assessment. This kind of interchange will help each party. However, when differences of opinion persist, the caregiver must maintain responsibility.

For example, a public health nurse may be teaching a daughter to give bed care to her elderly mother. After several sessions, the daughter believes that she is performing adequately. However, the public health nurse observes that the daughter is careless about keeping side rails up on the hospital bed, that provisions for washing the mother's genitals are lacking, that regular turning is not being carried out, and that foot support is not being used—all are lessons that have been taught. Whatever the daughter's reason, emotional or otherwise, for not giving essential care, the nurse is faced with a choice. One alternative is to find the basis for lack of learning and reteach the learner, weighing the likelihood that the learner will change against the relative adequacy of the care. The other is to suggest that the learner make other arrangements for care because the nurse is responsible for supervision of care. Sometimes the learner becomes hostile toward the nurse. It is a way of expressing a desire to get out of the situation. Evidence of positive change in the learners is rewarding for the teachers, as well as the learners.

The relationship between learner's competence and teacher's competence is entangled in evaluation. To some extent this relationship depends on which person is regarded as more responsible for learning. Sometimes it is obvious that a teacher cannot communicate or does not understand the subject matter. In this case the teacher needs to be helped to develop teaching skill. Teaching has the potential for being harmful as well as ineffective, and professional incompetence exists in this area of nursing or medicine, as well as in any other. Possible harmful effects include leaving the patient with incapacitating confusion, a loss of self-confidence, or an inability to accomplish necessary reintegration into a family or other social group.

Evaluation of teaching and learning also includes a perspective of the known limitations of teaching today—particularly in the area of motivating individuals. Knowledge of the determinants of behavior at the present time is both limited and fragmented, and a practical means of assessing the relative influence of each factor is virtually nonexistent. Therefore in a particular situation it is difficult to estimate how each factor that is already present is influencing particular behavior and how new factors might affect behavior. In many of the complex situations that require learning, reality factors, such as poverty, health, and family crisis, limit the effect that teaching can have. In such situations, small but important effects are characteristic even of the "good" programs.

One solution has been to use several complementary kinds of interventions (teaching may be one) in order to maximize the effect. Sometimes nothing seems to have an effect, and the individual or family does not recover from illness or achieve high-level wellness. Explanation may be sought through inquiry into the patient's perceptions, motives, values, intelligence, and grasp of relevant knowledge. It has also been suggested that the patient's situation might reflect a condition such as powerlessness, and his or her ability to learn may be only one of the behaviors affected.

Because behavioral syndromes exist, and because learning is a central means used by individuals and groups to adapt, learning should be affected on a regular basis. Teaching programs are affected by limitations in our knowledge of factors that affect learning, descriptions of the effects of such factors, and predictions that can be made about learning. The educational approach allows participants to accept, adopt, or reject learning. This approach may allow too much freedom for some objectives that are important to society. Institutional controls, although more difficult to establish, can be more effective in controlling behavior.

Thus evaluation during and at the conclusion of a segment of teaching-learning is a summation and interpretation of the results of measurement. It reinforces successful behaviors of learners and teachers. It also provides a time to analyze progress and to redirect activities.

Inevitably, if teaching fails, the same question is asked before beginning the process of teaching: Is the behavior change necessary? The answer may not be clear.

This question about proper patient behavior is never more unclear than in the affective domain. For parents of disabled children, a widespread, common-sense ideology of "acceptance" is used by both medical personnel and parents. "Gratefulness" and "self-help" are common themes in the journals, and there is frequently a lack of support for public disagreement with the official morality. The cost of "bucking the system" on this implied educational objective may be too high.

PROGRAM EVALUATION

A program has been identified by Cronbach and others[7] as a standing arrangement that provides for a social service. Increasingly, patient education services are being organized into programs of common goals: teaching and evaluation approaches for patients with similar conditions and learning needs.

Evaluation is a systematic examination of events occurring in and consequent to a contemporary program. Evaluation is initiated for many purposes: choosing the best prospect among several proposed lines of action, fine-tuning a program already in operation, or maintaining quality control. It is worth the effort if flaws in the program or in its underlying conception become evident or if documentation of the benefits of an excellent program might encourage wider application. Finally, evaluation is as much involved with political interaction as it is with the determination of facts. It has to be credible to the several groups who have a stake in the program.[7]

Several preconditions must be met to evaluate. If not, proceeding may not be worthwhile. For example, the instructional program must have a reasonable design that can produce observable effects. If the goals are not clearly defined or if the teaching intervention will not yield the goals, the program should be redesigned before an institution spends the resources that a thorough evaluation requires. For example, if the outcome of a program is to ensure patient compliance with a drug regimen and needs assessment shows low compliance in the target group, yet, the program's design only involves a pharmacist who hands out drug information sheets when he or she has time, it is unlikely that the program as designed can meet its goals. Effecting compliance requires more than drug information, and a delivery system that is haphazard, diffuse, or unclear will not be effective.

Evaluation is especially important in the initial implementation of a recently designed program, when problem areas have been identified in a refined program, or when the program is introduced at a new site.[19] If evaluative data are collected at all in patient education, they are frequently unorganized and collected as an afterthought. Remember that the purpose of evaluation is to assist in making a decision. It lies on a continuum with research, which demands that results be applicable beyond the study population.[33]

Ruzicki outlines a series of steps in conducting an evaluation and illustrates this process with the evaluation of a cardiac rehabilitation program at her hospital as an example. The target audiences for the evaluation were identified as the hospital's patient education committee, administration, cardiologists, and cardiac surgeons. Six evaluative questions were formulated: Does the program meet stated objectives for patient learning? Does it have an impact on changes in risk-factor behaviors after discharge? As a result of their participation in the program do patients believe that they can manage their own care after discharge? Which teaching techniques are viewed as most helpful by patients? Are physicians satisfied with the program and do they notice differences after discharge in patients who have participated? Are teaching staff members satisfied with the program and do they implement it consistently? It is essential to focus the evaluation through development of questions. Because resources for evaluation in this example were limited, questionnaires were used and sample patients were studied.

Results of the evaluation showed that overall the program was functioning as it should. However, it revealed that there was a lack of documentation and that the nurses were not familiar with some of the information they were to teach or with the closed circuit television films available. The evaluation clearly served as a management tool for improvement of the program.[33]

Administrators are frequently interested in cost data such as the cost per infection averted after a patient education program. In formulating data collection tools and in evaluating individual patient learning the same cautions apply. Homemade instruments may fit a particular program better; however, they will not permit comparison with other evaluations. Standardized instruments have an opposite set of benefits and concerns. Remember as well that results may reflect inadequate measurement and a need to improve the data gathering tools. Data can be gathered as part of routine administrative procedures or in a periodic survey.[19]

Some of Ruzicki's questions relate to evaluation of the outcomes of the program and some to process. Administrators are frequently interested in the cost per infection averted after a patient education program and in whether the program could be more cost efficient. Costs usually include personnel, equipment and depreciation, materials, other operating expenses, and sometimes a portion of overhead costs. The easiest way to get a sense of efficiency is to compare one program with another one that shows the same outcomes and utilization. However, competition among programs for survival does not encourage such comparisons. Insurance companies have been interested in efficiency in areas they reimburse for patient education programs.[3]

Sometimes evaluation of a clinical program shows the need for a teaching program. Whatley, Guthrie, and Turner describe a program of intravenous therapy in the home that uses right atrial catheters. Eighty percent of the catheters were removed because of potentially preventable complications. Some believed that the catheter removal rate could be reduced with an organized teaching program including practice for patients and staff, a protocol to prevent early patient discharge before teaching, and 24-hour home care service on discharge. Three years after initiation of the program, longevity of the catheters had improved significantly.[38]

An evaluation reported in the literature[15] provides good examples of several of the points made previously. For 4 years, staff conducted retrospective evaluations of teaching programs for patients with diabetes and patients with myocardial infarctions. These evaluations were done with questionnaires that assessed patient knowledge of disease. They also recommended changes of behavior such as diet or quitting smoking. It was found that 3 years earlier all coronary patients had reported climbing stairs, and many had reported attending coronary club meetings. However, in a recent survey only 89% were climbing stairs and none was attending coronary club meetings. Earlier, a clinical specialist had done coronary teaching, had spent considerable time with patients, and had given personal invitations to the club meetings.

Later, a staff nurse was coordinating the rehabilitation program along with other responsibilities, and several staff nurses were handling most of the teaching. As a result of the evaluation the program now gives patients a brochure about the club and reminders about the meetings.

The diabetes survey showed some strong points of the program. However, it also showed that 90% of the patients said that they stayed on their diet only sometimes. The program will now have patients plan their own menus while in the hospital. Results on foot care and rotation of injection sites were also unsatisfactory. The presentations on these topics were revised, and visual aids were added. Staff nurses began writing orders for foot care on patients' charts. These changes improved the evaluation. This description of one program shows use of historical data to determine whether results are satisfactory. It considers the delivery system an important element that can be altered to improve instruction. The yearly evaluations of these programs served to fine-tune the programs and maintain quality control.

An example of process, outcome, and, to a certain extent, efficiency outcome in a public health setting has been reported by Dignan and others.[10] The Forsyth County Cervical Cancer Prevention Project is a community-based health education program designed to encourage black women in the target population to obtain Pap smears on a regular basis and to return for follow-up care when necessary. Process monitoring is done to ensure documentation of program activities, such as distribution of printed materials and coverage of the target population. Those monitoring the process discovered that leaflets distributed in grocery stores were not reaching low-income women often enough. Thereafter, distribution of the leaflets was timed to coincide with receipt of Social Security payments. Interviewing members of the target population provided perspective about which materials and activities were having the greatest impact in raising awareness of cervical screening. In addition, morbidity and mortality data were used. Evaluation served to redirect and improve the campaign as it went along at a cost of 7% of the project's annual expenditures.[10]

Quality assurance

Evaluation of services given to groups of patients is usually carried out through quality assurance studies—most frequently, audits. Donabedian believes that quality is represented by the discernible improvements in health status.[11] Health care can be judged by medical efficacy, social acceptability, and economic efficiency.

Comparing the quality assurance methods for evaluation with the body of thought that supports program evaluation is useful. Quality assurance methods focus on the appropriateness and adequacy of services provided to program recipients. Program evaluation focuses on client outcome variables as they relate to the type of service, the level of staff effort, or the comparative cost-effectiveness of service modalities. Quality assurance relies heavily on peer review, on structural criteria derived from accrediting standards, and on consensus. In program evaluation greater emphasis is placed on scientific research methods and use of statistical methods. In quality assurance, standards of performance are established. Whenever levels of quality are judged inadequate, some means of improving care must be devised. Usually care is improved by provider-patient interaction through education or in the compliance of both in some aspect of the service setting. Quality assurance often uses some form of records review. Program evaluation requires systematic collection and analysis of data.[20]

A quality assurance program for a hospice provides an example of the necessary elements and illustrates how patient education is often an integral part of such programs. Ongoing quality assurance programs have been mandated for agency accreditation for hospices. The following are criteria for hospice patient education:

Patient and caregiver education

1. Hospice program has been discussed with patient and family.

2. The dying process has been discussed by patient and family.
3. Patient and caregiver understand management of symptoms for which there are complaints: pain, constipation, edema, shortness of breath, nausea, vomiting, etc., as indicated by
   - RN instructions given
   - Understanding demonstrated by family's appropriate questions, responses, and actions

Hospice patient education must conform to the criteria. Instructions for retrieving data include:

- Look for instruction and return demonstration at beginning of hospice service and each time medical/nursing orders change regarding symptom management.
- Look for documentation that patient and/or family indicated understanding of dying process at least 1 week before patient's death; look for such things as: *accepts appearance of patient near death, finds 24-hour medication acceptable, accepts patient's low energy and appetite, accepts patient's inability to interact with others, etc.*

Criteria must include percentages that mark the standard that the patient is expected to achieve. Current records should be audited.[34]

Audit studies of patient records frequently show serious difficulties with documentation of patient education. The experience of one committee when auditing records of cholecystectomy patients does not seem uncommon. They found the highest deficiency rate in documentation of patient knowledge on discharge. Subsequently, the following criteria for this group of patients were written:

Outcomes—cholecystectomy*[32]

1. Knowledge
   a. Patient verbalized knowledge of discharge diet as ordered by physician.
   b. Patient verbalized knowledge about returning to normal activities in 4-6 weeks.

---

*From Rinaldi LA, Kelly B: What to do after the audit is done. *Am J Nurs* 77:268-269, 1977.

2. Physical status
   a. Ambulates
   b. Afebrile
   c. Wound clean and dry

In a study measuring clinical performance of physicians with patients with hernia repair, two criteria were basic: Was the wound healed at the first outpatient visit? Was the patient educated about exertion, smoking, and obesity? Failure to educate the patient was the most frequent reason for low scores.[13] One hospital reported that it had wrestled with problems of inadequate documentation for years; however, observation proved that teaching was taking place. Staff were confused about how to document patient education, and previous teaching forms had been limited to one specific diagnosis. A new 8 × 11 inch foldover form was designed with a section generic to education for all diagnoses. It was placed on the Kardex and made part of the permanent chart. Audits made before and after initiation of the form showed that documentation had improved. Graphs of these results were displayed on stations as motivators. In the maternity unit, where repetitive teaching occurred, the medical staff successfully used brightly colored stickers to record relevant teaching.[26]

Sometimes the problem is not lack of documentation but absence of appropriate criteria. In an analysis of criteria used for 448 medical audits completed in the Minneapolis–St. Paul area from 1975 to 1979, it was found that 63% of the audits had no patient-education criteria. In the total number of audit criteria, 96% were diagnosis and treatment oriented, 4% were patient-education criteria, and 3% related to psychosocial history or impact of illness criteria.[2]

Outcome and process criteria are probably needed in evaluation of patient education. In other areas of care it has been found that outcome and process studies on the same patients do not correlate highly.[4] Sometimes health status at the end of the study period is dependent on the initial status, with process measure playing a small role. Process audit can provide some control over the quality of service, even though the process can become an end in itself.

Standards for evaluation and study design

The judgment involved in evaluation can be based on various standards: historical, normative, absolute, theoretic, negotiated, arbitrary, as well as other standards. Health education usually has used historical or normative standards.[16] However, significant areas of the practice of patient education exist where measurement has been insufficient or primitive, and the level of effect historically or across programs is not known.

Summaries of patient education outcome research are available. (See Appendix E for summaries of these meta-analyses.) As more research is done and good-quality summaries are produced, these findings will produce additional standards.

All studies have a study design: a description of the way subjects are chosen; the method for assigning interventions; the occasions when measures can be obtained; and the quality of the measures. As indicated earlier, evaluations fall on a continuum according to the rigor of their designs. Those with the most rigorous designs might be called evaluative research because they incorporate procedures and measures that conform to standards of research. They try to isolate the effect of the educational program. These research standards include study of a representative sample of the target population by randomly assigning individuals to control and to experimental groups and by using measures with a high degree of reliability and validity.

Appropriate study designs are described by Green.[17] The most common and least valid form of evaluation is the post hoc survey. In this survey people are asked about their health behavior and if they had been exposed to the educational message or treatment. These studies suffer from inaccurate reporting. In addition, those who say that they were exposed to education are usually either people who exposed themselves because they were already motivated or people who had previously adopted the behavior of interest and then were exposed to the message.

The midcycle switch design is useful for those who cannot afford two new programs for comparison groups but are concerned about the ethical implications of withholding patient education.

Experimental group	O	X	O		O
Control group	O		O	X	O

O = observation, X = treatment.

With random assignment, the design is strengthened.

Times of measurement and interpretation are important in light of other possible reasons for the effects obtained. Figure 9-4 shows some examples. Curve A illustrates the error that would be made in underestimating the impact of an educational program if the effect were measured as the difference between O_1 and O_2. This pattern can occur when the learner must go through an attitude change between the educational exposure and the actual change in behavior. Curve B illustrates the

overestimation of impact if observations at time 2 (O_2) were viewed as permanent. This backsliding effect is not uncommon with behavioral changes that are complex, such as stopping smoking, diet changes, and complicated medication regimens. Some educational effects are really only triggers to behavior that would have changed eventually anyhow (curve C). The gains at O_2 may be offset at O_3, so the net long-term gain is zero. This phenomenon is most notable in some mass media campaigns designed to recruit new patients to a screening clinic or a family planning clinic. The gains immediately after the broadcasts represent patients who would have appeared within a few months anyway. Curve D shows why control groups are important: apparent gains or losses may have been occurring already as part of general trends or extraneous events. Finally, curve E shows a relapse

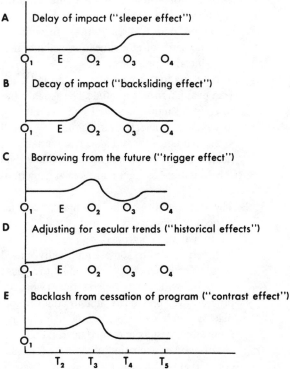

FIGURE 9-4. Points of observation relative to different educational inputs. (From Green LW: *Am J Public Health* 67:155-161, 1977.)

that can occur from premature termination of the educational treatment, such as in self-care, smoking, or diet programs.

More rigorous formal evaluation of patient education programs will become common. Examples of program evaluation appear that are politically sensitive and are using the strongest research design possible. One such example is a practical guide for evaluating child-life programming.[36] Such programs may be especially vulnerable because they do not generate a readily identifiable source of revenue and are relatively new (55% have been established since 1968). Although they do not evaluate in any rigorous sense, logs of the number and length of services offered and recordings of spontaneous patient responses are useful. The following evaluation steps measure child-life programming:

1. Describe the goals of the program, such as seeking to reduce psychologic upset among children and promoting normal growth and development.
2. Translate the goals into measurable indicators of goal achievement, including cost. For example, use the research literature on control of postoperative upset as a basis for showing reduced cost in care to families and to the hospital and increased benefits to the hospital in competing for patients.
3. Collect data on indicators for those exposed to the program and for an equivalent group not exposed, such as those on a different unit or before and after institution of the program.
4. Compare the data in raw form or by statistical tests and write the report. The report should read like a lawyer's brief; that is, it should advocate the program. Place particularly impressive results on specially prepared summary sheets or in the agency newspaper. Include in the report results of ongoing evaluation of the program (formative) to show efforts to improve it, changes or services not possible because of lack of resources or satisfactory conditions, and recommendations that would improve the delivery of services.

The ongoing monitoring of the program might have used a tool, such as the Goal Attainment Scale, for individual patients. A distribution of goal attainment scores for clients completing a program reveals those cases with very high or very low scores. These can be identified and studied for common traits. This monitoring allows the teacher to draw conclusions about the type of clients best served by the program.[25]

Studies done by external evaluators are likely to aim for a more objective tone than that suggested in item 4 in the preceding list. Evidence about a program is often mixed and can be presented with a negative or positive focus. The essential needs of the program include some standards for evaluation that are adequate to support the practice of a particular program—standards that are always presented in a more or less formal, nonbiased way. The administration usually makes decisions about programs, as do accrediting teams. These decisions are based on professional judgment and can often be strengthened with a base of empirical evidence. The following points, though in a formulative stage, are standards or guidelines for evaluation of a patient education program:

1. A combination of goal-attainment and goal-free evaluation is essential. The teacher has to consider unintended and intended effects, as well as the objectives in light of the overall goals patient education shares with all of health care—an intelligent compliance and rehabilitation to optimum social functioning.
2. The evaluation should summarize all instances of the service so that its quality can be known and controlled.
3. Comparison with some empirically based standards is necessary. At this time these standards will mostly be historical (what the program was previously able to attain). Normative standards should accrue as programs report their results and have instruments that are of good enough quality to allow for valid comparison.
4. The program should meet absolute standards in terms of medical safety. That is, the learn-

ing goals must represent at least minimum knowledge and skills for safe self-treatment. Also, evidence must show that every patient meets at least those minimum goals when exiting the program. If patients cannot meet the minimum standards, a noneducational therapy must be substituted.

5. Several evaluation methods and measurements should be used because each in itself is too limited to allow for generalization about the program.

6. An operational description of behavioral units to be attained should be formed for minimum and optimum patient education goals.

After the program has been launched and has been operating for a short period of time, formative evaluation (feedback) can be implemented; however, it need not be mandatory. Rapidly molding

the program to an acceptable level of effectiveness will conserve resources. This is a better option than letting the program function at reduced effectiveness because evidence is not available. Also, it is a far better strategy to develop a strong teaching program with sufficient potency for the job and to evaluate the worth of one or another element of the program by withdrawing it and studying the effect.[18] In a strong program the teacher intervenes when the motivation is high or the teacher creates motivation. Practice is always involved. A variety of learning modalities and levels of materials are provided, and teachers and environment are persuasive.

Special norms, especially guidelines 3 and 4 listed in the foregoing text, should probably be kept for different categories of patients as listed in the box below.

CLASSES OF PATIENTS FOR PATIENT EDUCATION BASED ON READINESS* AND ON BEHAVIORAL-DISTANCE-TO-TASK CAPACITY

Profound difficulty

Judged not to be amenable to educational therapy.

Maximum difficulty:

Months or years of continual training required. Cannot profit from highly verbal, mass methods or mass instruction.

In the meantime, cannot be counted on to do the task well enough to be self-sufficient.

Intermediate difficulty:

Learning distance is considerable, but patient learns well in several modes, although often requires help with synthesis of the ideas and application to reality.

Learning distance may be intermediate, but patient is able to learn well in only two modalities; motivation may be moderate.

Minimum difficulty:

Behavioral distance is small, and patient is successful at self-instruction.

Instruction can be given as normal part of care if it requires less than half an hour of nursing time.

Delayed:

Motivation not up to learning now—may be ready in the future.

Also includes periodic reeducation of patients with chronic illnesses.

---

*Readiness: motivation, skills already possessed, and learning skills.

**POSSIBLE ERRORS IN TEACHING-LEARNING PROCESS
IF GOALS ARE NOT BEING MET**

Readiness/motivation goals:

1. Did the learner ever accept the goals, or were you teaching only what *you* believed to be important?
2. What evidence do you have that the goals were appropriate?
3. Were the goals clearly written and understood by teacher and learner?
4. Were the goals broken into sufficient intermediate steps to provide guidance?

Teaching-learning:

1. Had teaching materials previously been tried with persons of ability similar to your patient and found successful?
2. If previous experience with the materials was not available, in what ways did their characteristics match the patient's readiness?
3. Were evaluative data gathered often during teaching, to give evidence of areas of success and lack of success?
4. Was teaching continued for sufficient time for learning to be thorough?
5. Were the data gathered for evaluation sufficiently valid and reliable to form an adequate basis for the evaluative decision?
6. Were baseline data obtained for measuring change? People rarely start with no knowledge or skill.

SUMMARY

Although evaluation is the final step in the process of teaching-learning, it is forward looking because its message redirects activity (box above). Information necessary for an evaluation of how well objectives have been met is gathered by various measurement techniques. A concerted effort is made to gather reliable information by perfecting measuring tools and by using them in conjunction with one another. This method provides a sounder basis for decisions about the competence of the learner to behave in the manner specified in the objectives.

STUDY QUESTIONS

1. You observe a nurse who has been teaching a patient how to give himself an injection. The nurse asks the patient the following questions as he goes through the procedure:
   Is it all right to give the injection with the syringe and needle you used yesterday without changing it?
   Review why you are wiping the skin a particular way.

   What would you do if the tip of the needle touched the table as you were picking up the syringe?
   What would you do if you touched the skin now (after it has been cleansed with the alcohol sponge and before the injection is given)?
   State the subobjective that the nurse is evaluating.

2. A public health nurse is teaching a wife and a daughter how to care for a bedfast elderly father and husband. The patient moves little but has not been incontinent. He has had no skin breakdown at the present time but according to the wife has been allowed to lie in one position for 4 hours. The main objective, which follows, is part of the more-encompassing objective: to avoid harmful consequences of bed rest.
   Main objective: To avoid decubitus ulcer formation.
   Subobjectives:
   a. To recognize any evidence of tissue breakdown by criteria of color, sensation, and response to massage.
   b. To reposition the patient at least every 2 hours so that the body is resting on the same surface only every fourth time.
   c. To keep all linen wrinkle free.
   d. To massage vigorously at every turning the skin that has been receiving pressure from body weight.
   e. To report to the public health nurse or physician evidence

of incontinence or skin breakdown within a day after it is observed.

Answer the following questions concerning this situation:

a. What methods of measurement might be used to evaluate the learning in such subobjectives?

b. During a subsequent visit the nurse found that both mother and daughter could identify evidence of skin breakdown in all five photographs shown. They could not identify areas reddened by sheet wrinkles on the patient's back as potential sites of breakdown. They reported that the patient had not been incontinent and that they usually turned him every 2 hours except when he put up a big fuss. What should the nurse do?

3. How is the notion of transfer used in evaluation?

4. You are trying to teach a mentally disabled youngster self-dressing skills, and he is inattentive and rebellious. It is obvious that he is showing lack of motivation to learn. List three possible factors that might be producing this behavior, and indicate the action a caregiver might take in response to each.

5. You are the teacher in a class for patients with diabetes, who make the following comments. What evidence does each question or comment give about the individual's understanding?

a. "Would blood sugar be the same for man, woman, or child?"

b. "I don't feel I'm really a diabetic because I don't have to take insulin." (Patient is a 19-year-old girl in whom pregnancy precipitated signs and symptoms of diabetes. The physician has ordered that her diabetes be controlled by diet).

c. Father whose 8-year-old son has newly diagnosed diabetes, talking to a college student who has been insulin dependent for 2 years: "Are you able to hunt?"

6. How useful is the tool at the top of p. 238,[37] given to patients for evaluation of educational booklets distributed at a health care setting?

7. Pp. 238 and 239 show portions of a perioperative teaching plan for craniofacial reconstruction.[24] How useful are the entries under "evaluation"?

8. Read the article by Frances Taira, "Individualized Medication Sheets," in Nursing Economics 9:56-58, 1991.[35] Study Table 3, Medication Knowledge Tool: Interview and Assessment. Do the test items adequately test the objectives? Would two different providers using this test come to the same conclusion about the patient's knowledge?

9. Read the article by Margaret Reuter, "Parenting Needs of Abusing Parents: Development of a Tool for Evaluation of a Parent Education Class," in Community Health Nursing 5:129-140, 1988.[31] Focus on the evaluation tool reproduced in the Appendix. Is this tool a measure of feelings, as indicated in the directions?

After you have read this booklet, you can help us improve our patient education materials by answering these questions.

PLEASE CIRCLE YOUR ANSWERS

1. Did you find the information in this booklet useful to you?
   Yes   No
2. Did you understand everything that is discussed in this booklet?
   Yes   No
   If no—what topics did you find hard to understand?

3. Did you find that the information in this booklet answered all of your questions?
   Yes   No
   If no—what questions do you have which are not answered by this booklet?
4. Do you plan to share this booklet with members of your family?
   Yes   No
5. Do you feel that you or your family members could use more information on the topic discussed in this booklet?
   Yes   No
   If yes—what additional information would be helpful?

From Tierney DO, Eisenberg MG: *Hosp Topics* 64(2):28-33, 1986.

PERIOPERATIVE TEACHING PLAN

Instructional content	Teaching activity	Evaluation
Craniosynostosis is a process resulting in the closure or obliteration of one or more cranial sutures. An overgrowth occurs parallel along the involved sutures and results in a misshapen skull. Increased intracranial pressure (ICP), along with mental retardation and developmental delays, can occur. As the child matures, more severe skull deformity becomes apparent.	The nurse reinforces, with diagrams, the information given to the parents by the physician. Also, printed information can be sent home with them to read.	The parents will have a better understanding of their child's deformity and the sutures involved.
Etiology is unknown.	The nurse reinforces that the parents are not at fault for their child's deformity. Local support group information is given, and parents are encouraged to participate.	The parents will begin to accept that their child's deformity is not their fault. They will gain support and reassurance.

From Kershner DD: AORN 44:564-569, 1986. Portions of the plan are shown.

PERIOPERATIVE TEACHING PLAN—cont'd

Preoperative

Evaluations include complete blood count (CBC), chest x-ray, developmental testing, ophthalmologic examination, and anesthesiology screening.

The nurse gives parents information about the screening process, phone numbers to set up appointments, and reinforces the importance of this process. The parents are also given information about the option to directly donate blood for their child.

The parents will understand and accept the importance of screening procedures. If parents are given a choice about donating blood, they will feel more in control in a situation where they may feel totally dependent on others for the well-being of their child.

The day of admission evaluations include a CBC, electrolytes, prothrombin time and partial thromboplastin time, type and crossmatch, and urinalysis. The surgeon does a history and physical and has the parents sign an informed consent, and an anesthesiologist's assessment is done. The patient is NPO for 6 hours before surgery and has a bath and shampoo the night before surgery.

The nurse explains preoperative laboratory work and the importance of NPO status. If the patient is older, the family and child are shown a teaching handbook that includes pictures of the holding room, OR attire, OR bed, OR room lights, anesthesia machine, tubing, mask, and electrocardiogram (ECG) monitoring pads. Play therapy can also be used.

The OR environment will be less frightening to the child.

Intraoperative

The procedure includes oral intubation, insertion of intravenous (IV) lines, head shave and scrub, and insertion of urinary catheter.

The nurse explains the IV tubing lines and reinforces their importance for monitoring and fluid replacement and explains the Foley catheter for bladder drainage and fluid status assessment. The nurse also explains that the child may be hoarse postoperatively because of the endotracheal tube.

The family will be less frightened at appearance of IV tubings and ECG wires.

The surgical procedure does not start until all IV and monitoring lines are in, and the head is shaved, scrubbed, and positioned.

The nurse explains to the parents that the length of the procedure varies for each patient and that calls will be made to the waiting room to inform them of progress.

The parents will be better able to handle the stress of waiting.

REFERENCES

1. Anderson LW: *Assessing affective characteristics in the schools,* Boston, 1981, Allyn & Bacon.
2. Berg JK, Kelly JT: Evaluation of psychosocial health care in quality assurance activities, *Med Care* 19:24-30, 1981.
3. Blodgett C, Pekarik G: Program evaluation in cardiac rehabilitation. IV. Efficiency evaluation, *J Cardiopulmonary Rehabil*7:466-474, 1987.
4. Brook RH, Appel FA: Quality-of-care assessment: choosing a method for peer review, *N Engl J Med* 288:1323-1329, 1973.
5. Brown SA: Quality of reporting in diabetes patient education research: 1954-1986, *Res Nurs Health* 13:53-62, 1990.
6. Budan LJ: Cardiac patient learning in the hospital setting, *Focus Crit Care* 10(5):16-22, 1983.
7. Cronbach LJ and others: *Toward reform of program evaluation,* San Francisco, 1980, Jossey-Bass.
8. Dershewitz RA, Posner MK, Paichel W: The effectiveness of health education on home use of ipecac, *Clin Pediatr* 22:268-270, 1983.
9. Devins GM and others: The Kidney Disease Questionnaire: a test for measuring patient knowledge about end-stage renal disease, *J Clin Epidemiol* 43:297-307, 1990.
10. Dignan MB and others: Use of process evaluation to guide health education in Forsyth County's project to prevent cervical cancer, *Public Health Rep* 106:73-77, 1991.
11. Donabedian A: The quality of medical care: a concept in search of a definition, *J Fam Pract* 9:277-284, 1979.
12. Ellsworth RA, Dunnell P, Duell OK: Multiple-choice test items: what are textbook authors telling teachers? *J Educ Res* 83:289-293, 1990.
13. Fernow LC, McColl I, Thurlow SC: Measuring the quality of clinical performance with hernia and myocardial infarction patients, controlling for patient risks, *Med Care* 19:273-280, 1981.
14. Garrard J and others: Psychometric study of patient knowledge test, *Diabetes Care* 10:500-509, 1987.
15. Gilliland MM: What patients can teach you, *Nursing* 11(12):52-53, 1981.
16. Green LW: Toward cost-benefit evaluations of health education: some concepts, methods, and examples, *Health Educ Monogr* 2(Suppl):34-64, 1974.
17. Green LW: *Research methods translatable to the practice setting: from rigor to reality and back.* In Cohen S, editor: *New directions in patient compliance,* Lexington, Mass, 1979, Lexington Books.
18. Green LW, Figa-Talamanca I: Suggested designs for evaluation of patient education programs, *Health Educ Monogr* 2:54-71, 1974.
19. Green LW, Lewis FM: *Measurement and evaluation in health education and health promotion,* Palo Alto, Calif, 1986, Mayfield.
20. Green RS, Attkisson CC: Quality assurance and program evaluation, *Program Eval* 27:552-582, 1984.
21. Grossman HY, Brink S, Hauser ST: Self-efficacy in adolescent girls and boys with insulin-dependent diabetes mellitus, *Diabetes Care* 10:324-329, 1987.
22. Heringa P, Lawson L, Reda D: The effect of a structured education program on knowledge and psychomotor skills of patients using beclomethasone dipropionate aerosol for steroid dependent asthma, *Health Educ Q* 14:309-317, 1987.
23. Howes DH: Knowledge of the ocular component to diabetes: a study of diabetic patients and their health care providers, *J Ophthal Nurs Tech* 2:67-68, 1983.
24. Kershner DD: Perioperative teaching plan, *AORN J* 44:564-569, 1986.
25. Kiresuk TJ, Lund SH, Larsen NE: Measurement of goal attainment in clinical and health care programs, *Drug Intell Clin Pharmacol* 16:145-153, 1982.
26. Kuehnel C, Rowe B: Patient education and the audit, *Superv Nurs* 11(12):15-19, 1980.
27. Lorig K and others: Development and evaluation of a scale to measure perceived self-efficacy in people with arthritis, *Arthritis Rheum* 32:37-45, 1989.
28. McSweeney M: Measuring the effect of patient teaching, *Diabetes Educ* 7(3):9-15, 1981.
29. Natriello G: The impact of evaluation processes on students, *Educ Psychologist* 22:155-175, 1987.
30. Nowacek GA, Pichert JW: An item bank of diabetes related test questions, *Diabetes Educ* 11(3):37-41, 1985.
31. Reuter MM: Parenting needs of abusing parents: development of a tool for evaluation of a parent education class, *Commun Health Nurs* 5:129-140, 1988.
32. Rinaldi LA, Kelly B: What to do after the audit is done, *Am J Nurs* 77:268-269, 1977.
33. Ruzicki DA: Evaluation: its what you do with what you've got that counts, *Promot Health* 6(4):6-9, 1985.
34. Stephany TM: Quality assurance for hospice programs, *Oncol Nurs Forum* 12(3):33-40, 1985.
35. Taira F: Individualized medication sheets, *Nurs Economics* 9:56-58, 1991.
36. Thompson RH: Showing them what you can do: a practical guide for evaluating child life programming, *Child Health Care* 10:29-36, 1981.
37. Tierney DO, Eisenberg MG: Evaluating patient health education printed materials, *Hosp Topics* 64(2):28-33, 1986.
38. Whatley K, Guthrie P, Turner WW, Jr: Developing a patient assessment and teaching program for right atrial catheters, *NITA* 7:529-530, 1984.
39. Wigal JK, Creer TL, Kotses H: The COPD self-efficacy scale, *Chest* 99:1193-1196, 1991.

CHAPTER 10

Delivery systems for patient education: program development and implementation

In the last 20 years patient education has developed from an interesting innovation to a required service in the delivery of health care. The tremendous expansion of activity in this field has been complicated by the nature of patient education. It involves a shift in the practice norms by most professionals. This means that program development and construction of systems of delivery for patient education have to be approached as institutional change. Lack of a clear reimbursement mechanism for patient education means that institutions lack strong reinforcements for developing and maintaining comprehensive patient-education programs. This chapter provides a view of strategies and structures for institutional planning and delivery of patient education. It also reviews in some detail the health conditions for which patient education programs are commonly developed.

DESCRIPTIONS OF DELIVERY SYSTEMS

During the past few years hospitals have been hit with serious cost containment. Until then systems for delivery of patient education in health care and community settings were evolving quite rapidly. The President's Committee on Health Education provided a view of the health education endeavor in this country in the early 1970s. The committee's report described the whole field of health education as fragmented, uneven in effectiveness, and lacking any base of operations. No agency in or outside of government was responsible for, or even assisted in, setting goals, maintaining criteria of performance, or measuring results. The effort

was underfinanced. The Department of Health, Education and Welfare's budget for health education was less than one quarter of 1%, and state budgets allotted less than one half of 1% for health education.[111] The health education budget contained an enormous expenditure for health information but relatively little for effective education (the extra component that would help people act on the information they had been given). The committee found only two instances of agencies seeking to evaluate the effectiveness of their materials. One insurance company was spending $2 million a year for materials they had not evaluated in 20 years. Among the 7000 hospitals in the United States the committee found that no more than four were doing an effective job of patient education. School health education was in total disarray in the United States.[134] The committee recommended a national center for health education with divisions for research in the following areas: health education, demonstration programs, communications in health education, community health education centers, and a clearinghouse for health information and education. One member of the committee showed concern about the apparent lack of commitment to the report from the professional health organizations.[111]

A 1976 survey deliberately sought out (by means of literature review, consultation with technical experts, and extensive discussions with health education evaluators) and studied programs that contained strong evaluations. The survey found that the ability of consumer health education programs to foster beneficial short-term impact on patient knowledge, attitudes, behavior, and health status had been reasonably demonstrated in a number of different settings. The programs addressed many different health problems and used various techniques. The report claimed that the long-term effects of consumer health education programs had not been measured, perhaps partly because most programs had not existed very long. A number of the programs seemed to operate over a period of 3 to 4 months. The study staff encountered few programs that had been in continuous operation for more than 2 years. Programs that existed were self-care programs, system-utilization programs, disease-control programs, and others. They had been sponsored and funded by hospitals, regional medical programs, public health departments, health maintenance organizations (HMOs), voluntary associations, and insurance companies.[9,136]

In almost all settings, hypertension, diabetes, and nutrition were prevalent topics in consumer health education programs. Hospitals had inpatient, outpatient, and community-oriented programs. The public health department's involvement in consumer health education was typically multifocused, short term, and nonintensive. Frequent topics focused on child care and nutrition education for young parents, education in health services and resources available, and common public health problems, such as drugs, venereal disease, and lead poisoning. Insurance companies were involved primarily in facilitation of program development rather than in front-line delivery of educational services.[9,136]

More recent data show considerable development of structure to support patient education programs (some merging with community and health promotion services in hospitals) and development of client education programs in diverse health care delivery sites. Despite these advances, full availability of education services for patients, families, and communities, and integration of education into all health care services is a goal not yet attained, partly because insurers have not responded with adequate coverage.

Education service by hospitals to nonpatients began in earnest in 1978. By 1981 more than 53% of hospitals had nonpatient community health promotion programs, initially oriented toward disease prevention. Now the focus has shifted to life-style and achieving optimum well-being. Target populations have included clerical staff or executives in local businesses, grandparents, frail elderly, or health-active older adults; single parents; police and fire personnel; discharged and home-bound patients; and children. Community health promotion programs include patient education outreach, such as· stroke clubs; behavior-change programs for smoking cessation or stress management; life-style and wellness education (low-calorie cooking); and self-care programs. In addition to the usual educational approaches, screening, health-risk assessment, camps, retreats, and health fairs are used. Sometimes these services are delivered through a separate corporate entity, such as a wellness center.[88]

The most recent survey of patient education programs in hospitals was completed in 1987.[6] It showed that 87% of hospitals responding offered inpatient education programs, 73% offered outpatient education programs, and 73% offered community health promotion programs. The survey also showed that hospitals considered outpatient education rather than inpatient education as a revenue-producing service. The nursing department or education department usually administered the education program. Twenty-one percent of responding hospitals, especially larger hospitals, reported having a consumer, health information library.

A survey of hospitals in Australia found that most hospitals conduct some education programs: diabetes education (80%); childbirth education (68%); and heart disease (52%). Reasons for not conducting patient education included a lack of trained staff and a lack of funds. Australia's national health insurance does not include special reimbursement for patient education. Programs are conducted mostly by nurses (95%). Almost half of all programs are not evaluated; therefore it is difficult for administrators to see the benefits of patient education.[37]

New forms of service that focus heavily on education have evolved in the last two decades. Health fairs now provide multiphasic screening and education to more than 3 million Americans every year, and a national organization offers assistance and certification to health fair sponsors.[17] In the past 20 years more than 100 drug information centers have been developed in the United States to provide consumers with reliable information about drugs and to promote appropriate drug use. Consumer concerns most often include drug abuse, withdrawal, identification of ingredients in drugs, dosage, efficacy, adverse reactions, and interactions with food and other drugs.[7]

Statewide coalitions and networks have also begun to deliver health programs with heavy emphasis on education. One example is the statewide network of all hospitals in Vermont delivering newborns. This network offers infant safety seat rental and education.[32] And in Minnesota a partnership between the International Diabetes Center and the Minnesota Department of Health has assisted six rural communities in developing diabetes education and services tailored to each community's needs and resources.[12]

Individual institutions

The programs described below are a few examples of the many individual health education programs in existence.

The Cooperative Care Unit at New York University Hospital opened in 1979 and is designed especially for treatment and education of acutely ill patients who face changes in life-style. These patients must have a care partner and must be able to get around independently or with the aid of a walker, crutches, or wheelchair. The patient may be admitted directly from home for a presurgical procedure such as cardiac catheterization or for a medical treatment such as radiation, or the patient may be admitted by transfer from the main wing of the hospital. The average stay is 5 days, and the cost is 40% less than the daily university hospital

charge. The unit has a homelike atmosphere and provides privacy for patient and partner; however, emergency care is always available by phone. Patients have schedules of appointments, and the education center is included in the list. It has 80 teaching plans and a permanent staff.[35]

Recent evaluation of this program found that it offers an alternative to traditional inpatient care. The program has significant educational and management advantages, it is less costly, and it is enthusiastically accepted by patients, families, and health care providers.[29]

Hartmann and others trace the evolution[57] of the Patient Education Advisory Committee at the Veterans Administration Medical Center in Milwaukee and inspect its role in promoting and governing the patient education program in this institution. The committee was formed in 1979 and during its first years evaluated existing programs. It subsequently developed working subgroups to focus on coordination, resources, new program development, and program evaluation. In more recent years the committee has focused on quality assurance, an inhouse patient education television channel, expansion of networking activities with the community, and closer cooperation with veterans' organizations.

Other institutions have responded to changes in reimbursement and length of stay by developing outpatient education programs.[102] Through its Community Nursing Center the Medical Center of Long Beach provided direct access to 2500 patients a month with programs such as: (1) a lactation service that educates and supports breast-feeding mothers; (2) a preoperative/preadmission education program; (3) an enterostomal outpatient service; and (4) a "Living with Lung Disease" program that focuses on self-care skills in training patients with lung disease. Patients pay for these services directly or through a third party.

In 1987 the University of Minnesota Hospitals and Clinics opened a learning center, featuring a lablike environment. At the center patients and families learn, practice, and demonstrate skills necessary for self-care. The lab is open 7 days a week and on holidays. The lab is staffed by RNs. The center offers these skill units: administration of intramuscular, subcutaneous, or intravenous medications; caring for tracheostomy or laryngectomy; caring for wounds and decubiti; providing self-catheterization; caring for colostomies and ileostomies; providing home intravenous nutrition, placing the tubes, and administering tube feedings; measuring blood pressure; performing diabetic survival skills, using electronic glucose monitors; caring for the patient who is bedbound; and caring for intravenous access devices. Among patients who need to learn several of these procedures, readmission is significantly lower for patients who have used the learning center. The simulation devices used in the lab are especially useful for patients who live in rural areas some distance from the medical center.[52]

One small hospital trains nurses to increase their expertise in a particular area of patient education. These nurses can act as resources for peers, patients, and families. This system has a significant influence on the quality of patient education in the hospital setting.[74] Another 115-bed hospital uses an RN patient education consultant to work with the head nurse and staff nurses to develop and improve patient education services.[140]

Because admission of most patients to a hospital the day before surgery is no longer economically feasible, one hospital has established a preoperative testing center to perform presurgical assessment and instruction for patients having elective surgery. Packaging the service through the center saved the hospital an estimated $500,000 in 1985. Nearly half of those served were outpatients who entered the surgery day care unit an hour and a half before surgery and left the same day. Only 7% were traditional inpatients.[33]

Each of these institutional programs represents a structure that has served to integrate patient education into an institution, or it represents the special way that educational services have been made available to patients. Innovations in delivery will continue as institutions search for more effective ways to reach patients and to provide these services during the times patients need them. Many health education services have not been autonomous, freestanding programs but were generally an integral part of other health programs.

Financing and marketing

Patient education repeatedly achieves cost savings that exceed the cost of the educational program. Recent examples include a diabetes teaching program in an air force medical center that showed savings because of a decrease in admissions and length of stay,[66] an outpatient diabetes regulation and self-care program offered as an alternative to hospitalization,[137] an outpatient teaching program for Hickman catheter care,[84] and a workplace health education program that helps employees make informed decisions about when to seek professional care at a physician's office or emergency room. This last program was offered through 22 California employers and resulted in a reduction of more than 7% in visits.[89]

A perceived major difficulty with patient education has been financing. In the past this service has not been recognized as a reimbursable expense by most insurance companies. Successful attempts to obtain reimbursement have included thorough documentation of the program, including evaluation and follow-up, evidence of cost effectiveness, qualifications of the patient educators, and the influential role of the patient-education committee. Approval of one carrier can be used to set a precedent with others. A critical element in procuring reimbursement lies in demonstrating that patient education is integral to care.

In 1984 the American Diabetes Association issued a position paper urging third-party reimbursement for outpatient education and nutrition counseling for persons with diabetes. The new prospective payment system for hospital service caused some to voice a concern that inpatient diabetes education programs might disappear.[4] Several states have taken action to make payment for diabetes education available. In 1984 the Iowa Legislature passed a bill requiring health care insurance providers to offer coverage under group policies for diabetes outpatient self-management education programs, with the Department of Health developing standards for certification of these programs.[65]

A more recent statement strongly encourages third-party reimbursement for outpatient diabetes education and counseling. The statement notes that numerous published studies have shown that education and self-care programs lead to reductions in costs associated with diabetes.[5]

California has passed similar reimbursement legislation.[122] After several years of demonstration of the benefits of Diabetes Education Centers in North Dakota, Blue Cross of North Dakota voted to provide coverage for diabetes education for persons attending these centers and for future centers that receive the endorsement of the American Diabetes Association, North Dakota Affiliate.[75] Maine, one of the 20 states under cooperative agreement with the Communicable Disease Centers to implement a statewide diabetes control project, established follow-up programs at hospitals and other health care facilities throughout the state to provide patients with diabetes with self-care capabilities. The major third-party payers agreed to support these programs if they met certain criteria.[120]

The Diagnostic Related Group (DRG) payment system for services has especially affected hospital-based patient-education services. Patient-education managers in hospitals report dramatic changes in the way that they must justify and support education services: (1) they must be able to articulate the role of patient education in decreasing costs, nonprofitable DRGs, or increasing appropriate admissions of profitable DRGs; (2) they must streamline programs to meet the need for survival skills for inpatients and move general disease management education and continued support to an outpatient status; (3) they must have fewer education staff members and make greater use of consultants and volunteers; and (4) they must generate revenue through program fees; contracts for services with health departments, physician's offices, smaller hospitals, home care agencies, and worksites; sales of educational materials and programs; and grants.

Education before admission and after discharge not only generates increased revenue but can also decrease inpatient hospital costs.[135]

Other strategies for increasing revenue and saving costs include use of patient education as part of risk management; more frequent use of group instruction; development of patient education consortia for shared services; use of early discharge programs, cooperative care, and care by parent units; and charge for educational services as part of the sale or rental of medical equipment for home use.

Marketing is a strategy and a conceptual approach that defines services that complement the usual patient-education planning point of view. A marketing strategy is an internally consistent plan of action dealing with product pricing, distribution, and communication.[108] A market analysis involves (1) defining important trends, (2) defining the people who constitute a particular market and the groups they represent (homogeneous groups), (3) assessing the needs of each segment, (4) assessing the degree of awareness people have of the product, (5) assessing the image of the organization and of its competitors, (6) determining how potential clients learn about the service and make decisions to apply, and (7) assessing consumer satisfaction. Resource analysis involves defining strengths and weaknesses of present resources and recognizing opportunities for using the resources. Mission analysis involves clarifying the type of business, defining the customers, determining the demands that need supplying, deciding which market segments to target, and electing competitive benefits to offer the target market.[81]

Marketing was developed in business contexts and has been extended to nonbusiness—concerns that have different benefits and costs for clients. Often, only weak personal benefits that do not reinforce or maintain longterm behaviors occur in health. Costs are usually measured in dollars and in time, inconvenience, and psychic burdens (although at times these can be considered benefits). That which constitutes a cost to an individual may be a benefit to a larger group. Most products are

TABLE 10-1. Benefit segmentation analysis

Segment name	Group with sense of urgency		Health-conscious group	
	The fire fighters	**The desperates**	**The worriers**	**The infertiles**
Benefits sought	Immediate solution to problem (pregnancy, breast lump, midcycle bleeding, etc.), reassurance, shoulder to lean on	Relief from feelings of desperation (I can't cope), financial stability, marital harmony, feeling of being in control of something for the first time	Security about health, relief from worry	Conception, birth, children
Category beliefs	Family planning may be able to solve my problem	Birth control will solve most of my problems	Good health means a better way of life for me and my children	Medical expertise will help solve my problem
Services sought	Health care, birth control testing, referral (especially abortion), counsel, education	Birth control, shoulder to lean on	Education, GYN services, counsel, testing and referral, total health care	OB-GYN health care, testing, referral, counsel
General description	Women of all ages—especially younger, lower income and education; have immediate problem	Couples with two or more kids, lower income and education, socially limited fatalistic outlook	Tend to be younger married, maybe 1-2 kids under 8 years; more hypochondriacal, self-oriented, cautious	Married couples of all ages who want children
Media habits	TV, radio, magazines, all types of info, newspapers	Not information seekers; TV, AM radio	TV, radio, magazines, newspapers	TV, radio, magazines, newspapers; high information seekers, especially "reputable" literature

Miaoulis G, Bonaguro J: *J Health Care Mark* 1:35-4, 1980.

intangible and cannot be shown in promotional materials. Some authors believe in a minimum level of latent demand for the issue or product. If an organization's mandate is to serve all of society, it must consider different strategies and behavior reinforcers for the various segments.[111]

An excellent example of the marketing approach in behavioral health care is available from a family planning agency.[94] This agency did marketing research by interviewing—in depth—160 users and nonusers of its service. This research, along with information and perceptions gathered from the

The rationals			
The marrieds I (want children)	**The marrieds II** (set against kids)	**The singles I** (with children)	**The singles II** (without children)
Freedom of choice, control, financial stability, health, marital harmony	Freedom of choice, financial stability, marital harmony	Pregnancy prevention for financial stability, avoid social stigma	Pregnancy prevention, to avoid stigma, to retain independence, for financial stability, to avoid hassles of unwed parent
Having control of life situations leads to a better life	I hate kids; kids are not worth the cost	More children will not allow me to care for me and my family adequately	It is wrong, inconvenient, expensive/a pain in the neck to be an unwed parent
Birth control, health services, counsel, education, information	Birth control, sterilization, referral, general health care	Birth control, counsel	Birth control, abortion referral
Rational, independent, decision makers, see selves as autonomous, tend to be younger, tend toward higher end of educational spectrum	Independent, rational, self-oriented, lower middle of age spectrum	Young, single, or divorced with kids; hectic life-style	Career-oriented, socially active (may be husband hunting), younger, single, working, all educational levels
Newspapers, magazines, TV, radio	Newspapers, news magazines, TV, radio	TV, AM radio	TV, radio, magazines, especially women's

staff, identified eight target populations. These populations were clustered in three major segments with enough internal consistency to permit the formulation of three marketing plans rather than eight. Segments were matched to agency resources (Table 10-1). The first major segment incorporates two subsegments: "fire fighters" and "desperates." Both of these segments believed they had problems and saw the family planning agency as a potential solver. Both had a sense of urgency. They were not routinely seeking information. When a crisis developed, they sought information and services.

They needed to perceive that their problems were being addressed immediately. The second segment was a health-conscious group described as "worriers" and "infertiles." They desired medical care that was not available at the clinic. They were therefore excluded from promotional strategies because they could be better served by private health care. The third major segment was labeled "rationals." They were information seekers. The marketing strategy developed for the first segment ("fire fighters" and "desperates") included the theme "got a problem? . . . We can help." This message was presented to them on broadcast media. Hotline and reception procedures were modified to identify this segment for quick access to staff. The strategy for the "rationals" included a theme: "A brighter future . . . Plan it now." Media used were nonbroadcast because this group had actively sought information. The marketing strategy apparently increased the number of individuals in the target population who used agency services.

The concept of segmentation is congruent with educational notions of individualization and with health planning notions of target groups. All methods are aimed at better effectiveness for lower cost by precisely matching strategies to need.

Use of marketing concepts is increasing in patient education practice, partly in response to the changed fiscal incentives brought about by prospective payment systems. Bills[18] reflects on the shift in patient education from inpatient to outpatient settings for persons with diabetes. She notes that the teaching sequence has changed from teaching anatomy and physiology first and skills last to teaching enough information to make patients safe at home. This teaching sequence is supported with written back-up material. It is an approach that fits more closely with the consumer-driven notion of marketing—a perspective that insists that the consumer's perceptions of his or her needs must be met. Practical information the patient can use directly, such as ways to modify favorite recipes or ways to interpret restaurant menus. is satisfying. Patients enjoy such classes.

Hospitals have used community health education to obtain preferred provider contracts, to change their image of being an institution that treats only the sick, and to instruct community members about the hospital's services and personnel. Health maintenance organizations have used health promotion and education programs to increase patient satisfaction and decrease disenrollment and no-show rates. Optometrists use newsletters as education tools and as tools to penetrate new markets. An enterostomal therapy services brochure presents and clarifies the services offered by the ET nurse and includes inpatient and outpatient services, such as referral methods and a fee schedule. This type of brochure can be sent to appropriate physicians, suppliers of ostomy equipment, ulcerative colitis and Crohn's disease support groups, home health agencies, nursing homes, and local chapters of ostomy and cancer associations.[139]

Paralleling the concept of product line management in business is service line management in health care agencies. Each service line coordinates the specific services relevant to the identified needs of clients. A high-risk maternity service line with coordinated nursing, laboratory, and other services differs from a program that offers the function- or discipline-oriented services separately. A service line manager would define services to be marketed. as well as geographic areas and populations to be served; assess the competition; and create marketing plans, including information systems, advertising plans, and new service development. He or she would also cooperate in resolving problems and issues in the delivery of services; define new services or changes to existing services to increase volume and patient satisfaction; coordinate development of standards of care; address quality practice issues; and provide continuous feedback regarding business opportunities and services development.[27]

A recent study has shown that more than two thirds of hospital education departments are now responsible for generating external revenue. Many do so by sponsoring programs for the community.[55] Consumer health information and education programs are used as marketing tools for hospitals. In turn, patient-education programs must also be marketed.

OBSTACLES TO PATIENT EDUCATION

1. Materials are not available for staff to use in patient education; there is no system to keep materials current.
2. Many times patients are too sick during hospitalization to become actively involved in a teaching program; they are often discharged unprepared to care for themselves.
3. Hospital staff end up reinventing the wheel because they are not aware of what has already been done in the area both inside and outside the hospital.
4. The patient population is not accustomed to seeing the hospital as a place where they go for preventive teaching or for learning how to take an active role in their health care management.
5. The acuity/staffing system does not adequately reflect the patient's educational needs.
6. There is lack of third-party reimbursement for outpatient education.
7. There is no mechanism or system established whereby staff can charge time spent in patient education activities, especially in departments such as pharmacy.
8. Space for patient education is extremely scarce.
9. The cost of implementing such a wide-scale program is high; risk is involved because physician support and patient acceptance are unknown.
10. Some professional staff members are not comfortable with the principles of teaching patients.
11. It is difficult to see a strong commitment to patient education in the individual department philosophies.

From Woodrow M: *Hospitals* 53(9): 1979.

STEPS IN DEVELOPING A PATIENT EDUCATION PROGRAM

1. Assess program need.
   This can be done by questionnaires and interviews with health professionals and clients, the medical records department and various community agencies (VNAs [visiting nursing associations] or associations for a disease such as diabetes). When requesting statistics from the medical records department, ask for the top five or ten admission diagnoses, including both primary and secondary diagnosis.
2. Obtain administrative and professional support.
3. Determine potential clients, sources of referral, and subsequent follow-up.
4. Plan program content with an interdisciplinary team (committee).
5. Determine program goals, objectives, and evaluative procedures.
6. Select learning strategies.
7. Determine and use available resources.
8. Recruit, motivate, train, and retrain teaching personnel.
9. Implement the program.
   Delay in implementation because of a small number of patients or other reasons can quickly lead to a decrease in interest and enthusiasm for the program.
10. Document teaching.
11. Do follow-up.
12. Evaluate teaching and program.
13. Revise program.

From Nemchik R: *Developing an education program.* In Guthrie DW, Guthrie RA, editors: *Nursing management of diabetes mellitus,* St Louis, 1977, Mosby–Year Book.

MANAGEMENT OF PATIENT EDUCATION PROGRAMS

A program can be defined as a standing arrangement that provides a social service. Programs in patient education have developed as services for groups of patients with particular disease entities or health problems. Over time several of these programs will evolve in an agency. Some will deliver services to patients sporadically and inconsistently. Many times agencies place all patient-education activities under a central coordination to prevent overlap and to improve services by standardizing and evaluating them. Home care and community health agencies are also attending to optimum organization of patient education services because a great deal of care is given in the community now.

Obstacles to patient education have remained the same for more than a decade. They are outlined by Woodrow[142] in the box at the top of p. 249. Steps in developing a new patient education program developed by Nemchik[100] can be seen in the box at the bottom of p. 249.

It might take a year for a program to be planned, gain support, and become operational. Increasingly, packaged instructional programs developed by health care institutions or by commercial firms are being used.

Hospital-wide management structures and processes

As noted earlier, to offer coordinated, quality patient-education programs, and to fulfill legal responsibility, many hospitals have developed an institution-wide multidisciplinary patient education committee charged with developing policy and coordinating and monitoring the quality of patient-education services. Frequently, a staff person with hospital-wide responsibility for patient-education consults, develops, coordinates, and evaluates the services under direction of the committee. Sometimes a patient-education department is established. Usually the actual development of programs is carried out by unit committees that prepare progress reports for the institution-wide committee. Figure 10-1 shows the structure used by the Texas Children's Hospital. In this hospital the hospital-wide committee members help to develop, implement, and evaluate programs. An executive committee sets policy, outlines priorities, and allocates funding. Task forces do the detailed work of planning education.[14] Discipline committees (nursing, medicine, and others) or service committees (pediatrics, surgery, and others) may be named. A wide range of involvement assists staff in acquiring a sense of ownership and commitment to the patient-education program.

Table 10-2 lists criteria used to assess patient education programs in Michigan hospitals. It shows the percentage of programs that reported the presence of these criteria.[103] Whether the presence of these structures and processes is related to comprehensive delivery of good-quality education to the target groups remains an unanswered question. Stanton found a statistically significant relationship between the presence of six management-level components (policy, patient education committee, coordinator, budget, audit, and evaluation) and the three instructional-level components of design, implementation, and evaluation.[125]

Several studies completed by Redman, Levine, and Howard[109] found that the degree of structure for implemtation (chart forms, procedures), provider perception of reinforcement for doing patient education, and perceived payoff from the program were significantly related to reported receipt of instruction by patients and delivery of instruction by providers.

Because of a changed financial environment, some hospitals have eliminated entire education or health promotion departments or individual education positions. Others have recreated patient-education coordinators or staff to manage expansion into ambulatory care areas.[49] Hospitals are the only sector of the health care system that has gathered relatively comprehensive data about patient education services. Their system for delivery of these essential services is in a great deal of flux.

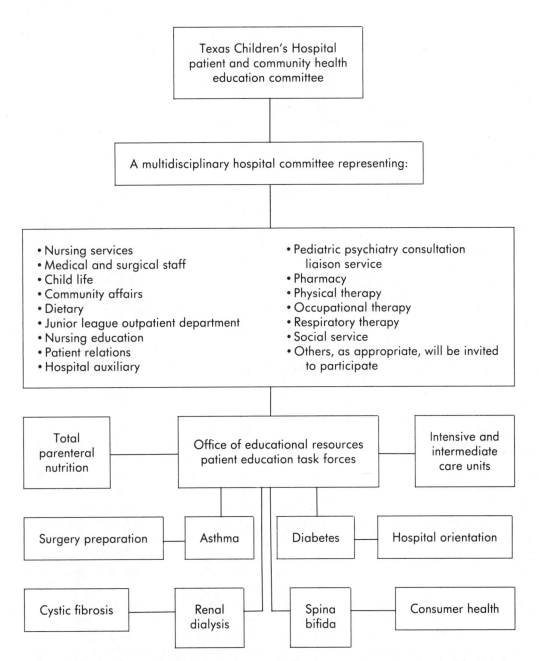

FIGURE 10-1. Structure of Texas Children's Hospital. (From Bartholomew LK, Ferry GD, *Texas Hosps* 41:26-29, 1985.)

TABLE 10-2. Percentage of 281 programs in 235 Michigan hospitals reporting presence of assessment criteria

Criteria	% Yes
Is there a coordinator for this program?	78
Is coordinator responsible for patient education?	74
Is there a planning or advisory group for this program?	61
Does program involve use of other agencies' services?	52
Does program have a written definition of potential target population?	62
Are there written program goals?	74
Does program evaluate extent to which program goals are attained?	44
Does the planning or advisory group receive evaluation results?	30
Is there a written outline of program covering major content areas?	79
Are there written learning objectives for program's target population?	57
Is there an educational assessment of patient's learning needs on entrance to program?	63
Are three or more of educational methods (discussion, AV, written, demonstration, role playing) used by the program?	90
Are there provisions made for adaptation of education methods or materials to learner's needs?	76
Is patient's progress with the program evaluated?	88
Is documentation of patient's progress with program part of permanent medical record?	69
In case of inpatients discharged prior to program completion, are arrangements made for additional patient education?	32
Is number of patients who have attained learning objectives documented?	53
Is the program specifically identified in a departmental budget?	72

From Pack BE and others: *Patient Educ Counsel* 7:345-358, 1985.

PERSONNEL FOR DELIVERY OF PATIENT EDUCATION

Health care professionals who deliver care directly to patients have an educative role inherent in their daily activities. An example is the nurse practitioner in a congestive heart failure clinic who was successful in markedly decreasing hospital days for this population. Her success was related to the considerable patient education inherent to her role and to her inclination to be available to patients. Patient education can also be delivered by education specialists. A single study comparing this delivery mode with delivery of education by the primary nurse found the latter to be more successful, presumably because the nurse was available and because the patient knew and trusted the nurse.[79] Patient education can also be delivered by an interdisciplinary team—a circumstance that is particularly common in rehabilitation settings where the patient needs to learn topics best known by individual members of the teaching team.

Nurses have the most direct contact with patients and are the largest resource for delivery of education. Getting nurses to deliver education has been a source of frustration for patient-education managers for some time. These difficulties have occurred in part because of deterrents to teaching, time constraints, feelings of inadequacy, and confusion regarding the nurse's role. One patient-education manager worked with a task force of staff nurses and nurse managers to write a new job description with an evaluative tool that was clear about the nurse's responsibilities for patient education (Figure 10-2).[123] Ruzicki, by assessing the needs among staff nurses in her institution, found that staff members were not aware or were uncer-

PATIENT TEACHING

Identifies the learning needs of patients and family members and meets these through the teaching-learning process. Documents teaching and evidence of learning in the patient's records.

% WEIGHT		PERFORMANCE RATING		TOTAL
$\boxed{5}$	×	$\square$	=	$\square$

UNSATISFACTORY - 1

□
_____
_____
_____
_____
_____
_____

MARGINAL - 2

□
_____
_____
_____
_____
_____
_____

GOOD - 3

□ Basic learning needs of each assigned patient are identified and individualized as evidenced by reports, documentation, or direct observation.

□ Each assigned patient is provided with appropriate and accurate basic health care information as evidenced by reports, documentations, or direct observation.

□ Existing resources on the unit are shared on an ongoing basis with unit staff.

□ Information given, patient/family input, and the learner response is documented on the medical record for each patient (i.e., "Ongoing Teaching and Discharge" Record).

COMMENDABLE - 4

□ Elicits patient and family feedback and degree of understanding regarding information taught for each assigned patient.

□ Collaborates with Clinical Specialists in the process of patient teaching.

□ Reinforcement of learning is given through consistent utilization of teaching aids.

□ Existing resources throughout the hospital are shared on an ongoing basis with hospital staff through interaction with peers, unit conferences, etc.

□ Evaluates and alters teaching as indicated by learner response.

DISTINGUISHED - 5

□ Indepth learning needs of each patient are identified and individualized to encompass the patient's disease process, misconceptions, physical limitations and other relevant factors.

□ Teaching is expanded to include indepth learning needs with each patient who requires adaptive life style changes.

□ Designs at least one relevant teaching aid which can be used by other staff in teaching.

□ Community resources are utilized to meet learning needs of patients and/or significant others as indicated.

COMMENTS: _____
_____
_____
_____
_____
_____

FIGURE 10-2. Performance evaluation tool. (From Speros C: _Patient Educ Counsel_ 8:86-89, 1986.)

tain about their responsibilities concerning patient education. Orientation programs and continuing education; patient education protocols, teaching, and documentation tools; frequent monitoring of staff teaching activity; and recognition and reinforcement for teaching were important.[118]

Although pharmacists also deliver considerable education in community and institutional practice, incomplete patient education is evident in that group as well. A survey sampling 400 community pharmacies in Michigan found that pharmacists were not routinely providing oral information to most of the patients to whom they dispensed medications. However, the pharmacists willingly provided advice to patients whom they perceived needed or wanted such information—particularly those who requested information.[10]

Patient education is also provided by interdisciplinary teams. The teams often need special preparation for working together and assistance in delineation of roles. A study of patient education in a women's hospital by Olive and Olive found strong disagreement between the nursing and medical staffs about issues of patient ownership. Although most physicians believed that they were providing adequate patient education, most nurses believed that physicians were not. Physicians believed that all medically oriented questions should be referred to a physician, while nurses strongly disagreed. The issue of nurses as the main educators in the hospital was also polarizing. Nurses strongly stated that educating patients was their function, but a majority of physicians disagreed.[102] Developing a truly collaborative practice would be worthwhile and is associated with better quality patient-provider interaction and health education.[80]

Patient education has become a specialty role. Formation of the American Association of Diabetes Educators, whose goals are to aid in professional development of individuals responsible for educating patients with diabetes, to foster communication among these individuals, to serve as a resource center for diabetes education, and to develop guidelines for diabetes education programs, occurred more than a decade ago.[39]

The childbirth educator is another example of a specialized patient education clinician who can work relatively autonomously. The incompleteness of currently available health care services and the important goal of trying to fit patients into medical-hospital structures with the least possible amount of resistance creates a need for this kind of practice. Sources of information, someone to talk with about personal concerns, and a way to gain skills for childbirth are needs that patients can only partially satisfy by reading. The childbearing period should also be used for growth-promoting activities. Learning to use touch, for example, is useful for childbirth and is also transferable to other realms, such as sexual functioning. Childbirth educators may operate in direct cooperation with local medical services or as an optional, independent addition to regular medical services.[56]

Competency statements (shown in the box on p. 255) have also been developed for the hospital-wide patient-education director.[145]

Patient-education councils have been growing across the United States since the middle 1970s when the first one was formed in Richmond, Virginia. By 1984, 30 such councils existed in 18 states. Councils encourage networking and formal education for coordinators in patient education.[70] More recently the International Patient Education Council has been formed.

With proper interest on the part of professionals, volunteers can play important roles in both delivery of patient-education services and support tasks (outlined in the box on p. 256).[86]

Similar work has been done with trained home health aides caring for persons with diabetes. In an 18-month intervention the patients showed decrease in fasting blood sugar levels, missed appointments, and emergency room use.[61]

SAMPLE AREAS OF PROGRAM DEVELOPMENT

Programs or efforts directed toward patient education often originate to satisfy the needs of a particular group of clients. This section will review a number of these areas. Each area includes specific

COMPETENCY STATEMENTS FOR PATIENT EDUCATION DIRECTOR

I. Policy development
    A. Develop goals and philosophy statements for the patient education service
    B. Establish appropriate policies and procedures that support recognized standards of legal cost and quality accountability for institution wide patient-education services
    C. Maintain current knowledge regarding local, state, and federal legislation policy and trends related to patient education

II. Management
    A. Manage institutionwide patient education services
    B. Provide sound fiscal direction of patient education service-related resources
    C. Use current media and technology to ensure optimum quality of patient education services

III. Coordination of institution-wide patient education services

IV. Consultation
    A. Provide consultation to individuals, groups, and organizations institution-wide and seek consultation with outside experts to achieve patient education goals

V. Training and continuing education
    A. Assess training needs of those responsible for patient education
    B. Develop specific program goals, objectives, content, and implementation strategies for each program

VI. Program development for target populations
    A. Identify patient education needs through data collection and analysis
    B. Develop specific program goals, objectives, content, and implementation strategies for each program
    C. Organize and develop multidisciplinary task forces for patient education programs for specific target populations
    D. Analyze behavioral theory and empirical evidence from research and make interpretations to the practice of patient education
    E. Direct the implementation of patient education services

VII. Evaluation of patient education services
    A. Design and manage the evaluation and revision of patient education programs and activities
    B. Advocate the development of greater accountability for and quality of patient education services.

VIII. Generic knowledge and skills (verbal and written communication, group meetings, liaisons, and cooperation)

From Young B, Johnson L: *Patient Educ Counsel* 6:19-24, 1984.

VOLUNTEER TASKS IN A GENERAL MEDICAL-SURGICAL FACILITY

SUPPORT TASKS

Project

Needs assessment surveys
Evaluation surveys
Visual aids—design and production
Dramatic aids—design and production
Materials collection

Long-term/ongoing

Clerical support
Routine material evaluation
Bulletin board displays
Patient reception

Fund-raising

PATIENT-EDUCATION TASKS

Community-wide

Health fairs
Topic lectures
Screening clinics

Program

Cancer
Childbirth
Diabetes
General orientation—pediatrics
Renal dialysis
Cardiac catheterization
Weight loss and nutrition
Smoking

Outpatient

Medication and physician's orders
Hypertension
Well-baby information
Birth control

From Lemons WL: *Family Community Health* 7(4):66-75, 1985.

lessons, common goals, and often particular patterns of readiness. The content and objectives depend on how much is known about treating the particular problem, the readiness patterns of patients, general public knowledge about the problem, and the skills that the treatment requires. All areas use common skills in the process of teaching and employ a wide range of teaching, assessment, and evaluation methods. Patients with unusual needs (not common statistically) need education developed on a one-to-one basis.

Acquired immunodeficiency syndrome

Most readers are aware that controlling the AIDS epidemic is dependent on educating people in ways to avoid becoming infected. Since the beginning of the epidemic the public has disagreed about the propriety of educational messages. The nation has yet to mount a comprehensive, intensive, and targeted program to prevent the disease.[44] Yet, some are amazed at evidence that suggests a dramatic reduction in powerfully reinforcing, habitual behavior, particularly among those homosexual populations and IV drug abusers who have received education about the virus.[16,124]

Because AIDS has been treated as a preventable public health problem, most educational approaches reported in the literature target specific populations. There is concern that there is little documentation that adolescent and young adult heterosexual groups and black and Hispanic populations are changing sexual behaviors that put them at risk.

Most agree that knowledge about the disease and about how it is transmitted is a motivator. However, knowledge alone is insufficient to bring about the behavior changes necessary. Individuals must become skilled in preventive behaviors, and those behaviors must be reinforced by their peers. They must have the materials they need, such as condoms. Most interventions have used social learning theory. In addition to education, people must have strong negotiating skills to maintain preventive behavior in pressured social relationships. They must be strongly tested to learn if they can maintain these behaviors. They must be confident in their ability to avoid risky behaviors.[13]

Experience in California[96] shows that the success of a program appears to depend on the staff's ability to locate and gain access to members of the specified target groups, to identify the appropriate type of educational intervention, and to determine whom to hire and how to train them to deliver the education. Gay men were contacted at home-based parties and at gay bars and resorts. However, it is difficult to reach minority gay, bisexual, or closeted men, especially in rural areas. To reach ethnic minorities, it is effective to employ ethnic staff members who understand the social networks in those communities. Intravenous drug abusers are best served by street outreach.

The education that must be done in clinical settings is much less well documented. When an individual is notified that he or she is HIV positive, counseling and education are crucial. These individuals must be helped to cope emotionally and should not be allowed to leave the notification session until they can repeat the information they have been given. They must know how to recognize important symptoms and how to avoid infecting others.[131]

Individuals with severe hemophilia (9.2%) have been exposed to the HIV virus through contaminated blood products. Regional networks of diagnostic and treatment centers provide instruction and support for these patients. The centers perform family-centered care, including sex education and family planning. Approximately half of the centers are using formal AIDS knowledge tests with patients and the patients' partners.[92]

AIDS education can and will be dramatically expanded for the public and in all treatment settings.

Cancer

Patient education helps patients detect cancer, as well as helps treat and rehabilitate patients with cancer.

Monthly breast self-examination (BSE), advocated for more than three decades to detect breast cancer early, is an example of detection activity. A summary of more than 33 intervention studies[67] shows that more than 90% of women are aware of recommendations to practice BSE, yet only 25% to 35% do so on a monthly basis. Although the profusion of BSE information has gained women's attention, it has not encouraged many to practice or to become proficient at BSE. Most women have not been taught to detect lumps in a silicone breast model; however, this method is being reviewed favorably. BSE education can be augmented if the learner practices the technique on her own breasts while the provider stands ready to monitor and correct. One program supplies a silicone model and a 10-minute videotape that demonstrates the correct technique for the learner to use at home.[46] Prompts and reminders seem to contribute to frequent, long-term use of BSE.

Teaching also uses other approaches in preventing cancer. For example, Josten, Evans, and Love[72] describe a cancer clinic that provides genetic and medical information for individuals who are at greater-than-average risk for developing the disease because of a family history of cancer. Patients want an objective assessment of their level of risk, information about specific actions they can take to reduce the risk, and tests that can lead to early diagnosis. In keeping with the increased emphasis on tools for self-management, a new method has been developed for detection of fecal occult blood. The method involves placing a chemically treated paper pad in the toilet bowl after a bowel movement and watching for color change on the pad. This technology eliminates gathering a stool specimen,[113] an unpleasant act to some patients.

Many patients with cancer are becoming active in decisions about treatment; therefore education is important to them. For example, women need information to choose among breast cancer treatment alternatives, an appreciation of their own values, and time to themselves before and during treatment. It has been documented that for obvious reasons many women have greater difficulty concentrating just before having a breast biopsy. Some authors have developed a test to assess knowledge of treatment options.[133] The areas of knowledge tapped by the Breast Cancer Information Test may be found in the box on p. 258.

Some educational programs are concerned with the particular sites of cancer and the usual treatment forms, such as muscle rehabilitation and prosthesis adaptation after mastectomy and ostomy care after bowel surgery for cancer. Programs to educate siblings about cancer and its treatment help them feel involved in the care of their brother or sister with cancer and provide an opportunity for them to discuss their feelings and concerns.[82] Many patients return home and administer their own chemotherapy orally or through long-line catheters; therefore compulsory instruction before discharge, continuing education, and follow-up are necessary.[33]

Relaxation training with guided imagery is useful in dealing with conditioned side effects to chemotherapy, such as nausea, vomiting, or appetite loss.[28] Rimer and others[112] have described an educational program to improve the cancer patient's pain control. The program, entitled "No More Pain," provides information about specific actions that will help avoid undertreatment for patients' pain.

Cancer is an acute and chronic disease with an ongoing series of crises that change the cancer patient's roles, needs, and financial obligations. Adult cancer education offers information, resources, and support in an organized manner. It helps the patient adjust to the course of the disease and to prescribed regimens, to recognize and to control side effects, to participate in and to develop control over the body, to prevent medical crises or to manage them if they occur, to prevent social isolation, to normalize life-style, to interact with others, and to use resources and options to control pain.[20]

A survey of cancer rehabilitation programs found patient education to be the most common feature in all institutions studied.[58] Some excellent model programs have been developed to help families care for cancer patients at home or to help patients cope with cancer. A study of one such program, "I Can Cope," found significant differences in anxiety, meaningfulness in life, and knowledge about cancer. Primarily, this program is a supportive educational one and includes eight sessions on learning about the disease, coping with daily health problems, communicating with others, liking oneself, living with limits, and locating helpful resources.[69] This program, as well as others, is being distributed nationally.

The "Reach to Recovery" Program uses postmastectomy volunteers to visit women with new mastectomies. The volunteers provide patients with a kit containing a temporary breast form and a booklet about adapting to the physical and emotional trauma of cancer diagnosis and surgery. Volunteers do not answer medical questions. Evaluation of this program showed that 60% of patients found the visit to be helpful as a source of support, especially for the availability of a role model and for shared understanding.[114]

Programs also need to be aimed at the issues of continuing care and remission, with its requirement for self-monitoring.

Pillon and Joannides[106] have described how to sustain such an educational and support group for a decade. The "Living With Cancer" program addresses the needs of a family from diagnosis through a disease-free state or until death occurs. In addition to an oncology nurse and a mental health nurse the program uses volunteers who have been screened with regard to their own bereavement and trained as group facilitators. Weekly staff meetings that include volunteers serve to solve the participants' problems and to provide mutual support. Because the needs of cancer patients and their families change quickly, group sessions are scheduled on a weekly basis. A several-week break is granted at the conclusion of the series to allow patients to separate from the group. Session topics include chemotherapy and radiation, relaxation techniques, mental imagery and visualization, nutrition, and

health insurance. The series of patient-education programs is usually marketed through oncologists' offices, other hospitals, newspapers, and radio.

Cardiovascular problems

Reported education programs in the cardiovascular area deal with topics that involve the alteration of risk factors (hypertension and Type A behavior), the decrease in time delay until treatment, the implementation of cardiac rehabilitation after myocardial infarction or cardiac surgery, and regimen maintenance.

In the last 20 years community-based interventions to control cardiovascular risk factors have been carried out in Germany, Finland, Australia, Switzerland, South Africa, the United Kingdom, and the United States. These programs are designed to address high blood pressure, smoking, high blood cholesterol levels, excess weight, and lack of exercise. The interventions frequently use a theoretical framework based on principles of behavior change, a community organization that involves voluntary cooperation, the training of indigenous leaders, educational self-help, and diffusion of the innovation through social networks in the community. A multi-media campaign is aimed at large audiences and is carefully segmented to influence individuals toward behavior change by using clear, repetitive messages. To change the risk factor each individual must traverse a motivational phase, skills training, and maintenance.

Education is a part of all these interventions. For example, the Pawtucket Heart Health Program is based on social learning theory. It teaches that an individual is a self-determining organism who interacts with environmental stimuli through mechanisms of reciprocal determinism and modeling. Spreading behavior changes in a person's social network is the key concept in this particular intervention. The program provides risk-factor screening with a strong teaching component and aggressive recruitment into risk-factor change programs. Newspaper articles in the community are a source of education. Programs such as "Quit Smoking" provide people with skills to alter risk factors. Involving the entire community and working through community organizations is certain to ensure large-scale participation in this prevention program.[41]

The North Karelia study in Finland was also based on social learning theory. It emphasized exposure to powerful models, external and self-reinforcement, and cognitive control. To help individuals change behaviors related to risk factors a program must provide preventive services to identify risk factors and information to educate people about the relationships between behavior and health. The program must use persuasion to motivate people at risk and to encourage their intentions to adopt the health action. Other necessary services include training to increase the skills of self-management and environmental control, social support to help people maintain the initial action, environmental change to create the opportunity for healthy actions and improve unfavorable conditions, and community organization to mobilize the community for broad changes that support adoption of the new life-style in the community. Communication of the behavioral changes through mass media and by individuals has to be able to overcome the conflicting messages that support maintaining well-established habits. New life-styles are innovations that in time diffuse through the natural networks of the community. They must be maintained through the complex network that exercises great influence over behavior and life-style in any community. As with previous interventions of this type the North Karelia study reports positive changes in smoking, dietary habits, and blood pressures.[107]

For high blood pressure control the Minnesota Heart Health Program uses direct education through adult extension classes, screening-education centers, media education, campaigns, and community organizations that have the leadership to establish a permanent framework for an ongoing prevention program. This project uses educational staging that involves alerting, educating, motivating for change, organizing for implementation, measuring community efforts, and maintaining community ef-

fects. A small benefit that affects many people may have a powerful effect in reducing disease.[19]

In the United States since the early 1970s the National High Blood Pressure Education Program has been administered through the National Heart, Lung, and Blood Institute. The program coordinates medical, public health, and voluntary health organizations that implement activities through their own constituencies. The lowering of blood pressure in all segments of the U.S. population between 1960 and 1980 has been well documented. This program's strategy was directed first at public education in simple behaviors: Have your blood pressure checked yearly; if it is elevated, seek treatment; if it is treated, maintain treatment conscientiously. Physicians were encouraged to take a more active role in detection and treatment. The response was striking and rapid.

In 1984 similar activity occurred. The National Cholesterol Education Program was initiated by the National Heart, Blood, and Lung Institute. A patient approach sought to identify and treat those at highest risk. A population approach sought to influence the public to alter current eating patterns, resulting in lower cholesterol readings. In 1990, 93% of those surveyed said they had heard of high serum cholesterol, compared with 77% in 1983 and 81% in 1986. In 1990, 65% knew that a cholesterol level below 200 was desirable—a marked contrast to 16% in 1986. By 1990 two thirds had had their own cholesterol level checked and knew the cholesterol level that is considered desirable.[119] Reaching population goals for lower blood cholesterol will require the efforts of individuals, the food industry, the mass media, health professionals, and many government agencies.[99]

In addition to these large, community-based programs a number of studies have tested similar interventions to decrease Type A behavior patterns that are often present in patients who have already had myocardial infarctions. Specific short-term goals derived from these interventions include the patient's speaking more slowly, interrupting others less often, using a time and place for relaxation, increasing the amount of positive self-talk, and reducing negative self-talk.[130] Type A behavioral counseling teaches participants to identify an array of overt manifestations of Type A behavior; to recognize exaggerated physiologic, cognitive, and behavioral reactions to stressful situations; and to develop competence in physical and mental relaxation and coping skills as an alternate response. Some of these studies have shown lower recurrence rates in the counseled groups than in control groups of nonfatal infarctions.[47]

Screening programs designed for those with hypertension has revealed information that has produced certain concerns. A 1971 study found that workers whose hypertension had been detected and labelled had greater absenteeism from work than did their nonlabeled co-workers. Although results of subsequent studies were not entirely consistent, labeling by itself may be harmful. Attribution theory could explain the labeling effect as mistaken attribution to hypertension of a host of "vague and transient symptoms" that accompany the arousal that is caused by being labeled hypertensive. Studies have also shown that the harmful effects of labeling can be prevented or at least alleviated by an intervention consisting of (1) a warm, empathetic, supportive, and available health professional; (2) an individualized instructional program that teaches patients what to expect, stressing their abilities to lead normal, active lives and explaining each new symptom as it occurs; and (3) a set of compliance-improving strategies of demonstrated effectiveness.[90] The labeling effect might occur in patients with other disorders in the absence of adequate instruction.

Devices for self-measuring blood pressure have become available in the form of portable home devices, stationary automated machines in shopping centers, and noninvasive ambulatory monitors. Self-measurement is beneficial in evaluating or in adjusting the efficacy of therapy. It reduces the number of visits to the physician's office. This equipment should be accompanied by complete educational material explaining its use and how to interpret the results.[64]

Many agree on the content of patient education programs for myocardial infarction, although far less clarity exists about the actual behavioral goals patients can reach and about the ability of programs to produce them. Areas of content for these programs include (1) nutrition (restriction of calories, fats, and, if necessary, sodium); (2) physical activity, including the rationale for early restriction related to the healing process, the concept of gradually progressing in activity, magnitude, and type of exercise prescribed, and the advantages of enhancing and maintaining fitness; (3) specific counseling about resumption of sexual activity; (4) advised cessation of smoking, methods suggested, and rationale explained; (5) general information about normal health function, coronary atherosclerotic disease, and myocardial infarction, emphasizing structural changes that occur during infarction and healing; (6) understanding information about all prescribed medications—name, purpose, dosage, detailed instructions for use, desired effects, and possible untoward effects; and (7.) the importance of control of associated diseases, particularly coronary risk factors. The patient should be instructed how to respond to new or recurrent symptoms, particularly chest pain or arrhythmia. The patient and the family should know early warning signs of infarction and should be taught to seek immediate medical care.

Over the past decade, cardiac rehabilitation has been established as a service for patients who have had heart surgery or myocardial infarctions. The goal has been to assist the patient in achieving a symptom-free life-style and to help modify risk factors.[77] Services have commonly included exercise programs that are based on the results of the patient's stress test and assistance with changing cardiac risk factors.

Runions[117] describes an approach to rehabilitation after myocardial infarction that begins in the coronary care unit and extends 12 weeks after discharge. The program is designed to help patients and spouses adopt behavior that leads to a sense of self-control and a mastery of the problems that accompany a heart attack. It teaches them how to avoid becoming irritable, tense, or excessively fatigued or distressed. It also teaches them how to prevent the deterioration of their marriages (many individuals experience this as late as a year after the infarction). In the coronary care unit, high anxiety may provide motivation for the swift learning of maladaptive patterns of behavior, such as phobic responses or avoidance behavior. A mental review of the experience of chest pain and its implications becomes repetitive. Intervention involves structuring opportunities for the patient to gain both cognitive and behavioral control of the situation by clarifying misconceptions. It also provides new information to help the patient appraise his or her physical condition. The program helps patients to describe, differentiate, and control chest pain, as well as to exhibit the proper responses to activity restrictions. Relaxation, imagery, diversion, and thought control are all useful techniques. The spouse's assistance with adjustment to the situation is another important goal. After transfer to the ward or clinic, patients focus on monitoring activity progression, using medications, and learning how and when to obtain medical assistance. Groups are organized to provide social support.

Dracup[40] describes using interactionalist role theory during cardiac rehabilitation. The theory is based on the assumption that both patients and spouses are in a period of role transition. Group work directed toward clarification of new roles and opportunities to role-play new behaviors and receive group support forms the core of the psychosocial intervention. Taylor and others[127] have developed an intervention to enhance wives' confidence in their husbands' cardiac capability by having the wives observe the husbands' treadmill exercise testing and participate in it themselves. The combined perception of patients and their wives concerning the patient's cardiac capabilities proved to be the most consistent predictor of patients' cardiovascular functioning at 11 and 26 weeks.

Some agencies have developed early heart attack programs for the first year after the patient experiences a myocardial infarction. In an emergency the patient calls the coronary care unit hot line and a nurse using standing orders tells him or her to transmit an electrocardiogram over the phone by means of a cardiobeeper. After assessing the strip the nurse may tell the patient to inject lidocaine into his thigh and may notify the rescue squad. The program's success depends on thorough patient education. The nurse calls regularly to review emergency procedures and to ask the patient to transmit an electrocardiogram.[132]

With the introduction of improved technologies and with insurance companies paying for hospital services by diagnostic related groups (DRGs), the length of stay in the hospital after myocardial infarction has been reduced from 3 weeks to 7.2 days, and 2 to 4 of these days are spent in the intensive care or cardiac care unit.[101] It is increasingly important to help patients continue their exercise regimens and to provide continuing education to help them cope with life-style changes and with disease progression. New treatments suggest the possibility that damage can be controlled if patients seek treatment early. However, the effects of campaigns to educate the public about the symptoms of heart attack have sometimes yielded a decrease in the length of time before the patients present themselves at the hospital, and sometimes not. For stroke victims the length of time until presentation is frequently quite long.[2,48,60,97]

The effects of cardiovascular disease are immense. Each year about 1.25 million Americans suffer a myocardial infarction. Depending on the criteria, 30% to 40% of adult Americans might be hypertensive. More than 20 million are now in treatment at a cost of $8 to $9 billion.[3]

Pulmonary disease

Pulmonary rehabilitation can be a beneficial and cost-effective mode of therapy for patients with chronic obstructive pulmonary disease. A basic component of the program is education that helps the patient understand the lung disease and learn skills such as abdominal and pursed-lip breathing. The program also provides patients with physical exercise to improve their level of activity, and it supports patients emotionally. The goal is to stabilize or reverse both the physiopathology and psychopathology of pulmonary diseases and to attempt to return the patient to the highest possible functional capacity allowed by the pulmonary handicap and his or her life situation. A recent study showed an improvement in physiologic parameters and a substantial decrease in the number of days of hospitalization. Postgraduate classes and a club are designed to reinforce and extend learning and to keep patients socially active.[143]

Approximately 10% of U.S. residents have asthma or wheezing at some time. Asthma, of all the chronic diseases of childhood, accounts for the greatest number of school absences. It is also a high-ranking reason for emergency room visits, especially in low-income groups. In the last 10 years approximately eight asthma education programs have been rigorously evaluated and found to (1) improve self-management; (2) reduce wheezing; (3) help families adjust to the demands the disease imposes on family life; (4) improve school attendance and performance; and (5) reduce emergency visits and hospitalizations.[30] These programs share common premises: (1) provider and patient are partners in management of asthma; (2) home environment and medical treatment are constantly changing; (3) at-home management must fit the family's life-style; and (4) children and families must learn by actively solving problems. All the programs teach the basic asthma self-management skills found in the box on p. 263.

The program's manuals guide health professionals through the teaching process and provide all necessary materials for conducting sessions. Even though they are described fully in the literature, particular effort is needed to disseminate the programs and make them available in many communities.[83]

Home care for ventilator-dependent patients also requires strong educational programs that describe the use and maintenance of equipment, cardiopulmonary assessment, and response to emergencies. Before the home care option was available, these patients were institutionalized.[62] As a final example, a home monitoring program of weight and gastrointestinal and pulmonary function of patients with cystic fibrosis is being used to develop early intervention criteria that can classify patients as improving, stable, or deteriorating. Strong educational programs that support these objective measures mark an improvement over subjective recall of symptom severity.[45]

Diabetes

Eleven million people in the United States have diabetes. Acute and chronic complications cost $20 billion annually.[5] Diabetes education is perhaps the most frequently offered patient education program. It is typically offered in the form of outpatient group programs. Topics covered commonly include the definition of diabetes, diet, oral agents, insulin types and actions, injection techniques, hypoglycemia and hyperglycemia, complications, foot care, urine and blood testing, exercise and diabetes, and sick day management.

BASIC ASTHMA SELF-MANAGEMENT SKILLS

Attack prevention

Recognizing early signs of asthma
Acting on early signs to ward off an attack
Identifying and avoiding triggers
Taking prescribed medicines properly and on time

Attack management

Resting and staying calm
Drinking liquids
Taking medicines as prescribed
Seeking assistance if necessary
Other steps as advised by the doctor

Social skills related to asthma management

Communicating with the doctor
Handling problems in school, at home, and with friends

From Krutzsch CB, Bellicha TC, Parker SR: *Health Educ Q* 14:357-373, 1987.

A summary of 82 studies of the effects of diabetes education showed a high effect for increase in patient knowledge, medium-sized effects for dietary compliance and urine testing skill, and lesser-sized effects for glycosylated hemoglobin and blood sugar.[25]

Most of the studies do not give in-depth descriptions of the interventions that were employed.[25] In areas of patient education the diabetes education field is the most structured and standardized, with accreditation available for programs and certification available for diabetes educators. However, programs might focus too much on development of a broad range of knowledge, with too little focus on the development of skills and judgment for daily management of the disease. Also, most available tests of diabetes knowledge do not measure the higher-level cognitive skills needed for successful disease management.

Recently, aggressive management programs that have included education have shown excellent outcomes. Glasgow and others[51] describe a program that works to reduce repeated admissions of a subgroup of children for diabetic ketoacidosis. These children are usually 14 to 15 years of age, are from poor, single-parent families with limited social support, and are not receiving needed insulin. Interventions by a team of providers formed a continuum and clearly explained that the patient's continual readmissions to the hospital were a result of missed insulin injections. They worked to fill knowledge gaps, confronted the patients, and encouraged them to take responsibility. They had parents assume responsibility for the administration of insulin, or they sent in home care nurses to do so. Finally, if all else failed, they got a court order. Readmissions were decreased by 47%.

In another center[54] children in chronically poor metabolic control were again dealt with in a hierarchical series of steps: (1) correcting educational deficiencies; (2) defining and negotiating family care roles so that the patients were not expected to assume too much responsibility; and (3) confronting families' perceptions of adequate care to enable them to achieve better control. Some families are dysfunctional and are incapable of altering their behavior with patients in dangerously poor metabolic control. Because such behavior can result in medical neglect, child protective services monitor compliance, and they will intervene on the child's behalf.

Pregnancy presents a formidable challenge to a woman with Type I diabetes. A successful outcome depends on her ability to manage her diabetes. Frequent blood glucose testing and strict diet are required to maintain acceptable blood glucose levels. Often, a change in insulin type and dose may also be required. The goal, of course, is to have a healthy baby, and these women can be helped toward positive feelings about successfully meeting this challenge. They can gain important skills and perspectives for lifelong diabetes management.[85]

Patients inevitably must adjust as new technologies become part of diabetes care. Pump clubs support and educate patients who are using insulin pump therapy. Self-monitoring of blood glucose (SMBG) was introduced some years ago. SMBG was expected to provide a crucial feedback loop in management of diabetes, including an ability to enhance patient education by providing real-life demonstrations of principles that could be learned in the classroom. However, some patients were apparently noncompliant and used the blood glucose data inadequately. Studies of SMBG revealed inaccuracies and technical errors; however, these were not necessarily related to impaired diabetes control.[144]

The field of diabetes management has incorporated patient education, and success clearly has been demonstrated. Yet, many questions remain.

Mental health

Educational interventions are becoming a customary part of mental health services. The lag in development of such interventions has occurred in part because it was assumed that patients might not be able to comprehend and use organized knowledge and that they might lack motivation to learn.

Perhaps the most frequent intervention is with patients who have mental dysfunctions and who are being treated in the community. The patients are educated in social skills, and their families are taught coping skills. Brown and Munford[26] describe training patients with chronic schizophrenia in interpersonal and instrumental skills, such as time management, nutrition, finance, and the use of community resources. Making daily activities less stressful is important because stressful life events have been found to correlate with psychotic relapses for chronic schizophrenics, even if they adhere to their medications.[26] Medication groups are also used to promote knowledgeable adherence to the regimen. A survey of academically affiliated lithium clinics found that two thirds of the clinics routinely provided patient education.[50]

Educational approaches are being tried for a variety of other goals in mental health. An orientation program to prepare low-income patients for psychotherapy focused on the roles and the responsibilities of therapist and patient and on the expected rate of progress during therapy.[1] In another setting phobic clients were educated about the physiology of their feelings in an effort to decrease their fears of dying during a panic attack.[11] Nutritional education has been used as an adjunct to psychotherapy in bulimia treatment. Patients can maintain their current weight in a nutritionally well-balanced diet worked out by the patient and the nutritionist. This built-in patient control can decrease anxiety, which is often considered the precipitating factor in the binge-purge ritual.[138] A series of classes on depression in the elderly was designed using the knowledge that these individuals are often reluctant to seek mental health services because they fear discovery of a pathology that may result in hospitalization. Each class developed a behavioral skill of mood monitoring and recording, and participants were assigned homework.[128]

In 1988 the National Institute of Mental Health launched a public education program, "Depression Awareness, Recognition, and Treatment." The program communicates that depressive disorders are common, serious, treatable, and frequently unrecognized. Like other public education campaigns, this one was preceded by educational efforts directed toward health care providers.[110]

Pregnancy and parenting

Pregnancy and parenting education programs are part of a continuum that begins before conception and extends through early parenting. This vision contrasts with the fragmented approach of conception counseling, followed by a small block of prenatal education in middle-to-late pregnancy and haphazard education about later parenting. Models of the behaviors and cognitive outcomes that this education will affect are complex and frequently are incomplete. For example, efforts to prevent unwanted adolescent pregnancy are usually based on the theory of underlying "cause." Prevention can involve teaching the interpersonal skills necessary for the patient to regulate intimacy and to experience the consequences of having a child. More recently, the discipline of marketing has been used to analyze the benefits various subgroups of preadolescents sought from pregnancy—exemplified in Table 10-3. This analysis is used to design services and communications.[95]

Preconception teaching may involve working with those with infertility problems. These patients may have difficulty recognizing and dealing with clinical uncertainty about how to treat their problem.

Childbirth education usually involves (1) teaching about physical happenings, emotional responses, hospital procedures, and medical intervention during birth; (2) facilitating skill in body relaxation and breathing techniques; and (3) helping couples work together. This education is usually delivered in 2-hour classes held during 6 to 8 weeks. The research base for childbirth education is still controversial. Critics charge that its effect results from selection bias because better-educated and older women are more motivated to attend the classes. Findings are inconsistent regarding the effect of prenatal education on the duration of labor;

TABLE 10-3. Summary of preadolescent (11 to 13 years) benefit segments

Segment name	Benefits sought
Goal-oriented	Conforming to adult expectations. Further enhancement of self-esteem, self-image reinforcement.
Just kids	Living day-to-day, my emotions are changing, my body is changing, that is all I wish to deal with.
Approval seekers	Approval, sense of belonging, fitting in, popularity, self-confidence. Keeping a boyfriend or girlfriend.
Innocents	Information, answers to questions. Validation of feelings.
Thrill seekers	Recognition by peers, father.
Avengers	Revenge, feelings of evening the score. Being seen as important/powerful. Seeking security and identity.
Security seekers	"Closeness," emotional security, emotional and physical comfort, parent substitute, warmth, affection. Sexual activity, not baby, is sought.
Love seekers	Emotional security through unconditional love, warmth, affection received from a baby.
Rite of passage	Feeling of being adult/rite of passage. Glamour, the Jerry Hall image. Becoming pregnant provides direction, sense of purpose.
Mother's daughters	Mother's approval through fulfillment of family expectations. Way to compete with mother in accepted manner.
Baby producers	Hope of keeping a boyfriend through giving the gift of a baby.
Macho males	Self-gratification, self-centered ego enhancement. Control that enhances self-image and power.
Controllers*	Sense of control, low self-esteem is overcome by controlling, having power over young girls, hero worship from younger girls.
Runaways	New living situation; physical escape and relief from home situation; attention, safety. Peer support from pregnancy.
Escapists	Escape from painful reality, relief from helplessness, pain relief.
Bail-outs	Financial independence. Not having to go to school. Baby by itself is not sought, but it is the course of least resistance.

From Miaoulis G: *J Health Care Marketing* 9:42-51, 1989.

*This group of male teenagers and adults is included because of their influence on preadolescent girls.

however, many studies document the mothers' increased awareness and ability to relate to their babies.[23] Topics commonly taught in childbirth education classes include growth and development of the fetus, well-being and nutrition during pregnancy, signs and symptoms of labor, methods of pain relief in labor, and complications of labor and delivery. Other sessions may cover breathing and relaxation techniques, cesarean sections, electronic monitoring of labor, infant feeding, characteristics of the newborn, and early infant care. Family adjustments to a new baby, marital adjustments during pregnancy, having sex during pregnancy and following birth, and new tests and procedures in obstetrics are also important topics for childbirth education. Teaching tools for these classes may include a film showing the birth of a baby and a tour of the maternity facilities.[91]

Increasingly, two other areas are being incorporated into prenatal education. Infant stimulation prenatally and postnatally can aid infant development. Frequently, parents do not know much about their infants' capabilities or how to stimulate them.[24] Efforts are being directed toward preventing preterm labor because its outcomes are costly. Education includes learning about the length of pregnancy, recognizing early symptoms of preterm labor, and distinguishing those symptoms from Braxton Hicks contractions and normal vaginal discharge.[8,21] Evidence of the effectiveness of these programs is still being assembled.

The perinatal period presents an opportunity to learn a great deal about the newborn: how to provide physical care and how to interact or communicate with the baby. In some institutions special emphasis is placed on lactation or breast-feeding counseling services. Postpartum follow-up is especially important because the mother's milk has usually come in by this time and the parents have been discharged and are feeling overwhelmed.[141]

Parenting education should be ongoing; however, it is frequently done intermittently, or it is undertaken to address a problem. At each child development stage parents may suffer from a lack of knowledge about the normal growth and development of children. Therefore parents can have unrealistic expectations of their children and lack the skills necessary to parent them. One extreme example is a program for abusive parents that was court ordered.[53] Often these parents were socially isolated and lacked good parenting models. Education was done in a peer group and focused heavily on developing parenting skills, including management of anger.

Preoperative and postoperative teaching

The operative experience, perhaps because it is stressful and occurs at a time when patients are in contact with health professionals, has been the focus of considerable patient education activity and research.

Providing information about sensory experiences the patient will have, encouraging relaxation, and rehearsing and practicing for events that will happen have been studied.[31] Personal control is a factor that modifies reactions to stressful experiences. One approach to enhancing personal control is to instruct patients to use coping techniques directed at controlling specific aspects of the expe-

rience. Another is to increase the patient's abilities to predict their experiences by providing them with a description of the impending experience. In a series of studies by Johnson, Christman, and Stitt preparatory information that focused on the concrete sensory elements of the experience was associated with the patient's rapid resumption of usual activities. Such information includes when events will occur, how long they will last, and what will be heard, smelled, seen, tasted, or felt during the event.[68] Some evidence suggests, however, that persons with high trait anxiety are not able to benefit from cognitive reappraisal treatment strategies.[121]

Effects studied include lung ventilation, the degree of urinary retention, the amount of postoperative vomiting, the amount of anesthesia and pain medication required, the rapidity of return to oral intake, and patient reports on the quality of sleep and anxiety. Fearfulness of their recollections about the operative event, length of the hospital stay, fear, anxiety, and mood state have also been included.[31]

A narrative hospital tour is the most commonly used preparation technique in the United States for children. The addition of an effective modeling session using a teddy bear puppet demonstrates all the situations a child is likely to encounter.[105]

Several formal reviews of a number of studies on preoperative preparation show consistent benefits in a shorter hospital stay and (less consistently) in the use of fewer analgesics. One reviewer, using quantitative techniques of research summarization, found that approaches that tended to offer emotional support and relieve anxiety were more effective than those approaches that were exclusively informational; a combination of both seemed clearly superior.[98] Devine and Cook,[38] studying psychoeducational interventions with surgical patients, found statistically reliable and positive effects on recovery, pain, psychologic well-being, and satisfaction with care. Positive, cost-relevant effects have been obtained across a wide range of patients, treatment providers, hospital settings, and historical periods.

Regimen adherence

Adherence to a regimen prescribed by a provider is a prevalent goal of patient education. Previously referred to as "compliance," the concept itself has come under some attack as moralistic and inappropriate in some patient-care situations, particularly when the regimen has to be adjusted to fit the patient's changing condition. Greater adaptiveness in compliance decisions on the part of parents was associated with better outcomes in a study of pediatric patients with asthma.[36] In a long-term medication regimen (frequently required with epilepsy), altering the patient's medication practice to suit his or her perceptions of the social environment can be called self-regulation.[34]

Errors in taking or not taking prescribed medications are widespread. In most studies at least one third of the patients failed to comply with instructions, and in some studies the rate of failure is 50% or higher. The type of action most commonly identified as noncompliance is the omission of doses. However, taking a medication for the wrong purpose or making errors in the dosage or the time of administration can also occur. Failure to have the prescription filled and premature discontinuation of the medication by the patient are special patterns of noncompliance. Contrary to expectations, noncompliance can also be a problem with patients who are hospitalized or under close supervision. The full effect of these situations is probably not known.

Clinical judgment is often unreliable for identifying the noncomplier because patients who are unreliable in one situation may not be in another. Patients are usually correct when they report that they are taking little or no medication; however, patients frequently overestimate when they say they are taking medicine regularly.[115] Factors related to patient nonadherence include severity of psychiatric diagnosis, sensory disabilities, forgetfulness, lack of understanding, competing concepts of disease and treatment, lack of social support, lack of resources, lack of overt symptoms in chronic conditions, lack of cohesive treatment delivery system, inconvenience, lack of supervision by or inadequate communication with health professionals, complexity of treatment regimen, side effects, and uncertainty regarding treatment efficacy.[93] Several of these causes are amenable to educative interventions.

Compliance with short-term treatments (less than 2 weeks) can be improved by clear instructions, by parenteral dosage forms, by special-reminder pill containers and calendars, or by simplified drug regimens. Compliance with long-term treatments is more difficult. Research has discovered no single intervention. A list of compliance-

---

A SHORT LIST OF COMPLIANCE-IMPROVING ACTIONS THAT HAVE BEEN SHOWN TO WORK

For all regimens
Information:
  1. Keep the prescription as simple as possible;
  2. Give clear instructions on the exact treatment regimen, preferably written;
For long-term regimens
Reminders:
  3. Call if appointment missed;
  4. Prescribe medication in concert with patient's daily schedule;
  5. Stress importance of compliance at each visit;
  6. Titrate frequency of visits to compliance need;
Rewards:
  7. Recognize patient's efforts to comply at each visit;
  8. Decrease visit frequency if compliance high;
Social support:
  9. Involve the patient's spouse or other partner.

From Haynes, RB, Wang E, Gomes MD: *Patient Educ Counsel* 10:155-166, 1987.

improving actions that succeed can be found in the box on p. 268.[59] Jones, Jones, and Katz[71] successfully demonstrated improvement in keeping follow-up appointments for patients with otitis media by using elements of the Health Belief Model. Information provided to patients was designed to stimulate their perceptions about susceptibility to complications and the seriousness of complications. It also taught them the benefits of keeping the follow-up referral appointment.

Children

Approaches used to prepare children for hospitalization and for procedures have evolved. These approaches are built on developmental theory and learning theory. For example, children 4½ to 7 years old can place tubes in or appliances on patient dolls. The children can discuss (postoperatively) their procedures and gain some mastery of the situation, clarifying the difference between fantasy and reality. Dolls (often custom made) are being used in many clinical areas. The Kelly Kidney doll has a zippered abdomen with enclosed organs, including a transplant kidney that can be removed. The doll also has a peritoneal catheter, a variety of hemodialysis access sites in her legs and arms with zippers that open to reveal color-coded arteries and veins, and incision lines that can simulate a flank nephrectomy and transplant incision. Dia-Lysa has a 1-liter transfer pack placed in her belly and allows transfer of peritoneal dialysis fluid.[76] Ostomy dolls with stomas have been described by Kirkland.[78] Letts and others[86] describe orthopedic dolls with traction pins, a miniature Thomas splint, and zippers that open to expose a fractured bone, a fracture that has been plated, a normal bone, or a roughened femoral head (to simulate Perthes disease). Little zippers over the ankles along with Velcro straps enable the foot to be positioned in any deformed position to show the effects of an Achilles tendon that has lengthened.[87] These dolls allow plenty of hands-on experimentation by children.

In a diabetes education program for children, a diabetic dog is used as a teaching model. Children learned how to identify the dog's symptoms during an insulin reaction and learned that his treatment was the same as theirs.[126] Books and games are also tools for teaching children. Books can be used for direct instruction and to establish rapport between the patient and provider. Rapport eases patients' confinements and also encourages them to ask questions they otherwise may be afraid to ask.

Some stories depict children with whom the child can identify. Others emphasize the humanity of health care personnel. Stories that deal with mothers and children can help keep the bonds tight. They can also help bridge the gap between parent and provider. Other stories openly deal with the child's feelings. All have the potential of facilitating discussion and dramatizing expected but unfamiliar experiences such as hospitalization. Games can be used as a tool to promote communication between provider and school-age children. The mechanics of the game give the children something to talk about. The children can size up the situation and decide whether they can relate to the providers.

Figure 10-3 shows an instruction sheet written especially for children.[63]

"Let's Pretend Hospital" is a mock hospital designed for schoolchildren to visit. It includes an admissions office and rooms for patients, surgery, radiology, and emergencies. Hospital volunteers dressed in various health care personnel use scripts to describe each area, including both procedural and sensory information, with coping strategies for fear and pain. The children go to the mock hospital in groups that include individuals designated to be the mother, the father, and the child patient. They have opportunities for hands-on experiences with medical apparatus.[42]

Just as play is a natural developmental tool with children, identification with a group of peers is the major developmental tool for adolescents. Brick[22] uses teen-life theater to teach sex education by offering a presentation planned around a scene, characters, and a conflict. She believes theater is an excellent way to teach emotion-laden material. Discussion about how a scene relates to the adoles-

---

St. Joseph Health Center child's sheet

Patient's name: _____ Date: _____

Instructions: You bumped your head.

You bumped your head, and we know it doesn't feel good. When you bump your head, sometimes it makes you feel sick all over.

"I BUMPED MY HEAD."

1. We want you to rest and not run around for a day or so. Read or color or watch TV until Mom or Dad says it's okay to get up.
2. You must not eat a lot. We told your Mom or Dad to give you only liquids for a day. This is so you won't get sick to your stomach.
3. Mom or Dad can give you aspirin or something if your head hurts a little. Ask them.
4. Ice in a little bag might make the bump feel better. Put it on your head off and on.

THINGS TO TELL MOM OR DAD:

1. Tell them if your head hurts real bad (if your headache gets worse).
2. Tell them if you can't see right—if things look blurry.

Hope you get better real fast.

Write your name _____

FIGURE 10-3. Instruction sheet written for children. (From Hughes MM: *JEN* 10:37-39, 1984.)

cents' own lives follows the play. It is a way for the young people to develop insight and possible application to their lives.

Health fairs for children are also excellent ways to educate them about issues such as looking at their bodies, sports injuries, poison control, and suicide prevention, as well as other topics.[15] Recently, strong emphasis has been placed on helping school-age children learn to take responsibility for their decisions—or at least involving them in the decisions. Figure 10-4 presents a structured interview guide used by health professionals to accomplish the involvement goal.[73]

Child life programs (also called children's activity programs, play therapy, pediatric recreation, and child development programs) were developed during the 1950s and 1960s in response to the serious and long-term consequences of children's adverse emotional reactions to hospitalization. The programs involve deliberate interventions to minimize stress and anxiety experienced by children and to ensure optimum growth and development. The interventions include (1) play; (2) preparation for hospitalization, surgery, and medical procedures; (3) emotional support offered in a receptive environment to parents and siblings; and (4) advocacy of the child's point of view to hospital personnel.[129]

SUMMARY

Providers have gained experience in designing and implementing delivery systems in patient ed-

Directions

1. Review the interview guide.
   A. Be able to verbalize the decision-making strategies identified.
   B. Gain an understanding of possible interaction responses.
2. Practice the strategies during interactions with school-age children.
3. Develop your own individual style of involving school-age children in health decisions.

Decision-making process

Strategy 1. Label the health concern.

Probe 1: "Tell me about why you came to see me today." If response is offered, proceed to Strategy 2. If no response, proceed to Probe 1A.

Probe 1A: Repeat question to clarify. Proceed to Strategy 2.

Strategy 2. Collect Data.

Probe 2: Collect subjective data: "Tell me what _____ feels like."

Probe 2A: Collect objective data: "I need more information and need to check _____."

Probe 2B: Data are summarized: "This is the information we have: _____, _____, _____, and _____. Now we have to make a decision about what to do.

Strategy 3. Review choices with the child.

Probe 3: "What is one thing we could do about _____?" (Fill in blank with child's label for health concern.) If response is offered, reinforce and proceed to Probe 3G. If no response, proceed to Probe 3A.

Probe 3A: Repeat question to clarify. If response is offered, reinforce and proceed to Probe 3G. If no response or unclear response, proceed to Probe 3B.

Probe 3B: "Have you ever had _____ before?" If response is offered, reinforce and proceed to Probe 3E. If no response or unclear response, proceed to Probe 3C.

Probe 3C: "Do you think someone in your family had _____ before?" If response is offered, reinforce and proceed to Probe 3E. If no response or unclear response, proceed to Probe 3D.

Probe 3D: "Would you like to know what some other kids tell me they do when they have _____?" Proceed to Probe 3F.

Probe 3E: "What is one thing you (they) did to make _____ better?" If response is offered, reinforce and proceed to Probe 3G. If no response or unclear response, proceed to Probe 3D.

Probe 3F: "One thing other kids did for _____ was _____," Proceed to Probe 3G.

Probe 3G: "What is something else you (your family, your friends, other kids) could do to make _____ feel better?" Continue to probe for choices with Probe 3G until the child's choices have been elicited. It is not necessary for every possible choice to be verbalized but the child should be aware of all important choices. Health professionals should fill in important choices if the child does not mention them. Proceed to Strategy 4.

FIGURE 10-4. An interview guide for helping children make health care decisions. (From Kaufman DH: *Pediatr Nurs* 11:365-367, 1985.)

Continued.

Strategy 4. Examine the positive and negative components of each choice.

Probe 4: "What do you like about _____?" (Fill in with first choice.) If response is offered, reinforce and proceed to Probe 4B. If no response or unclear response, proceed to Probe 4A.

Probe 4A: "Can you think of anything you like about _____?" If response is offered, proceed to Probe 4B. If no response or unclear response, proceed to Probe 4B.

Probe 4B: "What don't you like about _____?" If response is offered, reinforce and proceed to Probe 4D. If no response or unclear response, proceed to Probe 4C.

Probe 4C: "Can you think of anything you don't like about _____?" If response is offered, reinforce and proceed to Probe 4D. If no response or unclear response, proceed to Probe 4D.

Probe 4D: Repeat Probes 4 and 4B for each choice verbalized by the child and/or health professional. Proceed to Strategy 5.

Strategy 5. Review and summarize available choices and make final selection.

Probe 5: "What one of our choices seems the best to you?" If response is offered, reinforce and proceed to Probe 5D. If no response or unclear response, proceed to Probe 5A.

Probe 5A: Repeat question to clarify. If response is offered, reinforce and proceed to Probe 5D. If no response or unclear response, proceed to Probe 5B.

Probe 5B: "Tell me about the choice that would help you the most." If response is offered, reinforce and proceed to Probe 5D. If no response or unclear response, proceed to Probe 5C.

Probe 5C: "Would you like your parents or me to decide on the best choice?" Proceed to Probe 5E.

Probe 5D: "Tell me about why you chose _____." (Fill in with child's choice.) Proceed to Strategy 6.

Probe 5E: "Tell me about why you chose to have your parents (or health professional) make the best choice." Proceed to Strategy 6.

Strategy 6. Choice is maintained. Planning begins.

Probe 6: "Tell me about any reasons you wouldn't want to do _____." (Fill in with child's choice.) If response is offered, proceed to Probe 6B. If no response or unclear response, proceed to Probe 6A.

Probe 6A: Repeat statement to clarify. If response is offered, proceed to Probe 6B. If no response or unclear response, proceed to Probe 6B.

Probe 6B: "What is your final choice about what to do?" If response is offered, reinforce decision-making work and proceed to Probe 6D. If no response or unclear response, proceed to Probe 6C.

Probe 6C: Repeat question to clarify. If response is offered, reinforce decision-making work and proceed to Probe 6D.

Probe 6D: "O.K., what should we do next?"

FIGURE 10-4, cont'd. For legend see p. 271.

135. Weinrub H: The impact of prospective pricing on hospital health education: the New Jersey experience, *Patient Educ Counsel* 7:337-343, 1985.

136. Werlin SH, Schauffler HH: Structuring policy development for consumer health education, *Am J Public Health* 68:596-597, 1978.

137. Whitehouse FW and others: Outpatient regulation of the insulin-requiring person with diabetes (an alternative to hospitalization), *J Chron Dis* 6:433-438, 1983.

138. Willard SG, Anding RH, Winstead DK: Nutritional counseling as an adjunct to psychotherapy in bulimia treatment, *Psychosomatics* 24:545-551, 1983.

139. Willson SD: An enterostomal therapy services brochure— a visual aid, *J Enterostom Ther* 12:66-67, 1985.

140. Wilson VS: The RN consultant, *Nurs Success Today* 3(4):4-7, 1987.

141. Winikoff B and others: Overcoming obstacles to breast-feeding in a large municipal hospital: applications of lessons learned, *Pediatrics* 80:423-434, 1987.

142. Woodrow M: Cost-consciousness prompts three-phase education service, *Hospitals* 53(9):98-102, 1979.

143. Wright RW and others: Benefits of a community-hospital pulmonary rehabilitation program, *Respir Care* 28:1474-1479, 1983.

144. Wysocki T: Impact of blood glucose monitoring on diabetic control: obstacles and interventions, *J Behav Med* 12:183-206, 1989.

145. Young B, Johnson L: The development of hospitalwide patient-education director competencies, *Patient Educ Counsel* 6:19-24, 1984.

CHAPTER 11

Trends in patient education

In recent years significant changes have occurred in the financing and delivery of health care. Additional changes are likely. These changes have affected and will continue to affect the demand for patient education and the ways in which it is delivered. In addition, issues that deal with cost curtailment and patient-education ethics have surfaced. The discussion in chapter 11 considers the increase in home care and in self-care as still-evolving focuses of health care that will necessitate significant changes in the delivery of patient education. This chapter also contains a new section on the ethics of patient education.

HOME CARE

The home has become the site of prevention, follow-up, and long-term care, frequently involving the use of high-technology equipment. No special forms of delivery for patient education in home care have evolved. Education is a part of the flow of care as determined by the patient's physical illness. The expanding movement toward home care increases the possible number of instances in which failure of patient education can be serious and life threatening. Stress on caretakers can be considerable, sometimes resulting in the caretaker's abandoning the patient or, more frequently, in the caretaker's setting limits on the care that will be given.

In 1988, 8000 home care agencies were making 2 million home visits per week. Organized programs of *high-tech* home health emerged during the 1970s, encouraged by newly available insurance benefits, including home dialysis. Home total parenteral nutrition developed rapidly with the advent of third party coverage. In 1983 Medicare shifted to prospective payment. During the 1980s many for-profit home care providers appeared. The number of additional technologies now used in the home by patients and families include antibiotic and chemotherapy (using infusion pumps), ventilation, cardiac monitoring, and defibrillation. Marriage of the microcomputer and telephone is stimulating the design of electronic monitoring devices that can link a patient at home to a remotely located clinician. Visual display screens are used to give instructions and to issue reminders.[13]

Other changes in home care besides high-tech care are appearing. For example, computer links that can provide instruction and support to home caregivers are being explored. Because of budget cuts in the 1980s, public health nursing home visits were significantly diminished in scope and availability. A major service gap occurred, especially for low-income, isolated urban and rural families. The number of home visitor programs has increased—especially those designed to serve children and families with special needs. Home visitors may be professionals, paraprofessionals, volunteers, or paid individuals who provide a wide variety of support services in the home: social, health related, or educational.[7]

When hospitals discharge patients, they have a legal duty to protect those patients from forseeable harm. Medicare conditions of participation and other federal laws require hospitals to have discharge planning programs that are properly documented. Patients must be medically ready for discharge. A plan must be developed to meet the patient's needs after he or she is discharged. Patients must be able to understand the plan.[5] Also, proper documentation is necessary to ensure proper reimbursement for home care. Although reimbursable under Medicare, teaching in home care is frequently undocumented because it is done informally. Therefore reimbursement may be denied. Omdahl[24] identifies the kind of documentation needed to label teaching a skilled service: the patient must demonstrate a need to learn; the teaching must require the skills of an RN; and the impact of teaching on the patient's life must be shown. Omdahl's article provides specific examples of appropriate documentation.

Examples of home care services that specifically involve teaching can now be examined against this backdrop of historical development.

Education and support programs for caregivers of frail elderly persons are frequently based on the rationale that helping these individuals to function more effectively and efficiently will encourage and sustain caregivers. This arrangement naturally reduces reliance on formal (and expensive) systems of health care delivery. Many programs begin with a didactic session, perhaps dealing with practical concerns or legal questions, followed by a discussion period or group interaction for sharing feelings and reactions. Controlled studies of the effectiveness of these programs are sparse, and evidence is primarily impressionistic.[15]

Hospice home care nurses function as support persons and teachers, integrating crisis intervention techniques with teaching. Many situations can lead to crisis during the final stages of a terminal illness. For example, an episode of incontinence or increased pain or the realization of role changes can weaken the patient's denial by increasing his or her awareness of accumulated losses and lack of skills and knowledge to handle the change. The crisis event lowers barriers and defenses that previously inhibited learning and offers an opportunity for caregivers to grow and to feel that the situation is manageable. Self-determination and self-management are essential concepts.[8]

An aid developed to support home care can be seen in Figure 11-1. Total parenteral nutrition (TPN) involves infusion of nutrients into a central vein through an in-dwelling catheter. Patients must learn how to change the catheter dressing, irrigate the catheter, and infuse the solution. An excellent patient teaching aid, "Troubleshooting Complications," can be used to prepare the patient to manage common complications, some of which are emergencies.[32] Figure 11-1 shows a quality control check sheet for home intravenous therapy.[16]

Equipment designed for delivering phototherapy in the home for neonatal hyperbilirubinemia has become available in the past few years. Although the American Academy of Pediatrics believes that not enough information is available on the safety or efficacy of home phototherapy as compared with alternatives to warrant an endorsement of it, the Academy has issued preliminary guidelines for its use. Caretakers must be capable of following instructions. They must know how to use the equipment, how to provide adequate hydration during phototherapy, how to apply the eye patches correctly, and how to report problems promptly.[9]

Brooten and others'[4] studies of early hospital discharge and home follow-up of very-low-birth-weight infants have attracted a great deal of attention. Besides the tremendous cost of hospital care, studies suggest that the environment of the neonatal intensive care unit may have permanent adverse effects on the infant's hearing, vision, and motor coordination. In addition, prolonged hospitalization increases infants' chances of contracting infection and has been associated with a failure to thrive, with child abuse, and with parental feelings of inadequacy. In one study infants were randomly assigned to a control group discharged according to routine nursery criteria or to an early-discharge group. For 18 months families in the early discharge group had instruction, counseling, home visits, and daily on-call availability of a hospital-based nurse specialist. This intervention included promoting the parents' interaction with the infant; evaluating the parents' perceptions and concerns about the infant; teaching the parents how to bathe, soothe, and handle the infant, how to take his or her temperature, and how to prevent infection; and providing information about sleeping patterns and

Date _____   Time _____
Patient _____   Observer _____
Diagnosis _____   Age _____
Date I.V. home care started _____

A. Patient welfare and safety	Yes	No	N/A	Corrective action taken
1. Has the patient been evaluated for competency and comprehension of the particular I.V. therapeutic regimen?				
2. Do the patient and significant others understand all possible complications of the patient's particular treatment?				
3. Does the patient have written I.V. home care instructions?				
4. Can the patient and significant others return demonstrations of I.V. procedures and aseptic techniques?				
5. Do the patient and significant others feel secure in the home care setting?				
6. Has the patient been discharged with adequate supplies, medications, and solutions?				
7. During the site inspection of the home, is there an area in the home for clean storage of supplies and an appropriate area for using sterile supplies?				
8. Is the site of I.V. puncture in good condition?				
9. Are all connections fitted tightly together?				
10. Has the needle device been labeled with date, time, size and length of catheter, and initialed at the time of insertion directly on site?				
11. Has the I.V. solution been changed within the last 24 hours?				
12. Has the tubing been changed within the last 24 hours, dated, and initialed at time of replacement?				
13. Has the needle device been rotated every Monday, Wednesday, and Friday?				
14. Is all equipment clean?				
15. Has the subclavian cutdown dressing been changed every Monday, Wednesday, and Friday?				

FIGURE 11-1. Spartanburg General Hospital quality control check sheet for home IV therapy. (From Gardner C: *NITA* 9:193-201, 1986.)

A. Patient welfare and safety—cont'd	Yes	No	N/A	Corrective action taken
16. Is the dressing clean and dry?				
17. Has the infusion pump been set up correctly?				
18. Has the patient had appropriate home visits by the registered professional I.V. nurse and follow up care with the physician?				
19. Has the patient had advice and access to medical personnel on a 24-hour basis?				
20. Can the patient demonstrate emergency interventions?				
21. Is the I.V. equipment being discarded appropriately in the home care setting?				
22. Does the patient know the 911 number?				

Section A reference no.	Section A observer comments

B. Charting	Yes	No	N/A	Corrective action taken
1. Have written medical orders been countersigned by the physician?				
2. Is the home I.V. therapy teaching checklist on the patient's home care record?				
3. Has the consent form been signed by the patient and physician?				
4. Have the lab studies been done at appropriate intervals as ordered and placed on medical record?				
5. Have phone calls from the patient been documented?				

FIGURE 11-1, cont'd. For legend see opposite page.   *Continued.*

B. Charting—cont'd	Yes	No	N/A	Corrective action taken
6. Does the patient have written discharge instructions for his or her particular I.V. therapy?				
7. Is the documentation complete for each home visit by the I.V. Team nurse?				
8. Does the home care plan reflect the I.V. patient's needs?				
9. Is the history of all the patient's medications complete?				

Section B reference no.	Section B observer comments

FIGURE 11-1, cont'd. For legend see p. 280.

reportable signs and symptoms. Before discharge, parents were required to demonstrate these basic care-taking skills as well as a basic knowledge of any medications or special procedures required in the infant's care. One week before discharge the nurse specialist made a home visit to coordinate planning for the discharge and to evaluate the environment. Infants in the early-discharge group were discharged a mean of 11 days earlier, weighed 200 grams less, and were 2 weeks younger at discharge than infants in the control group. The two groups did not differ in the number of rehospitalizations and acute care visits or in measures of physical and mental growth. The mean cost of the home follow-up care in the early-discharge group was $576, yielding a net savings of $18,560 for each infant.[4]

Prenatal and postpartum nurse home visitation programs have also been designed for teenagers who are unmarried or of low socioeconomic status and who are bearing their first offspring. The goal is to prevent health and developmental problems in their infants. It was believed that office-based services did not reach those in greatest need. Nurses carried out three basic activities during their visits: parent education, enhancement of the women's information support systems, and linkage of the parents with community services. Positive effects on length of gestation and birth weight were found.[23]

Many opportunities exist to improve and prepare for home care. An example described by Cronin-Stubbs and others[11] suggests that those with therapeutic passes from inpatient psychiatric units should be encouraged to transfer skills learned in the hospital to the home and to the community. Using a rehabilitation model provides a clearer focus for therapeutic environment in the hospital rather than relying on an evaluation of the patients' ability to function away from the hospital.

Patient education to support home care probably will continue to expand and will require improved methods, delivery systems, and evaluations of patient education. Patients and their families will bear considerable responsibility.

SELF-CARE

Self-care has developed in two ways: (1) as a philosophic position aimed at giving individuals more tools to manage their health, regulate their bodily processes, and direct their use of the health care system and (2) as the reservation of responsibility to patients and families for kinds of care formerly provided by health professionals.

Some advocates of self-care believe that patient education is dominated by professionals who specify the information that patients must learn and that it is too heavily focused on compliance and cooperation. The self-care philosophy aims at correcting the imbalance in the provider-patient relationship, moving the patient from dependence to a more contractual arrangement. Available evidence indicates that a great deal of self-care is given but that it is often ignored by health practitioners or that it is considered "not real medicine," that patients' skills in self-care are not supported, and that their definition of the problem is believed to be unimportant.

Self-care involves the continuous substrate of behavior: the customs, life-styles, and discrete or episodic actions, such as self-diagnosis and self-treatment. In terms of health practices and health judgments, self-care practices are particularly prominent at the level of primary care. Some functions are complementary to those of a health care practitioner. Some are substitutive. Some authors believe that the legal base for self-care is not clear and that laws governing the licensing of professionals and the delivery of health care reflect the common assumption that medical care is synonymous with health professions. Medical practice acts often define practice of medicine and limit that practice to licensed individuals, overlooking the option of self-care.[1]

A number of educational programs for self-care and mutual aid groups have been launched. Examples include a self-care center for cuts or minor skin wounds in a college health program. The program was initiated because a self-care center for colds proved to be cost effective. The center comprises a supply counter and a set of instructions posted on the wall above the counter (Figure 11-2). The center provides students with a step-by-step approach to a self-evaluation of cuts or minor skin wounds, guidelines for self-treatment, or instructions for self-referral to a health professional, as well as the necessary supplies.[22]

A great deal of work remains to be done in the study of and the responsible support for self-care. The effective limits of professional care need to be known, just as the limitations of self-care models for specific individuals in some instances need to be recognized. Tools for self-care also need to be tested. Just as instruction may be incomplete, directions for self-care for a particular symptom may be unclear or incomplete.

Emerging issues related to medically directed self-care are definitions for negligent instruction and determining standards. Self-care programs have yet to develop a formal method for screening out those who cannot follow the system or for finding those who experience a drop-off in skills (requiring frequent follow-up) or for finding those who need help in retraining skills.[18]

Colleges also have developed self-care cold clinics[3] and portable self-instructional programs on stress management.[28] The self-care cold clinic provides information to help college students determine if their symptoms are cold related. The program also teaches them how to reduce discomfort associated with their symptoms, when to see a health care provider, and when to use self-treatment strategies. The program is self-guiding and inter-

① CONTROL BLEEDING

1) Place a sterile gauze pad over the wound
2) Put your whole hand over the gauze pad and press down firmly
3) Elevate the injured part above the level of the heart
4) Maintain direct pressure and elevation for 5 minutes*

While applying direct pressure and elevation, read ahead to PART 2: EVALUATION OF THE WOUND

*EXCEPTION: Allow puncture wound to bleed somewhat, as this washes bacteria and dirt out from deep in the wound.

② EVALUATION OF THE WOUND

Yes	No	
☐	☐	Does the wound still bleed freely after 5 minutes of direct pressure?
☐	☐	Is the wound on the face, chest, abdomen, or back?
☐	☐	Is it a deep puncture wound?
☐	☐	Is there yellow globular fatty tissue protruding from or visible in the wound?
☐	☐	Is there shiny white muscle tissue protruding from or visible in the wound?
☐	☐	Is there any numbness, tingling, or loss of movement in the affected area?
☐	☐	Is there foreign matter in the wound that cannot be removed by normal cleaning?
☐	☐	Is there a foreign object (glass, metal, etc.) embedded in the wound?
☐	☐	Is there difficulty in bringing the edges of the wound together?

If Your Wound Is Over 24 Hours Old:

☐	☐	Is there fever, pus, extensive redness, heat or swelling, or a red streak extending from the wound?

If Your Wound Is Very Deep or Dirty:

☐	☐	Has it been longer than 5 years since your last tetanus shot?

If you have answered YES to any of the above questions, please see the nurse or the security officer on duty for further evaluation.

If you have answered NO to all of the above questions, go on to PART 3: SELF-TREATMENT.

   Note: If a wound requires stitches, this must be done as soon as possible after the injury. If 6 to 8 hours has elapsed, it will not be sutured, due to the high probability of infection.

Rule of Thumb: WHEN IN DOUBT, CHECK IT OUT

FIGURE 11-2. Self-care for cuts. (From Mulvihill CJ: *J Am College Health* 32:121-124, 1983.)

③ SELF-TREATMENT

1) *Wash your hands,* so that you do not further contaminate the wound
2) *Flood the wound* with running water for 60 seconds
3) *Pour hydrogen peroxide* directly over the wound, separating the edges if necessary. This will help kill bacteria in the wound.
4) *Scrub the wound* with liquid soap, water and a 4 × 4 gauze pad for 60 seconds
   Rinse thoroughly with running water
   Blot dry with another gauze pad
5) *Bandage the wound*

Be sure to change your bandage whenever it becomes wet and soggy, or at least once a day.

Butterfly adhesive closures may be used to hold the edges of the wound together.

Choose a bandage

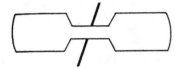

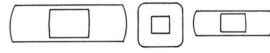

Bandaids

Applying a small amount of antibiotic ointment is optional

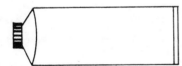

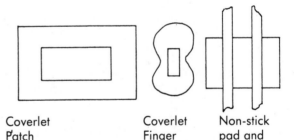

With or without it, a wound that is properly cleaned at the time of injury should heal without any problem.

Coverlet Patch

Coverlet Finger Bandage

Non-stick pad and tape

Sign the slip

④ SIGN THE SLIP

on the counter and check off the supplies used or taken for self-care. You may take enough for 4 or 5 bandage changes.

FIGURE 11-2, cont'd. Self-care for cuts.

Continued.

Watch for Complications

fever	redness and tenderness	pus
heat	swelling	red streak

These are signs of a wound infection. If any of these symptoms develop after the first 24 hours, please see the nurse for further evaluation and treatment.

Sign-in slip

SELF-CARE FOR CUTS (and Other Minor Skin Wounds)

Name _____ Date _____

Injury _____

Please check off the supplies used or taken for self-care. You may take enough for 4 or 5 bandage changes.

Bandaids:
☐ 1"   ☐ ¾"   ☐ patch

Coverlets:
☐ Finger bandage
☐ Patch

Gauze pads:
☐ Steri Pads
☐ Non-stick pads

☐ Butterfly adhesive closures
☐ Neosporin ointment
☐ Tape

Be sure to change your bandage whenever it becomes wet and soggy, or at least once a day.

Fever, redness, pus, heat, swelling, and a red streak are signs of a wound infection. If any of these develop after the first 24 hours, please see the nurse for further treatment.

FIGURE 11-2, cont'd. Self-care for cuts.

active. Supplies include a mirror, flashlight, and tongue depressor for self-examining throats. The program also provides photos of normal and abnormal throats for comparison. Thermometers are furnished, and trained student health aides can provide self-care information about colds, suggest treatment options, and give referrals. The stress management program maintains a series of stations where students learn to assess their responses to stress and see films about the nature of stress and its management through techniques such as cognitive restructuring and relaxation training. Stu-

dents are also given behavioral worksheets that help when practicing the various techniques.

Periodically, new studies are published that assess the individuals' and families' ability to manage symptoms of illness. During a 6-week period in Detroit, women averaged 17.9 symptomatic days while men averaged 13.2. Only 5% of women and 11% of men had no symptoms in that period. The most common symptoms related to musculoskeletal, respiratory, headache, and mental distress. People craft strategies of care over months and years and apply them when problems flare up.[31] A study of Swedish families during the winter months found that on average a health problem was recorded every fourth day. Measures were taken to handle health problems every sixth day. The professional health care system was contacted in less than one tenth of the cases reported during symptom days.[12]

In 1988 an estimated 14 to 16 million Americans belonged to one-half million self-help groups. These groups provided moral support, practical information, exchange of effective ways of handling problems, reduction of a sense of isolation, and increased self-esteem that members felt they could not get from existing social institutions. Many of the groups are "cause" oriented and focus on ideology or values that allow members to attain an enhanced sense of personal identity. However, potentially dangerous components of such groups include victim blaming, diverting attention from potential cures, and encouraging dependence.[26]

ETHICS RELATED TO PATIENT EDUCATION

The ethics of health care primarily have been undergirded by the field of bioethics. This field has addressed patient education only peripherally through the doctrine of informed consent. Patient education, an integral part of the health endeavor, also has ethical heritages that derive from the field of education, as well as from nursing. These traditions have always been unique and not totally dependent on those of medicine. No coherent discussion of the ethics of patient education has been offered. Instead, the education of patients has been viewed as an instrument for accomplishing a medical regimen, with little examination of the values underlying this assumption.

It is essential to address the ethics of patient education because of two interrelated trends. First, the examination of health care costs is leading to a broader discussion of issues related to distribution of limited resources. Questions about the usefulness of more extensive self-care education in meeting health care needs and questions about truly informed consent for limiting the use of health care

technology have arisen. Second, the explosion in information technology will further alter one of the heretofore unwritten and perhaps unarticulated assumptions of patient education: that health care knowledge belongs primarily to health professionals and that patient education consists of sharing that knowledge with patients toward a medically defined goal. As health care knowledge becomes freely available, will patient education turn (with the heritage from one of its parent fields) to focus more on helping individuals develop and become directors of their health over a lifespan?

From the perspective of nursing, other signs suggest that the present limited framework for considering the ethics of patient education is insufficient. Nurses are struggling to define a relational ethic of care, believing that the conventional scripts of biomedical ethics frequently fail to give character or essence to their clinical experiences.[25] Nurses also struggle with work situations that cause significant stress and ethical anguish because they bear the major responsibility for encouraging the patient to make moral decisions. The nurses' stress may be caused by inadequate skills with which to pursue the patient advocacy role required by their profession. Also, professionals other than physicians have not been able to use institutional mechanisms to review ethical issues; therefore the patient-education aspects of care are considerably thwarted.

The purpose of the following section is to describe facets of ethical practice in patient education.

Ethical patient education

Teaching is a fundamentally moral enterprise in which the teacher asks another person to change his or her thoughts or behavior. The authority of this request must be supported by certain standards of practice.

Access

The education of patients is considered an essential service. Licensing acts for health professionals and accreditation standards for institutions specifically list these services. In research protocols it is unethical to construct a pure control group, withholding education from patients. However, many people do not have access to the education service (even when it could make a significant difference in their lives), although they might have access to other health care services. An example may be found in a study by Mayo, Richman, and Harris.[21] The group studied involved adults with little formal education, who had previously required multiple hospitalizations for asthma attacks. A combination of vigorous patient education, provider accessibility, and flexible, intensive use of a few appropriate medications led to a sustained threefold reduction in readmission rate and a twofold reduction in hospital day use.

The research literature is filled with evidence of the efficacy of patient education and also with evidence that patients did not receive it. The general education system involves a public commitment to provide universal access to schooling. How to broaden that access to persons with limited learning skills and ability is a topic that is being discussed. Patient education is built on a different tradition, and the issue of access is not a matter of public concern. It is an issue that takes place primarily within a provider-patient relationship. In matters of public health, education is available through public channels and is limited in scope.

If education were commonly available, would better health care be delivered? Is our present system of limited and sometimes biased access to education ethical? A graphic answer to these questions is provided by Caplan, Callahan, and Haas,[6] who write about ethical issues in rehabilitation. The ability to learn is frequently important in the decision to initiate certain levels of rehabilitation as is an ability to judge appropriate levels of motivation and compliance for continuing treatment. Within this system of care, physicians have the power to decide whether to initiate or discontinue treatment, frequently with no formal or public set of criteria. Patients and families may not fully understand the kind of progress and rate of progress that professionals believe is necessary. Contri-

buting to the dilemma is an overwhelming demand and need for rehabilitation that outstrips resources.

Over the last 30 years physicians have made a dramatic shift in stated policies of disclosure to patients with such diagnoses as cancer.[2] If these policies continue to be carried out in practice, patients will have tremendous need for health education. The delivery and reimbursement systems for health care have not reflected a sensitivity to the ethical responsibility to provide education. This responsibility must be considered equally with all the efficacious services that deserve financial support. Individual health care providers must guide individuals to education services without bias and to the limit of resources available.

Competent Practice

The professional person's ethical practice must be competent. Competent practice in patient education might be considered in the following three ways: (1) the professional must be appropriately skilled in helping patients learn accurate content and behaviors; (2) the professional must be appropriately skilled in avoiding untoward side effects of education; and (3) the professional must know whether the right decisions about patient disposition (dependent on adequate learning) are being made.

Besides profound confusion, untoward side effects of education can include loss of self-confidence or the sense of self-efficacy, a sense of guilt for not having avoided a disease classified as "preventable," applying incorrect knowledge with disastrous consequences, or isolating oneself from a support group. Several examples are instructive:

- Home videotapes that teach children to protect themselves against sexual abuse must be evaluated to learn if they increase children's knowledge and promote the desired behavior of saying "no" and of telling a responsible adult.[20]
- It has been established that patients who are told they are hypertensive can perceive them-

derstanding of cleanliness, basic to asepsis, and of his manipulative skills.

3. Cognitive, knowing: To describe the way an ileostomy bag is used.

   Cognitive, application: To apply principles of physics in determining characteristics that a good ileostomy bag should have.

   Affective, valuing: To try to devise a more adequate design for an ileostomy bag.

4. Certain missing pieces of information from the study would greatly enhance the accuracy of the judgment to be made. For example, how many patients were involved in the study and how many responded? If all did not respond, how were those who did different from or similar to those who did not? What kinds of deviations were reported and to what degree were they serious? How well could the mothers deal with the deviations they found? Depending on the answers to these questions, it may be necessary to see that the patients and babies have good access to medical care. Also, a teaching objective regarding recognition of deviancy must be initiated and some simple treatment measures can be taught while the mother is in the hospital or during early follow-up. If such an objective already exists, what evaluative data indicate its effectiveness? Resources needed for the task can be estimated from the size of the group that seems to need help.

5. a. "As instructed" is unclear direction regarding measurements and the degree of accuracy desired.

   b. This is explicit if a clear definition of "low-sodium diet" is given.

   c. This is a good objective—assuming that the list of foods consists of those that are part of the general diet.

   d. The most obvious concern about this set of objectives is the assumption that after instruction the patient will comply. It would be more realistic to specify a percentage of a group of patients or degrees of compliance for individual patients and to project a reasonable increase over the degree to which these patients or others like them are presently complying. A second point is that "will know," in objective 1, is not behavioral. "Will explain" or "will state" would be a better choice. Subobjective 1e contains two content areas. Side effects could more probably be placed with 1f.

6. (1) b. In addition, note how nonspecific this goal is—increase what?

(2) a. This objective lacks clear criteria. What critical elements do the patients have to discuss in order to assure the provider that they understand their diets and how these relate to convalescence?

(3) c and e. This kind of objective is rarely useful.

(4) a. The major problem with this goal is that it is specific to a particular voiding sheet, with which others who work with this patient may not be familiar.

(5) c and e. A program with this goal may be difficult to justify in an economic crunch, since it lacks clarity about "deliverables."

(6) c. Is this a teaching objective or merely a statement of a desired action on the part of the caregiver? The last half of the statement is a rationale that does not usually belong in a statement of objectives.

(7) a. This is a good objective, although it does not indicate criteria for a good answer.

(8) c and b. This statement contains two goals, the first a teaching process goal and the second a teaching outcome goal.

Chapter 5. Learning

1. a. Establish baseline.
   b. Modeling.
   c. Setting up reinforcement; however, it would be useful to know if pennies for toys reinforce the child's behavior.
   d. Shaping.
   e. Contingent reinforcement.

2.

Behavior	Possible rationale
A first response to this illness was anxiety and a frantic search for a "cause" of the illness as a way to control the disease by eliminating the cause.	This may be part of the disbelief stage, depicting a lack of readiness to accept oneself as vulnerable to the illness.
Some patients had an urgent need for rigid definition by the physicians about the correct way and extent of exerting themselves during convalescence and later—a kind of bargaining for control of the symptoms.	Learners will seek resolution of ambiguity. This may also reflect the anxiety that accompanies the convalescent phase of adaptation.

Behavior	Possible rationale
Some patients wished to remain confused about their understanding of the illness.	This may be indicative of disbelief or a way to maintain power over one's illness.
Other patients sought to identify with others who they knew had suffered a coronary occlusion. This helped to decrease the ambiguity they experienced in the early stages of the illness because, by following the pattern of the convalescence of their colleagues, they were able to structure some expectations for their own future.[2]	A model to imitate is a powerful learning tool. In addition, learners will try to structure and attach meaning to their experiences.

3. There is an assumption here that parents are interested in and ready to take this approach. If this is not so, parents may not feel success from such an approach. Even if there is some readiness in parents for this objective of self-determined and self-evaluated parenthood, the leader has to be careful not to deprive people of the support of standards defined by groups of people.

4. a. Everyone searches for a reason or an explanation for what is happening to him or her and, in the absence of one based on *scientific* evidence, makes up an explanation. The emotional, vague assumption of wrongdoing is sometimes the only alternative that can be imagined if alternatives are not known.

   b. This finding should be used as an interesting, early hypothesis to which new evidence can be added through research and clinical experience.

5. a. That patients said they understood the explanations and that they asked no questions are not valid indicators of patient understanding of informed consent.

   b. Illness experiences may teach very little unless they are explicitly educative.

Chapter 6. Teaching: definition, theory, and interpersonal techniques

1. a. The terms and concepts suggest that the learner would need at least a high school education with a science background and a familiarity with anatomic terms.

   b. Saran Wrap sticks together and pleura should not; therefore the analogy can create confusion. The comparison of a leaky valve to a warped door seems less confusing, since it does portray the concept of a flat piece of material covering an opening in which the fit is more or less perfect, the moving of the piece occurring only by means of force. The analogy breaks down in obvious ways: the door can be opened from both sides, whereas the valves cannot; no corollary in the valve to the latch mechanism present on most doors exists, and the amount of warping occurring on most doors would seem to have considerably less effect on their fit than would the damage on the diseased heart valves. If the learner can be told in what ways the valve is like the door, the analogy is not so likely to be overinterpreted.

2. Clearly, a combination of didactic and group interaction strategies is necessary. The didactic strategy provides information in efficient form. The parents' need to personalize the information for their child and to work through the feelings that arise as the topic forces them to face the whole pattern of adjustment to the retardation itself are permitted and sustained in the group by the leader.

3. Another way of saying this is, "Have you ever had a doctor or nurse drain urine from your bladder with a tube?"

4. a. Repetition will increase the amount of time on task (practice) and also assist with retention of information.

   b. Physician feedback corrects inaccurate learning and provides focus for correct learning.

   c. Physician attention was probably perceived as a reinforcer, thus increasing patients' motivation to learn and retain information and their satisfaction.

5. No. While the content is highly visual, the teaching methods are highly verbal. This pattern may reflect a lack of prepared material for patient education in this field.

6.

Teaching problems	Teaching interventions
a. Acceptance of respiratory therapist treatments to remove mucus from lungs	a. Analogy with clogged drain and use of a plunger
b. Refusal to eat	b. Nonreinforcement of undesirable behavior
c. Refusal to take enzyme supplement	c. Vividly visual analogy with a game Harry knew
d. Reluctance to tell friends he had cystic fibrosis	d. Role-reversal interaction

7. The procedure does contain many of the basics, although more focus on practice is needed. Perhaps more important is the question of whether the skill will be incorporated into self-care. This step requires that patients be taught judgment skills about when to use the nebulizer. They must possess a sense of self-efficacy in carrying out the treatment.

Chapter 7. Teaching tools: printed and nonprinted materials

1. Objectives to which the pamphlet on chronic cough may contribute:
   a. To define the characteristics of the chronic cough in terms of length of time present, frequency of coughing, and relationship of cough to smoking.
   b. To list four diseases that are the most likely causes of chronic cough.
   c. To seek medical aid for a chronic cough that is accompanied by pain and bloody phlegm; or, more likely (depending on the learner's state of readiness), to agree that medical care may be necessary for a cough that continues for more than 1 month and that produces pain or bloody phlegm.
   d. To state that cough medicine only relieves the cough without removing the cause.
   e. To agree that only a physician can determine the cause of the cough.
2. Terms and suggested alternative terms:
   Maternity care
   a. Menstruation—period, monthly
   b. Father's role—how father feels or fits in
   c. Adjustment to parenthood—how it feels to be a parent
   d. Uterus—womb
   e. Episiotomy care—care of stitches

   f. Signs of illness in pregnancy—list of symptoms for each illness
   g. Fetal growth—growth of baby before birth
   h. Conception—how pregnancy occurs
   i. Antepartum—before the baby comes
   j. Postpartum—after the baby comes
   k. Mood swing—how your feelings change
   l. Anesthesia—medications during labor and delivery
   Infant care
   a. Layette—clothing and supplies for the baby
   b. Genitals—baby's bottom or private part
   c. Weaning—weaning from breast or bottle
   d. Immunizations—baby shots
   e. Growth and development—what to expect
   Child care
   a. Sibling rivalry—jealousy between brothers and sisters
   b. Enuresis—bed wetting or night bed wetting
   c. Communicable disease—childhood disease
   d. Peer relationships—relationships with other children
   e. Socialization—how your child is with other children and adults
   Family planning
   a. Birth control—family planning
   b. How to control pregnancy—planning your pregnancy
   c. IUD—coil
   d. Condom—rubbers
   e. Anatomy and physiology—how men and women are built, inside and out.[2]
3. Readability is seventh grade, which is one grade above recommended level for handout material. The explanation about why the patient feels better but must continue to take the medicine is likely to be plausible to patients. This information sheet covers only some of the standard points for teaching about medications. It leaves out the very important mention of possible side effects, as well as how to store the medicine and how to take it. If other directions (such as the label) are not clear, the patient may still take the medicine incorrectly. The study that used this sheet found differences between use of the sheet (experimental group) and no sheet (control group) in compliance (measured as physical count of the remaining dosage units at time of the interview) significant at 0.05 level. The single-impact message may well have been best, although the study did not measure other aspects of compliance.[1]

4. Other possible reasons for no improvement in learning with the cartoons include these: (1) the cartoons did not add any information or at least did not add to the information tested; (2) the cartoons did add information, but these patients were of the educational level to learn from text alone; (3) everybody knew all the material before reading the booklet—no pretest was given to check this possibility; (4) other?

Chapter 8. Teaching: planning and implementing

1. All these goals may be met by nurse participation with patients in taking the health action and interpreting the meaning of various situations to them in several visits over a period of time. For the patient with more learning resources, a single teaching episode that is verbal as well as audiovisual (using demonstration-redemonstration tools) could be used. These two teaching approaches, based on patient motivation, represent ends of a continuum from more abstract, short-term learning to concrete, prolonged learning.

2. The nurse can suggest that the mother place green peas, cereal bits, apple slices, and other similar foods on the baby's food tray to provide practice of skills he or she needs to develop. Explanation of the organizing idea should also be given to the mother to show ways in which she can aid the baby's development. The U. S. Department of Agriculture has simple large-print booklets on this subject that can be read by mothers with limited literacy. The nurse can directly facilitate learning through modeling play and vocal games with the infant during visits and through his or her own expression of pleasure.[1] All three of these strategies can be used. If this learning goal is needed by a number of mothers, consider developing a group teaching situation.

Chapter 9. Evaluation of health teaching

1. To comprehend the means of attaining asepsis in giving an injection.

2. a. The following methods of measurement might be used to evaluate the learning:
   Subobjective A: Written or oral questions with use of photographs for color and response to massage.
   Subobjective B: Observation of behavior when turning to learn alignment and body mechanics. If possible, nurses should observe whether turning is carried out every 2 hours; however, they will usually have to rely on questioning and evidence of skin breakdown. Persons doing the turning should be questioned about the schedule of turning and why it must be done.
   Subobjective C: Observation of behavior and written or oral questioning regarding the importance of this measure and ways to keep linen wrinkle free.
   Subobjective D: Observation of massaging. The nurse has to rely to some extent on oral questioning and evidence that skin breakdown is not occurring to assess the adequacy of massage.
   Subobjective E: The action required by this objective may occur with varying frequency. Oral questioning plus observation of the skin to determine whether action was taken when it was appropriate are probably the best measures.

   b. Instruction for subobjective A appears to have been remiss if the teacher expected the goal to have been met by viewing photographs without using real skin. Even if the teacher included instruction on real skin, apparently it was not effective. Because this subobjective is a crucial item, it must be retaught. Observation of the skin is in order, as is further questioning about how often the patient is turned and why he or she complains about being turned. The suggested evaluation for other subobjectives should be carried out because some are crucial to the main objective or essential to the welfare of the patient.

3. Transfer is involved every time the evaluation task is different from the learning tasks. Such is the case with all levels of the taxonomy with the possible exception of knowledge. It is possible to index the degree of transfer of which the learner is capable by systematic testing of a wide variety of situations that require varying degrees of transfer (on a continuum from those tasks that are very much like the original learning task to those that are very little like it).

MEDICATION INFORMATION CARD PROCEDURE

Purpose

To provide the patient/family with concise information and directions for administration of new prescriptions being ordered at time of discharge.

Implementation

1. When a *new prescription* is written for discharge, the Health Unit Secretary or the nurse discharging the patient will obtain a Medication Information Card for each *new prescription*.
2. The nurse will complete the Discharge Summary Plan (per procedure) which will include instructions for taking the new prescriptions. To provide for easy identification by the patient/family, the nurse will place a check mark (√) to the left of each new prescription on the Discharge Summary Plan.
3. Prior to discharge the nurse will give the patient/family the Discharge Summary Plan, Medication Information Card(s), and a Wallet Medication Card. (Keep Discharge Summary Plan intact).
4. The nurse will instruct the patient/family to write the patient's name, dose, and directions for administration of the new prescriptions (those that are checked) from the Discharge Summary Plan in the space on the Medication Information Card.
5. The nurse will check the Medication Information Card(s) for accuracy prior to discharge.
6. If the patient/family refuses to complete the Medication Information Card prior to discharge, the nurse will encourage them to complete it at home and then have it checked by the physician.

Documentation

7. The nurse will document on the Discharge Summary Plan that the patient has accurately completed the Medication Information Cards or that the patient has not completed the Medication Information Cards and should have them checked by the physician at the next office visit.
8. The nurse will give the patient/family the patient copy of the Discharge Summary Plan.
9. The nurse will also explain the purpose of the Wallet Medication Card; she/he will encourage the patient/family to complete it at home and to ask the physician to check it at the next office visit.

Note

If you have concerns about the patient's ability to follow the medication regimen at home, consult with your pharmacist about possible strategies. You can encourage the patient/family to purchase a daily/weekly medication storage box (available in the SHMC Gift Shop or retail pharmacies) or develop other individualized methods to encourage or remind the patient to take medications as prescribed. A referral to a home health agency may be warranted.

Additional Medication Information cards may be provided to the patient for medications ordered to resume at home based on assessed teaching needs. Follow the above directions for completing the dose and administration instructions on the Medication Information Card.

From Ruzicki DA, Bettesworth LG, Steele JM: *Patient Educ Counsel* 7:311-319, 1985.

PARENT CHECKLIST

Dear Parents:

The following is a list of topics about which many parents of 2-week-old babies have questions. Please check off the areas you would like to discuss today with a nurse.

SOLID FOODS	WATER	CIRCUMCISION CARE
FORMULA	SPITTING, HICCUPS	NAVEL CARE
TYPES	BABYSITTER USE	RASHES
PEPARATION	OTHER CHILDREN	DIAPERS
AMOUNT	SLEEPING, SCHEDULE	HOW TO TAKE A TEMPERATURE
FREQUENCY	CRYING	BOWEL MOVEMENTS
BREAST-FEEDING	BATHING	OTHER
SUPPLEMENTATION	LAUNDRY DETERGENTS	
SCHEDULE		

From Smith LF: *MCN* 11:256-258, 1986.

POST-TEST FOR PARTICIPANTS: BEHAVIORAL OBJECTIVES QUESTIONNAIRE

Answer true or false:

1. Excessive urination is polydipsia _____.
2. Patients who have diabetes insipidus are very seldom thirsty _____.
3. Patients with diabetes insipidus should immediately notify their doctor or nurse if they cannot balance their fluid intake or fluid output _____.
4. Patients with diabetes insipidus may become dehydrated if their fluid intake and fluid output is not balanced _____.
5. The lack of or deficiency of the anti-diuretic hormone vasopressin causes central diabetes insipidus _____.
6. The water deprivation test, the vasopressin test, and the hypertonic saline infusion test are three tests used to diagnose central diabetes insipidus or nephrogenic diabetes insipidus _____.
7. Alcoholism is a cause of central diabetes insipidus and nephrogenic diabetes insipidus _____.
8. Infections, tumors, neurosurgical operations, bleeding, and head injuries may cause central diabetes insipidus _____.
9. Nephrogenic diabetes insipidus is acquired or may be inherited by male children _____.
10. It is always necessary to call your doctor or nurse if you have any problems or questions about your medications or your disease _____.
11. Insulin is the hormone that is deficient or to which the cells of the body are nonresponsive in diabetes mellitus _____.

Answers to post-test:

1. False		7. False
2. False		8. True
3. True		9. True
4. True		10. True
5. True		11. True
6. True		

From Graham O, Schubert W: *Patient Educ Counsel* 7:53-64, 1985.

8. "Change" could be more clearly focused on awareness of lesion characteristics such as asymmetry, border irregularity, color, and diameter. In addition, visible changes in pigmented lesions may occur so slowly as to be imperceptible to the individual; both pictures and a method of visually mapping the shape and size of one's lesion should help.

9. First, the authors are to be commended for focusing on actual use of knowledge rather than just knowledge acquisition. Second, the most valid measure of the instructional goal would be to watch and talk to patients managing actual side effects. Failing that, simulated case questions are useful, although they are often highly verbal. It might be useful to show video segments that would portray the patient's indecision and his or her process of interpreting symptoms and approaching the health care practitioner. These particular questions use fairly ordinary language and long sentences. It would also have been better to add some questions in which the right answer was not to call the doctor, since patients may well catch on to this consistent "right answer." What other suggestions do you have to improve the evaluation of patient's ability to recognize and make decisions about digoxin side effects?

10. Patients and families often cannot recall anything the physician says as he or she tells them about the diagnosis. An audiotape allows them to replay the physician's presentation to gain more information from it. Furthermore, patients may not be able to concentrate sufficiently after an emotional shock to gain information from reading a book. They are likely to learn more easily by watching a tape that can be shared with their families.

11. Education will be even more important to enable patients to make informed choices about the pregnancy, including use of new technologies for prenatal diagnosis and perhaps genetic screening and fetal surgery. In addition, health care practitioners will be even more at risk for liability if they omit teaching or teach improperly about these diagnostic and treatment benefits and their risks to the mother and the fetus.

12. *Teaching-Learning Principle*
    (a) Patients learn only when they are ready to learn, physically and motivationally.
    (b) Focusing teaching on clear outcomes enhances the probability of achieving useful learning.
    (c) Visual teaching techniques accompanying verbal explanations are more likely to be effective.
    (d) Rewards reinforce learning.
    (e) Environmental cues are important learning and memory aids.
    (f) Complex tasks are frequently best learned in simple steps.

13. First, look for corroborating findings from other studies. I could not find similar studies. If you are managing a patient-education program, pay special attention to structure (because it guides providers in busy and distracting work settings) and to staff reinforcements. The rewards may involve offering recognition from the health care agency and colleagues through a patient-education appreciation week, providing enhanced advancement opportunity through excellence in patient education, or calling attention to expressions of thanks from patients and families for the education they have received.

Client education standards

This sample of client education standards was developed by the Alberta Association of Registered Nurses* in December, 1986. Members of the Subcommittee to Develop Standards for Client Education included: John Abbott-Brown, public representative; Sandra Hirst; Illa Maher, Chairperson; Ida Sansom; Merriel Thoms; Marjory Lally; Ann Fisk, nursing consultant—Education. These standards are approved and address the education process related to adult learners. They do not address other specific age groups or certain client populations. In such circumstances the educational process includes the client and adult caregiver or legal guardian, who is a responsible adult.

Terms used in the standards need to be clearly defined:
- *Client*—individual, group, family or community
- *Client education*—formal and informal educational activities undertaken by nurses in cooperation with clients to assist clients in acquiring knowledge, changing their attitudes, or developing the skills required to achieve and maintain their highest level of well-being

INTRODUCTION

The purpose of this document is to identify minimum standards for client education to ensure that the process is an integral part of quality health care. These standards are intended to provide direction for nursing practice in client education and are based on **Client Education: Position Statement and Guidelines.**[5] It is recognized that the standards have a broad applicability and that further delineation may be needed for specific client populations.

ASSUMPTIONS

These standards are based on the assumptions that:
1. The nursing profession adheres to core beliefs de-

scribing the individual, family, society, health, education, and nursing itself.
2. The nursing profession is committed to integrity and knowledge in service, life-long learning, and accountability for personal action.[4]
3. Standards are developed in collaboration and consultation with nursing personnel and other members of the health care team, including the client.[15]
4. Client education programs are developed in response to the dynamic learning needs, values, and beliefs of the client.

PRINCIPLES OF LEARNING

The principles of learning are from the document **Client Education: Position Statement and Guidelines.** It states that learning occurs in the cognitive, psychomotor, and affective domains[10] and is influenced by internal factors such as knowledge, life experiences, physiologic and psychologic state, readiness to learn, and motivation. Physical and/or emotional stress may affect the degree to which learning occurs. Learning is also influenced by external factors such as physical environment, privacy, timing, the educator, teaching strategies, and resources.

The following principles are fundamental to learning:
- learning occurs in response to a need perceived by the learner
- active participation in the learning process is fundamental to its success
- reinforcement of desired behavior increases movement towards desired outcome
- immediate feedback following each teaching/learning episode reinforces learning
- progression from the known to the unknown promotes learning.
- progression from the simple to the complex promotes learning
- opportunities to practice new skills increase the rate of learning.[19,26]

---

*From Alberta Association of Registered Nurses.

STANDARDS
Structure

Standards in regard to structure relate to the human and material resources, including the administration and management of the health care agency. Nurses in both staff and administrative roles should contribute to the development and implementation of these standards.

Standard 1

The health care agency has a philosophy, goals, and objectives that reflect its mandate and provide direction for client education.

Guidelines

The philosophy includes:

- recognition of the individuality of the client, the client's right to information and planned education, and the value of client education as an integral part of quality health care.
- identification of the relationship between the client, the nurse, and other members of the health care team
- consideration of the society and community in which client education is provided
- collaboration with members of the health care team and client representatives
- a written format that is interpreted at the time of staff orientation and as necessary.

Standard 2

Client education is integrated into all areas of nursing practice in the health care system.

Guidelines

1. Client education responsibilities are outlined in all nursing job descriptions and evaluated in performance appraisals.
2. Nursing personnel serve as members of appropriate committees involved in client education within the health care agency and the community.

Standard 3

The nursing department of the health care agency takes an active role in developing a comprehensive plan for client education.

Guidelines

The plan includes:

- the specific objectives for client education and the systematic process that will ensure that they are achieved
- the expectations for the client, the health care agency, departments within the agency, and personnel within each department

- identification of nursing personnel responsible for client education within the agency's organizational structure
- agency support of ongoing individual professional development in the area of client education
- a report of the material, human, and financial resources in terms of needs, availability, and implications
- a mechanism for its periodic review and evaluation.

Standard 4

An individual/department is designated the responsibility of facilitating and coordinating matters pertaining to client education.

Guidelines

1. There is rationale given for the identification of the individual/department responsible for client education.
2. The individual/department should have appropriate educational and experiential background in client education.
3. The individual/department has responsibility for decision-making with regard to client education in collaboration with all professionals involved.
4. The individual/department is responsible for assisting in interpreting the agency's philosophy in matters pertaining to client education to all members of the health care team.
5. The individual/department assists in and directs the planning, implementation, and evaluation of client education within the agency.
6. The individual/department provides continuing education for nursing personnel in such areas as principles of teaching-learning and adult education.

Process

Process standards outline the criteria by which client education is delivered. The educational process includes the same steps as the nursing process.

Standard 1

The primary focus of the educational process is the client.

Guidelines

The educational process:

- provides for client participation
- assists clients to understand their lifestyle, condition, treatment, and care
- assists clients to understand their responsibility for participation in self-care in order to achieve and/or maintain optimal well-being.

Standard 2

An educational assessment is done by the nurse in collaboration with the client.

Guidelines

1. The collection of data is systematic and continuous.
2. Assessment data are communicated to appropriate members of the health care team.
3. To complete an education assessment, the following should be considered:
   * the client's beliefs, attitudes, cultural/ethnic influences, and experiences regarding health and illness
   * the client's language preference
   * the client's physical or mental limitations to learning
   * the client's existing knowledge and self-assessed health status
   * the client's level of literacy and comprehension
   * the client's motivation and readiness to learn
   * the client's acceptance of and adjustment to the condition
   * what the client wants to learn.
4. The findings of the assessment are validated with the client.
5. On the basis of the data, a nursing diagnosis of the knowledge deficit(s) is formulated (NANDA).
6. In conjunction with the client the educational needs are prioritized.

Standard 3

The nurse demonstrates planning in the educational process.

Guidelines

1. The plan for client education will:
   * establish specific, measurable, realistic objectives that delineate expected outcomes
   * provide a list of objectives in sequential order based on priorities and increasing complexity
   * identify current, approved material resources
   * identify the appropriate educational method(s)
   * identify the personnel to implement the teaching process.
2. The educational plan is individualized to meet the specific needs of the client.
3. The educational plan includes goals formulated in collaboration with other health care team members.
4. The educational plan is validated with the client and other members of the health care team.

5. The proposed educational plan will be recorded in the permanent health care record.

Standard 4

The nurse applies the principles of the educational process in the implementation of client education.

Guidelines

The implementation of client education:
* provides a climate conducive to learning
* is initiated according to the client's readiness and receptivity
* provides a means whereby the client and nurse can assess the learning that has occurred
* provides a means to reinforce what is taught
* provides opportunities for additional learning experiences for the client
* demonstrates that principles of adult learning are applied in the educational process where appropriate.

Standard 5

A written outline of the educational process is available as a communication tool, a resource to health professionals, and as a record.

Guidelines

1. Documentation includes the educational plan.
2. Communication with appropriate family members, health care team members, and agencies include recommendations to ensure continuity of the educational process.

Outcome

Outcome standards are the criteria by which the results of the educational process are measured.

Standard 1

The nurse evaluates the educational process.

Guidelines

1. The evaluation of client education:
   * identifies what has been learned by providing opportunities for client feedback
   * provides opportunities for the client to indicate the level of satisfaction with the educational experience
   * assesses the format, content, teaching-learning activities, environment, media, client satisfaction, time, cost, and resources of the educational plan.
2. The evaluation of the educational plan is documented in the permanent health record.
3. The client's progress directs reassessment, reordering of priorities, new goal setting, and revision of the teaching plan.

31. The documentation of the educational experience includes:
    a. Preprogram assessment
    b. Patient education plan
    c. Content, dates delivered, instructors identified
    d. Postprogram assessment
    e. Plan for follow-up

Standard

The role of each education team member shall be clearly defined, and the intercommunication between each shall be documented in the patient's record.

Review criteria

32. Members of the diabetes patient-education staff have written job descriptions that state their responsibilities for patient care and patient instruction.
33. Education team members use the patient's permanent record to communicate about the patient's diabetes education.

Standard

There shall be written evidence of coordination between different care settings.

Review criterion

34. On completion of the education program, and with the patient's permission, the patient's permanent medical or educational record is made available to other health care settings. On request, a copy of the educational record is also given to the patient.

V. PATIENT ACCESS TO TEACHING STANDARDS

It should be the policy of the institution to facilitate access to patient-education for the target audience specified in the plan. This is promoted by a commitment to inform patients and staff routinely about the availability and benefits of patient self-care programs. Diabetes patient education should be regularly and conveniently accessible, and the instructional program should be able to respond to patient-initiated requests for information. The program permits referral by health professionals, health care agencies, or individual patients. The instructional design encourages active patient participation.

A. Facility
Standard

The facility shall have a policy to inform patients routinely about the benefits and availability of patient education.

Review criterion

35. See criterion 29.

B. Program
Standard

The program shall be regularly and conveniently available.

Review criteria

36. For health care institutions, individualized education services at diagnosis or times of crisis are available.
37. Diabetes patient education programs are offered at least quarterly or as the caseload warrants.

Standard

The program shall be responsive to patient-initiated requests for information and/or participation in the program's activities.

Review criterion

38. A person is designated within the program to be responsible for receiving and answering patient-initiated requests during business hours.

VI. CONTENT/CURRICULUM STANDARDS

The individual needs assessment provides the basis for the instructional program offered to each patient. The assessment should be documented and should include all relevant information regarding the patient's treatment, education, and support systems. Responsibility for various facets of the assessment can be divided among the instructional team members. Curriculum and instructional materials should be appropriate for the specified target audience, taking into consideration the type and duration of diabetes and the age and learning ability of the individual. Both curriculum and available community resources should be reviewed and updated periodically. The institution should provide the program with adequate space, personnel, budget, and materials.

A. Facility
Standard

The facility will provide space, personnel, budget and instructional materials adequate for the program.

Review criterion

39. Space, personnel, budget, and instructional materials are available in the institution to support each content item identified in Content/Curriculum (VIB).

Standard

The facility shall periodically assess the availability of community resources.

Review criterion

40. The applicant, at least once every 3 years, assesses public, private, and nonprofit health agencies within the service area for their potential contribution toward improving diabetes education. This assessment includes the name, address, and telephone number of each identified resource.

B. Program
Standard

The program shall be capable of offering information on each of the following content items as needed:

a. General facts
b. Psychologic adjustment
c. Involvement of the family
d. Nutrition
e. Exercise
f. Medications
g. Relationship between nutrition, exercise, and medication
h. Monitoring
i. Hyperglycemia and hypoglycemia
j. Illness
k. Complications (prevent, treat, rehabilitate)
l. Hygiene
m. Benefits and responsibilities of care
n. Use of health care systems
o. Community resources

Review criterion

41. Each program content area has written and measurable behavioral objectives, a content outline, a designated instructional method, instructional materials, and a means of evaluating the achievement of objectives.

Standard

The applicant shall specify the mechanism by which the curriculum shall be reviewed, approved, and updated.

Review criterion

42. The curriculum is annually reviewed and approved by the advisory committee and modified accordingly.

VII. INSTRUCTOR STANDARDS

Qualified personnel are essential to the success of a diabetes patient education program. Each institution should be responsible for identifying and evaluating its instructors. Instructors should be skilled professionals with recent experience and training in both diabetes and educational principles. The number of instructors should be proportional to the caseload requirements.

A. Facility
Standard

The facility shall identify appropriate instructional personnel and ascertain their competence.

Review criteria

43. Instructors are health professionals who either hold a current valid license or registration. In addition, certification or a health-related degree from an accredited educational institution is desirable.

44. Primary instructional personnel must complete a diabetes education program (minimum of 24 hours) that includes educational principles.

Standard

The numbers of personnel identified shall be suitable for the diabetic caseload within the institution.

Review criterion

45. Appropriate resources are provided to support the case mix (See criteria 2-4).

Standard

Instructors shall be allotted sufficient time to accomplish the educational objectives.

Review criterion

46. The number and type of instructors are appropriate to the case mix, with adequate time for teaching provided. The teaching process must include program planning, implementation and instruction, documentation of the patient educational experience, and participation in program development and evaluation.

B. Program
Standard

A comprehensive diabetes patient education program has instructors skilled in teaching the curriculum of the program.

Review criteria

47. (See criterion 32.)

48. Instructors annually complete a minimum of 6 hours of continuing education in diabetes and educational principles.

VIII. FOLLOW-UP STANDARDS

Follow-up services are important because diabetes requires a lifetime of proper care. The facility should provide follow-up services that include periodic reassessment of the patient's knowledge and skills and offer supplementary educational services when warranted. Written communication between the program staff and the primary care physician is essential for ongoing identification of the patient's needs. This is especially appropriate in regard to referral for early diagnosis and treatment of the complications of diabetes. Referral to community resources may also provide ongoing support for long-term psychosocial needs and behavior-modification skills. If a patient changes care settings, the institution should request the patient's permission to send his/her records to the new health care setting.

A. Facility

Standard

The facility shall transmit the educational record to other appropriate health care settings when a patient transfers his/her care responsibilities.

Review criterion

49. (See criterion 34.)

B. Program

Standard

The program shall provide follow-up services for those patients who wish to maintain continuity of education within the institution. These services shall include:

  a. Periodic reassessment of knowledge and skills

  b. Timely reeducation based on reassessment

  c. Communication with the primary-care provider about the need for professional and nonprofessional services

Review criteria

50. The applicant informs and encourages the patient to use education follow-up services.
51. Patients who return for follow-up receive knowledge and skill reassessment.
52. Follow-up services/education needs are communicated to the primary-care provider.

IX. EVALUATION STANDARDS

The facility should review the educational program periodically to ascertain that it continues to meet the national standards. This review should be conducted by the advisory committee. The results of this review should be used in subsequent program planning and modification. An assessment of each patient's needs and progress should also be conducted at regular intervals.

A. Facility

Standard

The applicant shall review periodically the performance of the instructional program and ascertain that it continues to meet national standards.

Review criterion

53. The advisory committee and appropriate institutional officials conduct and record a yearly internal review of the program.

B. Program

Standard

The program shall conduct and record an individualized assessment of each patient's original needs and progress at regular intervals.

Review criteria

54. (See criteria 5, 6, 30, and 31.)

Standard

The program shall be reviewed continually for both process and outcome, and the results of this evaluation shall be used in subsequent planning and program modification.

Review criteria

55. Program process measures used for ongoing evaluation include but are not limited to:
  a. Yearly review of the curriculum
  b. Program description
  c. Target population
  d. Number of participants.
56. Program outcome measures of patient knowledge and skills are based on the program's stated objectives.
57. Results of process and outcome evaluations are utilized in program modifications.

X. DOCUMENTATION STANDARDS

Program planning and evaluation should be documented to provide the basis for future program development and modification. All information about the patient's educational experience should be documented in the patient's permanent medical or educational record, as should communication among treatment and education professionals.

A. Facility

Standard

All aspects of the evaluation program shall be recorded by the facility and reviewed periodically to ascertain that national standards are being maintained.

Review criterion

58. (See criterion 53.)

B. Program

Standard

All aspects of the educational program offered to each patient shall be recorded in that patient's permanent medical or educational record as maintained by the facility.

Review criteria

59. (See criteria 6, 7, 30, and 31.)

APPENDIX I

Standards of oncology education

I. PATIENT AND FAMILY EDUCATION*
A. Oncology nurse
Standard

The oncology nurse at both the generalist and advanced practice levels is responsible for patient/family education related to cancer.

Review criteria

The oncology nurse:

1. Applies the ONS/ANA *Standards of Oncology Nursing Practice* to patient/family care.
2. Applies teaching-learning theories to the development, implementation, and evaluation of patient/family educational experiences.
3. Values potential outcomes of education on the knowledge, skills, and attitudes of patients and families facing cancer.
4. Assesses the accuracy and applicability of cancer information prior to endorsement and dissemination.
5. Respects the religious, social, cultural, and ethnic practices of patients and families.

B. Resources
Standard

Resources are adequate to achieve the objectives of patient/family education related to cancer care.

Review criteria

6. An environmental conducive to learning is maintained.
7. Educational materials and supplies specific to health promotion and cancer care are available.
8. Educational materials are appropriate for individuals of varied age, sex, race, creed, culture, education, physical and cognitive ability levels, and health beliefs.

9. Personnel resources are sufficient to implement the patient/family education programs.

C. Curriculum
Standard

Knowledge, skills, and attitudes related to the management of human responses to cancer are reflected in the educational program for the patient/family facing cancer.

Review criteria

The patient/family education program includes:

10. Accurate and current information about cancer prevention, detection, diagnosis, treatment, rehabilitation, and supportive care.
11. Accurate and current information about alternative treatment methods.
12. Criteria to evaluate unproven cancer therapies.
13. Cognitive, psychomotor, and affective skills needed for problem-solving, decision making, and self-care.
14. Methods to modify health behaviors for health promotion, cancer prevention, detection, and control.
15. Signs and symptoms of potential physical and psychosocial responses related to cancer and/or treatment.
16. Signs and symptoms of potential responses related to cancer and/or treatment which should be reported to the health care team.
17. Psychosocial strategies to facilitate the adaptation of the patient/family to the cancer experience.
18. Legal and ethical rights of persons with a diagnosis of cancer.
19. Community resources available to the patient/family for health promotion and cancer care.

*From *Oncol Nurs Soc,* Pamphlet, 1989.

D. Teaching-learning process
Standard

Teaching-learning theories are applied to the development, implementation, and evaluation of learning experiences related to cancer care.

Review criteria

The nurse:

20. Collects data systematically from the patient/family and other sources to assess learning needs, readiness to learn, and situational and psychosocial factors influencing learning.
21. Analyzes assessment data to identify cognitive, psychomotor, and affective learning needs.
22. Develops a teaching plan in collaboration with the patient/family that includes:
    a. Behavioral objectives based on identified learning needs,
    b. Content to meet identified objectives,
    c. Teaching strategies and learning experiences that promote active participation by the patient/family,
    d. Environmental adaptations to promote learning, and
    e. Methods and criteria for evaluation
23. Implements the teaching plan in an environment conducive to learning.
24. Collects data from the patient/family and other sources to evaluate achievement of learning objectives, effectiveness and efficiency of instruction, and the need to revise the teaching plan.
25. Modifies teaching-learning process based on evaluation data.

E. Learners: the patient and family
Standard

The patient/family apply knowledge, skills, and attitudes to management of actual or potential human responses to the cancer experience.

Review criteria

The patient/family:

26. Describe the illness, goals and plan of therapy, potential risks and benefits, and available alternative therapies.
27. Assume an active role in decision making, and identification of needs with respect to the development, implementation, and evaluation of the plan of care.
28. Describe behaviors that promote a level of independence appropriate to age, developmental stage, learning ability, resources, personal preference, prognosis, and physical ability.

29. Demonstrate psychomotor and coping skills required for self-care.
30. Describe methods to modify behaviors for health promotion and cancer prevention, detection, and control.
31. Describe signs and symptoms which should be reported to the health care team.
32. Discuss affective and interpersonal responses to cancer treatment and care.
33. Identify community resources available for health promotion and cancer care.

II. PUBLIC EDUCATION
A. Oncology nurse
Standard

The oncology nurse provides formal and informal cancer-related public education commensurate with personal education and experience.

Review criteria

The oncology nurse:

34. Identifies strategies for health promotion and cancer prevention, detection, and control.
35. Demonstrates competence in applying teaching-learning theories to the development, implementation, and evaluation of educational experiences designed for the public.
36. Values the potential influence of public education on the promotion of healthy lifestyles of individuals and groups.
37. Values the potential outcomes of public education on cancer prevention, incidence, morbidity, and mortality.
38. Practices health behaviors consistent with health promotion as a role model for the public.
39. Respects the religious, cultural, and ethnic practices of individuals or groups.
40. Provides leadership in development and evaluation of public education materials.

B. Resources
Standard

Resources for public education related to cancer prevention, detection, and control are adequate and appropriate to achieve program objectives.

Review criteria

41. An environment conducive to learning is maintained.
42. Current educational materials specific to health promotion and cancer prevention, detection, and control, are available.

43. Educational materials are appropriate for individuals of varied age, sex, race, creed, culture, education, physical and cognitive ability levels, and health beliefs.

C. Curriculum
Standard

Knowledge, skills, and attitudes related to the physical and psychosocial aspects of cancer prevention, early detection, and control are included in public education programs.

Review criteria

The public education program includes:

44. Accurate and current information about principles of carcinogenesis and genetic, environmental, and lifestyle risks for cancer.
45. Methods to modify health behaviors and practices for cancer prevention and health promotion.
46. Signs and symptoms of common cancers.
47. Strategies to improve the accessibility, use, and evaluation of cancer prevention, detection, and control programs.
48. Criteria to evaluate unproven and alternative cancer therapies.
49. Community resources for health promotion and cancer-related information and services.
50. Legal and ethical rights of persons at risk for cancer.
51. Religious, ethnic, and cultural values and beliefs that influence health.

D. Teaching-learning process
Standard

Teaching-learning theories are applied to the development, implementation, and evaluation of learning experiences related to cancer education for the public.

Review criteria

The nurse:

52. Collects data systematically from the learner and other data sources to assess learning needs, readiness to learn, and situational or psychosocial factors influencing learning.
53. Analyzes assessment data to identify cognitive, psychomotor, and affective learning needs.
54. Develops a teaching plan in conjunction with the learner that includes:
    a. Behavioral objectives based on identified learning needs
    b. Content to meet identified objectives
    c. Teaching strategies and learning experiences that promote active participation by the learner
    d. Environmental adaptations to promote learning
    e. Methods and criteria for evaluation
55. Implements the teaching plan in an environment conducive to learning.
56. Collects data from the learner and other sources to evaluate achievement of learning objectives, effectiveness of instruction, and the need to revise the teaching plan.
57. Modifies teaching-learning process based on evaluation data.

E. Learners: the public
Standard

Personal behaviors and public policy related to cancer prevention, detection, control, rehabilitation, and supportive care are influenced by formal and informal cancer public education.

Review criteria

The public reached by cancer education:

58. Demonstrates positive attitudes about cancer and individuals experiencing cancer.
59. Describes lifestyle choices that minimize personal risks for cancer and promote health.
60. Participates in cancer screening activities.
61. Identifies a course of action for early detection when signs and symptoms of cancer are discovered.
62. Identifies sources of cancer information, care, rehabilitation, and supportive care in the community.
63. Describes the political process for accomplishing social change to minimize environmental and lifestyle risks for cancer and to benefit individuals experiencing cancer.

GLOSSARY

Advanced Practice Level: Level of practice for a nurse with a masters degree, doctorate, or post-doctoral education who applies theoretical knowledge in a specialized field.

Alternative Treatment: Scientifically accepted treatment options considered in clinical decision making.

Cancer Control: Arrest of the growth or spread of cancer.

Cancer Cure: Eradication of cancer and restoration of the client to normal life expectancy.

Cancer Detection: Performance of tests to make a diagnosis of cancer in symptomatic clients.

Cancer Prevention: Strategies to minimize client exposure to substances known to increase the risk for cancer or to promote optimal client exposure to substances known to decrease the risk of cancer.

Cancer Rehabilitation: A process by which individuals within their environment are assisted to achieve optimal function within the limit imposed by cancer.

Cancer Screening: Strategies designed to detect cancer in asymptomatic clients

Carcinogenesis: The production or origin of cancer.

Client: The individual, family, group, or community for whom the nurse provides formally specialized services.

Domains of Learning: Cognitive: knowledge and intellectual abilities; Psychomotor: physical skills; Affective: attitudes, values.

Education: The process of inducing measurable changes in knowledge, skills, and attitudes through planned learning activities.

Family: Persons who are related or who represent a significant support group for the client.

Generalist Level: Level of practice for a registered nurse who possesses general knowledge and skills applicable to diversified health concerns of clients.

Health Promotion: Strategies to achieve a dynamic state in which the well-being and health potential of clients are realized to the fullest extent.

Nursing: The diagnosis and treatment of human responses to actual or potential health problems (ANA, 1980).

Nursing Diagnosis: A description of actual or potential health problems that nurses by virtue of their education and experiences are capable and licensed to treat (Gordon, 1976).

Oncology Nursing: Nursing care of clients with an actual or potential diagnosis of cancer from prevention of disease to rehabilitation or terminal care.

Outcome Criteria: Description of the desired end results of specific actions.

GLOSSARY—cont'd

Palliation: Control of symptoms when disease is beyond cure.

Process Criteria: Description of the major sequence of events and activities required to obtain desired outcomes.

Public: The people of an organized community.

Standards: A norm that expresses an agreed-upon level of practice that has been developed to characterize, measure, and provide guidance for achieving excellence.

Structure Criteria: Description of the environment and resources needed to achieve desired outcomes.

BIBLIOGRAPHY

1. American Cancer Society; Oncology Nursing Society: *The master's degree with a speciality in oncology nursing*. Pittsburgh, Pa, 1988, Oncology Nursing Society.
2. American Nurses' Association: *Nursing: a social policy statement*. Kansas City, Mo, 1980, ANA.
3. American Nurses' Association: *Standards for continuing education in nursing*. Kansas City, Mo, 1984, ANA.
4. American Nurses' Association: *Standards for professional nursing education*. Kansas City, Mo, 1984, ANA
5. American Nurses' Association; Oncology Nursing Society: *Standards of oncology nursing practice*. Kansas City, Mo, 1987, ANA.
6. Gordon M: *Nursing diagnosis: process and application*. New York, 1982, McGraw-Hill.
7. Gordon M: Nursing diagnosis and the diagnostic process. *AJN* 76(8):1298-1300, 1976.
8. McNally JC, Stair JC, Somerville ET, editors: *Guidelines for cancer nursing practice*. Orlando, Fl, 1985, Grune & Stratton.
9. Oncology Nursing Society: *Continuing education approver program providers manual*. Pittsburgh, 1987, ONS.
10. Oncology Nursing Society. *Scope of oncology nursing practice*. Pittsburgh, 1988, Oncology Nursing Society.
11. Ziegfeld CR, editor: *Core curriculum for oncology nursing*. Philadelphia, 1987, WB Saunders.

Index

Page numbers in *italics* indicate boxes and illustrations.
Page numbers followed by *t* indicate tables.